The Consultation Guide

The Consultation Guide

PAUL W. LADENSON, MD
John Eager Howard Professor of Medicine
Director, Endocrinology and Metabolism
The Johns Hopkins University School of Medicine
Baltimore, Maryland

Donated by
Dr. Carl Ogas

LIPPINCOTT WILLIAMS & WILKINS
A **Wolters Kluwer** Company
Philadelphia • Baltimore • New York • London
Buenos Aires • Hong Kong • Sydney • Tokyo

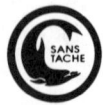

Editor: Tim Hiscock
Managing Editor: Keith Murphy
Marketing Manager: Daniell Griffin
Project Editor: Jennifer D. Weir

Copyright © 1999 Williams & Wilkins

351 West Camden Street
Baltimore, Maryland 21201-2436 USA

Rose Tree Corporate Center
1400 North Providence Road
Building II, Suite 5025
Media, Pennsylvania 19063-2043 USA

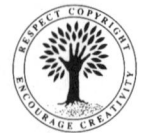

All rights reserved. This book is protected by copyright. No part of this book may be reproduced in any form or by any means, including photocopying, or utilized by any information storage and retrieval system without written permission from the copyright owner.

The publisher is not responsible (as a matter of product liability, negligence, or otherwise) for any injury resulting from any material contained herein. This publication contains information relating to general principles of medical care which should not be construed as specific instructions for individual patients. Manufacturers' product information and package inserts should be reviewed for current information, including contraindications, dosages and precautions.

Printed in Canada

Library of Congress Cataloging-in-Publication Data

Ladenson, Paul W.
　　The consultation guide / Paul W. Ladenson.
　　　p.　　cm.
　　Includes bibliographical references and index.
　　ISBN 0-683-30525-5
　　1. Medical consultation—Handbooks, manuals, etc. 2. Internal medicine—Handbooks, manuals, etc. I. Title.
　　[DNLM: 1. Referral and Consultation handbooks. 2. Internal Medicine. W 49 L154c 1998]
　　R727.8.L33　　1998
　　616—dc21
　　DNLM/DLC
　　for Library of Congress　　　　　　　　　　　　　　　　　　　　　　　98-23835
　　　　　　　　　　　　　　　　　　　　　　　　　　　　　　　　　　　　　　　CIP

The publishers have made every effort to trace the copyright holders for borrowed material. If they have inadvertently overlooked any, they will be pleased to make the necessary arrangements at the first opportunity.

To purchase additional copies of this book, call our customer service department at **(800) 638-0672** or fax orders to **(800) 447-8438.** For other book services, including chapter reprints and large quantity sales, ask for the Special Sales department.

Canadian customers should call **(800) 665-1148,** or fax **(800) 665-0103.** For all other calls originating outside of the United States, please call **(410) 528-4223** or fax us at **(410) 528-8550.**

Visit Williams & Wilkins on the Internet: http://www.wwilkins.com or contact our customer service department at **custserv@wwilkins.com.** Williams & Wilkins customer service representatives are available from 8:30 am to 6:00 pm, EST, Monday through Friday, for telephone access.

　　　　　　　　　　　　　　　　　　　　　　　　　　　　　　98 99 00 01 02
　　　　　　　　　　　　　　　　　　　　　　　　　　　1 2 3 4 5 6 7 8 9 10

In memory of Dr. Roland Ladenson, the consummate generalist and consultant.

Preface

> When thou arte callde at anye time,
> A patient to see;
> And doste perceave the cure too grate,
> And ponderous for thee;
>
> See that thou lay disdeyne aside,
> And pride of thyne owne skyll;
> And thinke no shame counsell to take,
> But rather wyth good wyll
>
> Gette one or two of experte men,
> To help thee in that nede;
> And make them partakers wyth thee,
> In that worke to procede.
>
> Dr. John Halle (1529–1566)
> *Goodlye Doctrine & Instruction*

Physicians have long consulted their colleagues to provide the best care for their patients. As the volume of medical knowledge and need for procedural expertise have grown, specialty referral has become an even more essential aspect of medical practice. A majority of patients now expect that consulting specialists will contribute to their care if their illness is puzzling, complex, or unresponsive. Physicians and health systems that frustrate this expectation often disappoint and distress their patients.

In addition to its clinical importance, the economic impact of specialty care is substantial. There are more than 15 million specialty consultations each year in the U.S.; two out of every five patients have been referred. And specialists more often request high-cost diagnostic procedures and prescribe expensive treatments for managing the more complex cases they are referred. For each dollar in healthcare expenditures generated by a primary care physician in the care of patients who will be referred, it has been estimated that two dollars are spent for the specialist's care and another four dollars for services provided by the consultant's health system.

To ensure that necessary specialty consultation remains available and affordable, the practice of consultation must be efficient. Patients should be referred for the right reasons to the right consultant at the right time. Primary care physicians should order appropriate tests before consultation, so results will be available for the consultant's consideration with the patient's clinical findings at the first visit. Conversely, excessive pre-consultative testing delays delivery of care and increases the risk of adverse events and costs. Once patients are referred, consultants should be empowered to proceed expeditiously with further needed tests and treatments whenever possible. Primary care physicians, consultants, and patients should all have an initial expectation of how many visits the consultant will typically need for following up on a given problem. When these optimal referral practices do not occur, the results can be missed or delayed diagnosis, disease progression, unnecessary visits to both consultants and primary care physicians, and inappropriate tests and procedures. These consequences translate into suboptimal patient care, dissatisfaction for all parties involved, and added healthcare costs without added value.

Many physicians have had the good fortune to practice in communities where sound consultative practices were second nature. An advance phone call to a known specialty colleague confirmed that the indications for referral were correct, the consultant was prepared to care for the patient, certain tests would be obtained in advance, and contingencies for additional testing and follow up by the consultant were discussed. Good generalist–specialist relationships facilitated subsequent referrals, and consultants often taught primary care physicians how to handle straightforward problems themselves. Unfortunately, a number of trends in medical practice have diminished the quality of cooperation between generalists and specialists: the pace of daily work; size of practice groups and communities; mobility of physicians; closed panels of specialists; required pre-authorization by payers; and a necessary, but sometimes too single-minded, commitment to control healthcare costs.

The Consultation Guide has been created to restore communication between primary care physicians and their consultants about the best practices for referral. This knowledge base provides recommendations for almost 500 of the most common clinical problems requiring consultation in ambulatory patients. These include symptoms, signs, diagnoses, test findings, and other clinical circumstances encountered in outpatient medical practice. For each, *The Consultation Guide* specifies why and when to consult, whom to consult, which tests to do and not to do before the first consultation, and what testing and follow up are appropriate to pre-authorize at the consultant's discretion. *The Consultation Guide* also provides a directory of clinical practice guidelines relevant to specialty consultation and references to germane medical literature.

The Consultation Guide's recommendations are based on the knowledge and experience of almost 100 contributing generalists and specialists. The primary criterion for selection of these panelists and reviewers was their reputation for clinical wisdom. Each of them has been recognized by their peers as a clinical leader in their discipline, institution, and community. The settings where they work in 44 states range from large faculty groups in metropolitan centers to solo private practices in small towns. The work done by these experts occurred at panel meetings, which were convened for each of eleven covered specialties of adult medicine. These meetings were typically attended by six to eight panelists equally divided between primary care and specialty medicine. It was essential for *The Consultation Guide's* recommendations to be developed by both generalists and specialists; and in the majority of cases, their perspectives proved to be remarkably complementary. Of course, primary care physicians and their consultants do not always agree on precisely how responsibility should be shared. On one occasion, a frustrated generalist exclaimed, "You don't want to see the patients I want to send you." When such differences of opinion arose, they were settled with rational argument supported by evidence and common sense.

Preparation for each panel meeting began with selection of the clinical problems to be covered. The most common indications for referral in a given specialty were identified by the frequency of diagnostic codes assigned by consultants at two large referral centers. These referral indications were reviewed in advance with the panel members, who added their own topics. In every specialty, a number of issues commonly prompting referral were not easily categorized by diagnostics codes, particularly those relating to clinical circumstances. Examples include "My patient's partner has AIDS," and "My patient with lung disease wants to know if airplane travel is safe." Special priority was given to problems for which diagnostic or therapeutic errors could have serious consequences and for which practice inefficiencies were perceived to be common. The goal was to identify the most important 50 to 70 clinical problems prompting referral in each specialty. These are the issues to which consulting specialists devote more than 90% of their time.

In advance of each panel meeting, an attempt was made to identify all relevant practice guidelines articulated by federal agencies and professional societies. This was accomplished by a search of the MEDLINE, HSTAT, and HSTAR databases; contacting specialty societies; and interviewing panelists. In general, there was remarkably little in the way of guidelines specifically related to the process of specialty referral. Some of what did exist was poorly supported by evidence or developed solely by specialists whose motives could, fairly or not, be called into question. In addition, a literature search identified clinical trials addressing many issues; studies defining the specificity and sensitivity of diagnostics tests were of particular interest. These practice guidelines and medical literature materials were distributed to the panel members in advance of their meeting.

After each of the eleven panel meetings, the participants' views were synthesized by *The Consultation Guide's* editorial staff. These draft recommendations were sent back to the panelists for their revision and comments. Then the proposed guidelines were sent to an additional set of four to six distinguished generalist and specialist peer reviewers, who were chosen with an eye toward ensuring geographic and practice setting diversity. Finally, the recommendations were reviewed by 81 practicing internists (52 in general internal medicine and 29 in specialty practices) participating in the guideline review network of the Internal Medicine Center to Advance Research and Education (IMCARE), an independent foundation created by the American Society of Internal Medicine.

PREFACE

Some may question the validity of clinical recommendations that are based on expert opinion, even when the process to ascertain them has been a rigorous one. While evidence from prospective randomized clinical trials would be preferable to guide physicians' decisions about specialty consultation, such evidence simply does not exist for the majority of issues covered by this knowledge base. Indeed, it has been estimated that only 10 to 20% of all medical practices are evidenced based. Furthermore, the time and cost required for widespread development of data-based guidelines development has proven to be prohibitive. While guidelines based on clinical outcomes would also be desirable, the information infrastructure for their widespread development is, with few exceptions, not yet in place.

We simply cannot wait for perfect evidence to preserve and enhance the value of specialty consultation. Health systems must move beyond simple cost containment and begin to define the roles of primary care physicians and specialty consultants in a clinically logical way. This set of referral indications and recommended test patterns is designed to initiate a dialogue between generalists and specialists by suggesting referral indications, facilitating diagnostic teamwork, and expediting patients' access to specialty care. *The Consultation Guide* is a good place to start a process that can optimize consultative practice.

Paul W. Ladenson, MD

Acknowledgments

Just as no one physician can master all aspects of clinical medicine, no editor could have created *The Consultation Guide* alone. The recommendations in this book reflect the clinical wisdom of almost one hundred distinguished generalists and specialists who generously contributed their knowledge, experience, and insights. This project was supported through the vision of Dr. Mark Leavitt and MedicaLogic, which has incorporated the Guide in its electronic medical record. Dr. Jane Scott provided valuable advice that shaped the concepts underlying *The Consultation Guide*. Dr. Mitchell Cahan, James Astrachan, Jonathan Pine and Keith Murphy at Lippincott-Williams & Wilkins, Carol Maggio, and Genevieve Polk have all made important contributions to the project. Finally, Cyndi Lemmon, *The Consultation Guide's* nurse-manager, has been responsible—more than any other contributor—for the successful completion of this work. Her intelligence, commitment, and spirit have kept us all on track and on time.

Contributors

Allergy and Immunology

N. Franklin Adkinson, Jr, MD
Clinical Director, Division of
  Allergy and Immunology
Professor of Medicine, Johns
  Hopkins University School
  of Medicine
Baltimore, Maryland

Daniel Ein, MD, FACP
Practice of Allergy and Immunology
Clinical Professor of Medicine
  and Allergy,
George Washington University
  School of Medicine
Founder and President, Capital
  Physicians Network
Past President, Medical Society of the
  District of Columbia
AMA Delegate, American Academy of
  Allergy and Immunology
Washington, DC

Phil Lieberman, MD, FACP
Practice of Allergy and
  Immunology
Chief, Allergy-Clinical Immunology,
  Baptist Memorial Hospital
Clinical Professor of Medicine,
  University of Memphis
Chairman, Medical Scientific Council,
  Asthma and Allergy Foundation of
  America
Memphis, Tennessee

Richard F. Lockey, MD
Practice of Allergy and Immunology
Professor, University of Southern
  Florida
Tampa, Florida

D. William Schlott, MD
Practice of Internal Medicine,
Johns Hopkins Hospital
Philip A. Tumulty Associate
  Professor of Medicine,
Johns Hopkins University School of
  Medicine
Lutherville, Maryland

Edward H. Wagner, MD, MPH
Director, Center for Health Studies and
  MacColl Institute for Healthcare
  Innovation,
Group Heath Cooperative of Puget Sound
Professor of Health Services,
University of Washington School of
  Public Health and Community Medicine
Seattle, Washington

Burton Zweiman, MD
Chief, Allergy and Immunology Section,
Hospital of the University of Pennsylvania
Professor of Medicine, University of
  Pennsylvania School of Medicine
President, American Academy of Allergy
  and Immunology
Past Editor, Journal of Allergy and
  Clinical Immunology
Philadelphia, Pennsylvania

Cardiology

Adolph M. Hutter, Jr, MD, FACP, FACC
Practice of Cardiology
Physician, Massachusetts General
  Hospital
Associate Professor of Medicine, Harvard
  Medical School
Past President, American College of
  Cardiology
Boston, Massachusetts

CONTRIBUTORS

Suzanne B. Knoebel, MD, DSc (Hon), FACC
Attending Physician, Indiana University Medical Center Hospitals
Herman C. and Ellnora D. Krannert Professor of Medicine,
Indiana University School of Medicine
Associate Director, Krannert Institute of Cardiology
Past President, American College of Cardiology
Editor-in-Chief, ACC Current Journal Review
Indianapolis, Indiana

Daniel B. Mark, MD, FACP, FACC
Co-Director, Cardiac Care Unit, Duke University Medical Center
Associate Professor of Medicine, Duke University Medical School
Durham, North Carolina

Joseph V. Messer, MD, FACP, FACC
Practice of Cardiology
Rush-Presbyterian-St. Luke's Medical Center
Professor of Medicine, Rush Medical School
Chicago, Illinois

Roger B. Rodrique, MD, MPH
Practice of Family Practice
Vice Chairman, Department of Family Medicine,
Medical Center of Delaware
Wilmington, Delaware

Harry P. Selker, MD, MSPH, FACP
Chief, Division of Clinical Care Research
Director, Center for Cardiovascular Health Services Research, New England Medical Center
Associate Professor of Medicine, Tufts University School of Medicine
Boston, Massachusetts

John Sotos, MD
Practice of Cardiology
Clinical Systems Developer
San Francisco, California

Endocrinology and Metabolism

David C. Aron, MD, FACP
Associate Chief, Medical Service,
Cleveland Veterans Administration Medical Center
Director, Endocrinology Fellowship Program
Professor of General Medical Sciences,
Case Western Reserve University School of Medicine
Cleveland, Ohio

John P. Bilezikian, MD
Chief, Division of Endocrinology
Professor of Medicine and Pharmacology,
College of Physicians & Surgeons, Columbia University
Editor, Endocrinology
Executive Editor, Trends in Endocrinology and Metabolism
Editorial Board, Journal of Women's Health
Associate Editor, Principles and Practice of Endocrinology and Metabolism,
President, American Society for Bone and Mineral Research
New York, New York

Richard D. Clover, MD, FAAFP
Professor and Chairman, Department of Family and Community Medicine,
University of Louisville School of Medicine
Louisville, Kentucky

Sheldon Greenfield, MD, FACP
Director, Primary Care
Outcomes Research Institute,
New England Medical Center
Professor of Medicine, and Chief,
Division of Health Services
    Research,
Tufts University School of Medicine
Academic Director, Managed
    Care Institute of the Tufts Associated
    Health Plan
Principal Investigator, Diabetes Patient
    Outcome Research Team
Boston, Massachusetts

Michael D. Hagan, MD
Professor and Chairman,
Department of Family Medicine
University of Kentucky School of
    Medicine
Lexington, Kentucky

Anne Klibanski, MD
Chief, Neuroendocrine Unit,
Massachusetts General Hospital
Professor of Medicine,
Harvard Medical School
Attending Physician, Massachusetts
    General Hospital
Co-Director, Mallinkrodt Clinical
    Research Center
Boston, Massachusetts

Philip Levy, MD
Practice of Endocrinology
Chairman, Endocrine Society
Clinical Initiatives Committee
Phoenix, Arizona

Helena Rodbard, MD
Practice of Endocrinology
Board of Directors, American
    Association of Clinical
    Endocrinologists
Washington, DC

Robert Vigersky, MD
Practice of Endocrinology
Past Chairman, Endocrine Society
Clinical Initiatives Committee
Washington, DC

Gastroenterology

William Banfield, MD
Practice of Internal Medicine and
    Gastroenterology
Easton, Maryland

Stephen B. Hanauer, MD, FACP
Co-Director, Inflammatory Bowel
    Disease Research Center
Professor of Medicine and Clinical
    Pharmacology
University of Chicago
Chicago, Illinois

H. Franklin Herlong, MD
Associate Professor,
Medicine, Johns Hopkins
    University School of Medicine
Associate Dean for Student
    Affairs
Baltimore, Maryland

Laura Mumford, MD
Practice of Internal Medicine
Active Staff, Johns Hopkins Hospital
Associate Professor of Medicine, Johns
    Hopkins University School
    of Medicine
Baltimore, Maryland

Daniel K. Podolsky, MD
Chief, Division of Gastroenterology,
Massachusetts General
    Hospital
Professor of Medicine,
Harvard Medical School
Boston, Massachusetts

J. Sanford Schwartz, MD
Executive Director, Leonard Davis
   Institute of Health Economics
Robert D. Eilers Chair in Health Care
   Management and Economics
Professor of Medicine, University of
   Pennsylvania School of Medicine
Professor, Health Care Systems,
The Wharton School
Past President, American Federation for
   Clinical Research
Past Director, American
   College of Physicians' Clinical Efficacy
   Assessment Project
Editor, Health Policy Perspectives
Forum, Journal of the
   American Medical Association
Philadelphia, Pennsylvania

Kathleen M. Weaver, MD
Practice of Internal Medicine
President, American Society of Internal
   Medicine
Portland, Oregon

Hematology

Richard Cohen, MD, FACP
Chief-of-Staff and Chief of
   Oncology/Hematology
Children's Hospital and
   Adult Medical Center
Research Associate,
Cancer Research Institute
University of California
   Medical Center
Clinical Professor of Medicine
University of California
School of Medicine
San Francisco, California

Jane F. Desforges, MD
Senior Physician and Hematologist, New
   England Medical Center
Distinguished Professor of Medicine
Emerita, Tufts University School of
   Medicine
Member, Institute of Medicine
Past President,
American Society of Hematology
Past Associate Editor, New England
   Journal of Medicine
Boston, Massachusetts

Thomas P. Duffy, MD
Attending Physician and Chief, Klatskin
   Medical Firm, Yale-New Haven
Hospital Director,
Hematology Fellowship Program
Professor of Medicine, Yale University
   School of Medicine
New Haven, Connecticut

Michael A. Hattwick, MD, FACP
Practice of Internal Medicine
Annandale, Virginia

Robert Jacobsen, MD
Private Practice of Hematology
West Palm Beach, Florida

Jerry L. Spivak, MD
Past Director, Division of Hematology,
Johns Hopkins Hospital
Professor of Medicine and Oncology,
Johns Hopkins University
School of Medicine
Baltimore, Maryland

Infectious Diseases

Marjorie A. Bowman, MD, MPA
Professor and Chair, Department of
   Family and Community Medicine,
Bowman Gray School of Medicine of
   Wake Forest University
Associate Editor,
Year Book of Family Practice
Advisory Board,
Health Management Quarterly

Editorial Board, Journal of the American
   Medical Association
Winston-Salem, North Carolina

William E. Dismukes, MD, FACP
Director, Division of Infectious Diseases
Professor of Medicine and Microbiology
Vice-Chairman, Department of Medicine
University of Alabama School of Medicine
Associate Editor,
American Journal of Medicine
Member, Committee on Microbial
   Threats to Health, Institute of Medicine
Birmingham, Alabama

Adolf W. Karchmer, MD, FACP
Chief, Infectious Disease Division, New
   England Deaconess Hospital
Professor of Medicine,
Harvard Medical School
Editorial Board and Section Editor,
Infectious Diseases in Clinical Practice
Boston, Massachusetts

John J. Mann, MD
Practice of Internal Medicine and
   Infectious Diseases
Associate Professor of Medicine
Johns Hopkins University
School of Medicine
Baltimore, Maryland

Patrick A. Murphy, MB, ChB, PhD
Chief, Infectious Diseases, Johns
   Hopkins Bayview Medical Center
Professor of Medicine and Microbiology,
Johns Hopkins University School of
   Medicine
Baltimore, Maryland

Edward J. Septimus, MD, FACP
Practice of Infectious Diseases
Clinical Professor of Internal Medicine,
University of Texas
Health Center at Houston

President, Texas Infectious
   Diseases Society
Houston, Texas

Martin F. Shapiro, MD, PhD, MPH, FACP
Chief, Division of General Internal
   Medicine & Health Services Research
Professor of Medicine
University of California—Los Angeles
Los Angeles, California

Nephrology

David M. Abbey, MD
Practice of Internal Medicine
Assistant Clinical Professor, University of
   Colorado Health Sciences
President, Colorado Society of Medicine
Fort Collins, Colorado

Sharon Anderson, MD
Chief, Nephrology Section, Portland
   Veterans Administration Medical Center
Associate Head, Division of Nephrology
   and Hypertension,
Oregon Health Sciences University
Past Chairman, Council on
   Complications, American Diabetes
   Association
Portland, Oregon

Daniel W. Coyne, MD
Director of Hemodialysis, Kidney Center,
Barnes Hospital
Assistant Professor of Medicine,
Washington University School of
   Medicine
St. Louis, Missouri

James A. Delmez, MD
Medical Director, Kidney Center, Barnes
   Hospital
Associate Professor of Medicine

Washington University School of Medicine
Assistant Editor,
American Journal of Kidney Disease
St. Louis, Missouri

Leslie S.-T. Fang, PhD, MD
Physician and Firm Chief, Bauer Medical Firm, Massachusetts General Hospital
Assistant Professor in Medicine, Harvard Medical School
Clerkship Director, Core Clerkship in Medicine, Massachusetts General Hospital
Boston, Massachusetts

Laura Mumford, MD
Practice of Internal Medicine
Associate Professor of Medicine, Johns Hopkins University School of Medicine
Baltimore, Maryland

Eugene S. Ogrod II, MD
Practice of Internal Medicine
Clinical Instructor, University of California—Davis
Past President, American Society of Internal Medicine
President, California Medical Association
Sacramento, California

Daniel G. Sapir, MD
Practice of Internal Medicine and Nephrology
Associate Professor of Medicine, Johns Hopkins University School of Medicine
Baltimore, Maryland

Andrew Whelton, MB, BCh, BAO, DSc (Hon), FACP, FCP
Clinical Director, Division of Nephrology, The Johns Hopkins Hospital
Professor of Medicine, Johns Hopkins University School of Medicine
Chairman, Maryland Commission on Kidney Disease
Baltimore, Maryland

David W. Windus, MD, FACP
Director, Acute Dialysis Unit and Renal Outpatient Services, Barnes Hospital
Associate Professor of Medicine, Washington University School of Medicine
St. Louis, Missouri

Neurology

Edward L. Langston, MD
Director, Memorial Family Practice Residency Program, Memorial Hospital Southwest
Associate Professor, Department of Family Practice and Community Medicine, University of Texas Medical School at Houston
Advisory Board, The Family Practice Resident Magazine
Houston, Texas

Eric Larsen, MD, MPH
Professor of Medicine, University of Washington School of Medicine
Medical Director, University of Washington Medical Center
Immediate Past President, SGIM
Seattle, Washington

Martin A. Samuels, MD, FACP
Neurologist-in-Chief, Brigham and Women's Hospital
Professor of Neurology, Harvard Medical School
Boston, Massachusetts

George H. Sands, MD
Director, Department of Neurology, Queens Hospital Center
Attending Neurologist, Mount Sinai Medical Center
Assistant Professor of Neurology, Mount Sinai School of Medicine
Member, Task Force on Access to Health Care, American Academy of Neurology

Member, Editorial Advisory Board,
American Family Physician
New York, New York

Sidney Starkman, MD
Practice of Emergency Medicine
University of California—Los Angeles
Los Angeles, California

Jerry W. Swanson, MD
Practice of Neurology, Mayo Clinic
Professor of Neurology,
Mayo Medical School
Rochester, Minnesota

Howard D. Weiss, MD
Practice of Neurology
Assistant Professor of Neurology, Johns
   Hopkins University
School of Medicine
Clinical Associate Professor of Psychiatry,
University of Maryland
School of Medicine
Baltimore, Maryland

Oncology

Martin D. Abeloff, MD
Director, The Johns Hopkins
Oncology Center
Professor of Oncology and Medicine,
Johns Hopkins University
School of Medicine
Baltimore, Maryland

Charles P. Duvall, MD, FACP
Practice of Internal Medicine
Clinical Professor of Medicine,
Georgetown University
Past President,
American Society, Internal Medicine
Chairman, Internal Medicine Section
Council, American
   Medical Association
Washington, DC

Daniel G. Haller, MD, FACP
Associate Chief for Clinical Affairs,
Division of Hematology-Oncology,
Hospital of the University of
   Pennsylvania
Professor of Medicine, University of
   Pennsylvania School of Medicine
Associate Editor, Annals of Internal
   Medicine
Associate Editor, Oncology
Editor-in-Chief, PDQ: National Cancer
   Institute Database for Physicians
Philadelphia, Pennsylvania

Robert Mayer, MD, FACP
Director, Medical Oncology
Dana Farber Cancer
Professor of Medicine
Harvard Medical School
Past President, Association of
   Subspecialty Professors
Boston, Massachusetts

Alvin I. Mushlin, MD, ScM, FACP
Co-Director, Technology
   Assessment Group,
Department of Community and
   Preventive Medicine, University of
   Rochester
Professor, Community and Preventive
   Medicine, University of Rochester
Consultant, US Preventive
   Services Task Force
Member, Agency for Health Care Policy
   and Research,
National Advisory Panel to the Cardiac
   Arrhythmia PORT
Chair, Design Committee,
New York State Department of Health
   Task Force on Clinical Guidelines and
   Medical Technology Assessment
Chairman of the Board, Rochester
   Healthcare Information Group
Rochester, New York

Ann B. Nattinger, MD
Associate Professor of Medicine & Health Services Research Director, Health Services Research,
Division of General Internal Medicine
Medical College of Wisconsin
Milwaukee, Wisconsin

Pulmonary

Jeffrey Glassroth, MD, FACP
Chairman, Department of Medicine
Professor of Medicine
President-elect,
American Thoracic Society
Univerisity of Wisconsin
Madison, Wisconsin

Wishwa N. Kapoor, MD, MPH, FACP
Chief, Division of General Medicine
Vice-Chairman, Department of Medicine
Co-Director, Center for Research on Health Care
Falk Professor of Medicine,
University of Pittsburgh School of Medicine
Professor of Health Services Administration,
University of Pittsburgh Graduate School of Public Health
Past Chair, Steering Committee,
Federated Council of Internal Medicine (FICM)
Pittsburgh, Pennsylvania

Wendy Levinson, MD, FACP
Assistant Chief of Medicine and Associate Director, Internal Medicine Residency Program,
Good Samaritan Hospital and Medical Center
Professor of Medicine, Oregon Health Sciences University
President, Society of General Internal Medicine
Associate Editor, Journal of General Internal Medicine
Co-Editor, Primary Care and General Internal Medicine
Portland, Oregon

Steven A. Schonfeld, MD, FACP
Practice in Internal Medicine, and Pulmonary and Critical Care Medicine
Director, Pulmonary Disease Division, Sinai Hospital of Baltimore
Associate Director, The Johns Hopkins Sarcoidosis Clinic
Assistant Professor of Medicine, Johns Hopkins University School of Medicine
Baltimore, Maryland

Deborah Shure, MD
Associate Professor of Medicine,
Washington University School of Medicine
President-elect, American College of Chest Physicians
Associate Editor, Angiology
Editor, Pulmonary Perspectives
St. Louis, Missouri

Mark Silverstein, MD, FACP
Consultant, Mayo Clinic
Associate Professor, Mayo Medical School
Editorial Board, Mayo Clinic Health Letter
Rochester, Minnesota

Gordon L. Snider, MD
Chief, Medical Service, Boston Veterans Administration Medical Center
Maurice B. Strauss Professor of Medicine, Boston University School of Medicine
Past President, American Thoracic Society
Boston, Massachusetts

CONTRIBUTORS

Robert A. Wise, MD
Associate Director, Division of
  Pulmonary and Critical Care Medicine
Director, Pulmonary Function
  Laboratory
Associate Professor of Medicine, Johns
  Hopkins University School of Medicine
Associate Professor of Environmental
  Health Services,
Johns Hopkins University School of
  Hygiene and Public Health
Editorial Board, Respiratory
  Medicine
Baltimore, Maryland

Rheumatology

Frank Arnette, MD, FACP
Director, Division of Rheumatology and
  Clinical Immunogenetics,
University of Texas Health Science
  Center
Professor of Medicine, University of
  Texas at Houston
Past President, Arthritis Foundation
Board of Directors
Houston, Texas

Richard A. Deyo, MD, MPH, FACP
Professor of Medicine, University of
  Washington School of Medicine
Principal Investigator, AHCPR Back Pain
  Outcome Assessment PORT
Co-Director, Robert Wood Johnson
  Clinical Scholars Program, University
  of Washington
Seattle, Washington

Ira T. Fine, MD
Practice of Internal Medicine and
  Rheumatology
Chief, Division of Rheumatology,
Sinai Hospital of Baltimore
Assistant Professor of Medicine,

University of Maryland School of
  Medicine
Instructor of Medicine, Johns Hopkins
  University School of Medicine
Baltimore, Maryland

Thomas J. Hirsch, MD
Practice of Internal Medicine and
  Rheumatology
Assistant Medical Director,
Dean Medical Center
Clinical Assistant Professor of Medicine,
University of Wisconsin
Madison, Wisconsin

David E. Kerns, MD
Co-Director, Division of General Internal
  Medicine,
Johns Hopkins Bayview Medical Center
Associate Professor, Johns Hopkins
  University, School of Medicine
Director, Community-Based Practices,
Johns Hopkins Bayview Physicians
Baltimore, Maryland

**Clement B. Sledge, MA, MD,
ScD (Hon)**
Chairman, Department of Orthopedic
  Surgery, Brigham and Women's
  Hospital
Professor of Orthopedic Surgery,
Harvard-MIT Division of Health
  Sciences and Technology
Past President, The American Academy
  of Orthopedic Surgeons
Member, Institute of Medicine
Boston, Massachusetts

Fredrick Wigley, MD
Director, Division of Molecular and
  Clinical Rheumatology, Johns Hopkins
  Hospital
Professor of Medicine, Johns Hopkins
  University School of Medicine
Baltimore, Maryland

Contents

CHAPTER 1

Allergy and Immunology

Allergen Disease, Environmental Controls for 2
Anaphylaxis or Anaphylactoid Reactions, History of 3
Beesting Allergy 4
Common Variable Hypogammaglobulinemia 5
Dermatitis
  Atopic 6
  Contact 7
  Occupational Contact 8
Drug Reactions
  Allergic 9
  Assistance with Desensitization 10
  Idiosyncratic 11
Eosinophilia 261
Food and Additive Reactions
  Allergic 12
  Nonallergic 13
Immunoglobulin A Deficiency ... 14
Insect Sting Allergy 15
Latex Sensitivity 16
Mast Cell Disorders 17
Multiple Chemical Sensitivity Syndrome 18
Nasal Polyposis 19
Pneumonitis, Hypersensitivity, Episodic 20
Postnasal Drainage, Perennial 21
Pruritus 22
Pulmonary Infections, Recurrent . 23

Rhinitis
  Seasonal 24
  Perennial 25
Rhinorrhea, Refractory 26
Urticaria and Angioedema
  Acute Episodes 27
  Chronic 28
Vasculitis with Cutaneous Lesions 29

CHAPTER 2

Cardiology

Aneurysm, Ventricular 33
Aortic Valve, Bicuspid/Calcified .. 35
Atrial Fibrillation 36
Atrial Flutter 38
Bradycardia 39
Cardiomyopathy 40
Cerebrovascular Accident (CVA) or Transient Ischemic Attack (TIA), Possible Cardiac Source of Embolus 42
Chest Discomfort
  Anginal 43
  Non-Anginal 45
  Possible Angina 47
Conduction Defect
  Left Bundle Branch Block 49
  Right Bundle Branch Block ... 50
  Left Anterior Fascicular Block . 51
Coronary Artery Disease, History of Previous Coronary Bypass Grafting, or Percutaneous Transluminal Coronary Angioplasty 52

CONTENTS

Coronary Artery Bypass Grafting or Percutaneous Transluminal Coronary Angioplasty—Second Opinion. 54

Dyspnea
   Chronic 56
   Episodic 57
   Nocturnal 58

Edema, Dependent 59

Electrocardiogram (ECG)
   Abnormal 60
   Abnormal Stress 62

Fenfluramine/Dexfenfluramine Use, History of 64

Heart Block
   First-Degree Atrioventricular . 65
   Second-Degree Atrioventricular, Mobitz 1 66
   Second-Degree Atrioventricular, Mobitz 2 67
   Third-Degree Atrioventricular . 68

Heart Failure
   Etiology Uncertain, New Onset 70
   Management 72

Heart Murmur
   Aortic 74
   Diastolic 75
   Mitral 77

Hypotension, Orthostatic 79

Lightheadedness/Near Syncope . . 80

Mitral Annulus Calcification 82

Mitral Valve Prolapse
   Click-Murmur/Suspected 83
   Echocardiographically Confirmed 84

Myocardial Infarction (MI)
   Recent, Uncomplicated 85

Silent/Electrocardiographic Evidence of 87

Palpitations 89

Pericardial Effusion 90

Pericarditis 91

Premature Ventricular Complexes (PVCs) 92

Preoperative Evaluation 93

Q-T Interval Abnormality 94

Syncope 95

Tachycardia
   Supraventricular 97
   Ventricular, Nonsustained 99

Valve Replacement, Postoperative Management 101

Wolff-Parkinson-White (WPW) Syndrome 102

CHAPTER 3

Endocrinology and Metabolism

Acromegaly 105

Adrenal Insufficiency 106

Adrenal Mass, Radiologically Detected 108

Amenorrhea, Secondary 109

Anovulatory Syndrome, Chronic . . 110

Carcinoid Syndrome 111

Cushing's Syndrome 112

Delayed Puberty
   Female 114
   Male 115

Diabetes Insipidus 116

Diabetes Mellitus, Glycemic Control 117

Diabetes, with Gastrointestinal
    Complications 119
Diabetic Nephropathy 120
Diabetic Neuropathy 122
Empty Sella Syndrome 123
Flushing 124
Galactorrhea 125
Glucocorticoid Taper 126
Goiter, Simple/Diffuse 127
Gynecomastia 128
High Density Lipoprotein (HDL)
    Cholesterol, Low 129
Hirsutism 130
Hyperaldosteronism, Primary 131
Hypercalcemia 132
Hypercalcemia, Low PTH 133
Hypercholesterolemia 134
Hyperparathyroidism 135
Hyperprolactinemia 137
Hypertension 138
Hyperthyroidism (see *Thyro-
    toxicosis*) 172
Hypertriglyceridemia 139
Hypoaldosteronism 140
Hypocalcemia 141
Hypocalcemia with
    Elevated PTH 142
Hypogonadism, Male 143
Hypoglycemia
    Fasting 144
    Reactive 145
Hypoparathyroidism 146

Hypopituitarism 147
Hypothyroidism 148
Impotence 149
Menopausal Hormone
    Replacement 150
Menopause, Premature 151
Multiple Endocrine Neoplasia I . . 152
Multiple Endocrine Neoplasia II . 153
Obesity 154
Osteodystrophy, Renal 155
Osteomalacia 156
Osteopenia 157
Osteoporosis 158
Paget's Disease 160
Pheochromocytoma 161
Pituitary Tumor 163
Polycystic Ovaries 165
Sella Turcica, Enlarged 166
Thyroid Nodule 167
Thyroid Ophthalmopathy 168
Thyroid, Painful 169
Thyroid Function
    Tests, Abnormal 170
Thyroiditis, Subacute 171
Thyrotoxicosis 172

CHAPTER 4

Gastroenterology

Abdominal Mass
    Epigastric 177
    Left Lower Quadrant 178
    Mid-Abdominal 179
    Right Lower Quadrant 180
Abdominal Pain, Chronic 181

CONTENTS

Alkaline Phosphatase, Elevated ... 182
Ascites ... 183
Barrett's Esophagus and Gastroesophageal Reflux ... 184
Chest Pain, Atypical, Possible Gastrointestinal Origin ... 185
Cirrhosis
    Etiology Unknown ... 186
    Primary Biliary ... 188
    With Complications ... 189
Colitis
    Infectious ... 190
    Ulcerative ... 191
    Ulcerative, History of, Currently Asymptomatic ... 192
Colon Cancer, Family History of ... 193
Colorectal Cancer, History of ... 194
Constipation ... 195
Crohn's Disease
    Colitis ... 196
    Regional Ileitis ... 197
Diarrhea, Chronic ... 198
Diverticulitis ... 200
Dyspepsia/Indigestion ... 201
Dyspepsia, Nonulcer and *Helicobacter pylori*-Positive ... 202
Dysphagia ... 203
Duodenal Ulcer, Recurrent ... 204
Esophagitis ... 205
Flatulence, Persistent or Recurrent ... 206
Gastric Ulcer, by Upper Gastrointestinal Series ... 207
Heartburn ... 208
Hematochezia ... 209
Hemochromatosis ... 210
Hepatic Cyst
    Multiple ... 211
    Solitary ... 212
Hepatic Mass, Solid, on Imaging ... 213
Hepatitis
    Autoimmune ... 214
    Exposure to ... 215
    Hepatitis B ... 216
    Hepatitis C ... 217
    Hepatitis D ... 218
Hepatomegaly/Abdominal Mass, Right Upper Quadrant ... 219
Hyperamylasemia ... 220
Irritable Bowel Syndrome ... 221
Jaundice/Hyperbilirubinemia ... 222
Liver Disease in the Alcohol Drinker ... 223
Malabsorption ... 224
Melena, Tarry Stools, Recent History of ... 225
Nausea, Persistent or Recurrent ... 226
Odynophagia ... 227
Pancreatic Mass
    Cystic, on Radiograph ... 228
    Solid, on Radiograph ... 229
Pancreatitis, Chronic or Recurrent ... 230
Peptic Distress, on Nonsteroidal Anti-Inflammatory Drugs ... 231

CONTENTS

Peptic Ulcer Disease
   Helicobacter pylori-Negative,
      Persistent Symptoms 232
   Refractory 233
Polyps, Family History of 234
Right Upper Quadrant Pain,
   Intermittent 235
Sclerosing Cholangitis 236
Splenomegaly, Abdominal Mass,
   Left Upper Quadrant 237
Steatorrhea 238
Tenesmus 239
Transaminase Elevation 240
Vomiting, Persistent or
   Recurrent 241
Weight Loss, Despite
   Good Appetite 242
Wilson's Disease, Personal or
   Family History 243

CHAPTER 5
Hematology

Anemia 247
   Aplastic 248
   Hemolytic 249
   Hemolytic, Hereditary 250
   In Chronic Renal Failure 251
   In Pregnancy 252
   Macrocytic 253
   Microcytic 255
   Normocytic, Elevated Corrected
      Reticulocyte Count 257
   Normocytic, Normal or Low
      Corrected Reticulocyte
      Count 258
   Sickle Cell, Management 259
Bleeding Disorder 260
Eosinophilia 261

Folate Deficiency 263
Glucose-6-phosphate
   Dehydrogenase (G6PD)
   Deficiency 264
Hematocrit, Elevated 265
Hypercoagulable State 266
Hyperglobulinemia 267
Hypersplenism 268
Iron Deficiency 269
Leukemia
   Acute Lymphocytic,
      History of 270
   Acute Myelogenous,
      History of 271
Leukocytosis 272
Leukocytosis in Pregnancy 273
Lupus Anticoagulant, in
   Nonpregnant Patient 274
Lymphocytosis 275
Lymphoma 276
Monocytosis 277
Myelodysplastic Syndromes 278
Myeloma, Multiple,
   Management 279
Neutropenia 280
Pancytopenia
   Elevated Reticulocyte Count .. 281
   Normal or Low
      Reticulocyte Count 282
Paroxysmal Nocturnal
   Hemoglobinuria 283
Polycythemia Vera 284
Porphyria, Acute, Intermittent ... 285
Splenomegaly 286

Thalassemia 287
Thrombocytopenia 288
Thrombocytosis 290
Vitamin B$_{12}$ Deficiency 291

CHAPTER 6

Infectious Diseases

Adenopathy
   Cervical 295
   Generalized 296
Carbuncles or Boils, Recurrent ... 297
Cough, in HIV-Positive Patient ... 298
Dementia, in HIV-Positive
   Patient 299
Diarrhea
   In HIV-Positive Patient 300
   History of Recent
      Foreign Travel 302
Dysphagia or Odynophagia in HIV-
   Positive Patient 303
Dysuria, Nonpyuric 304
Fatigue
   Chronic, Afebrile 305
   Chronic, Febrile 306
Fever
   Of Unknown Origin (FUO) ... 308
   With Rash 310
Headache, in HIV-Positive
   Patient 311
Hepatitis Serology, Positive,
   Rejected by Blood Bank 312
Herpes Zoster, Chicken Pox,
   Shingles Exposure 313
Human Immunodeficiency
   Virus Infection, Diagnosis
      Indeterminate Western Blot .. 314
      Positive Western Blot 315

Lower Leg Ulcers, Poorly
   Resolving 316
Lyme Titer
   Positive 317
   Positive, Typical
      Clinical Syndrome 318
Needlestick 319
Partner
   Is HIV-Positive 320
   With Gonorrhea,
      Asymptomatic 321
   With Herpes Simplex 322
   With Syphilis 323
Pneumonia, Recurrent 324
Pyuria 325
RPR Test, VDRL Test, Positive .. 326
Rubella Exposure 327
Sinusitis
   Persistent 328
   Recurrent 330
Soft Tissue Infection
   Poorly Resolving 332
   Recurrent 333
Sore Throat
   Recurrent 334
   Severe, *Streptococcus*-
      Negative 336
Tick Bite 337
Tuberculosis (TB) Skin Test
   Positive, Uncertain
      Duration 338
   Recent Conversion (Less
      Than 2 Years) 339
Urethral Discharge 340
Urinary Candidiasis 341
Urinary Tract Infections
   Recurrent 342
   With Indwelling Catheter 343

CONTENTS

CHAPTER 7

Nephrology

Acidosis, with Renal
    Insufficiency 347
Creatinine Elevation 348
Glomerulonephritis
    History of 349
    In Scleroderma 350
    In Systemic Lupus
        Erythematosus 351
Hematuria
    Gross 352
    Microscopic 354
Hyperkalemia 356
Hypertension
    In Diabetes Mellitus 357
    Labile/Paroxysmal 358
    Renovascular 359
    Rule Out Secondary Cause 360
Hypokalemia 361
Hyponatremia 362
Kidneys
    Enlarged, Bilateral 363
    Enlarged, by Ultrasound,
        Computed Tomography,
        or Magnetic Resonance 364
    Small, Unilateral 365
Medullary Cystic Disease 366
Nephritis
    Chronic Tubulointerstitial 367
    Chronic Tubulointerstitial,
        Drug-Induced 368
    Chronic Tubulointerstitial,
        Industrial Exposure 369
Oliguria 370
Polycystic Kidneys
    History of, Abnormal Renal
        Function 371

    History of, Normal Renal
        Function 372
    Incidentally Detected 373
Polyuria 374
Proteinuria
    Trace to 1+ Positive 375
    Nephrotic Range 377
Pyelonephritis, Chronic 379
Red Blood Cell Casts 380
Renal Parenchymal
    Calcification 381
Renal Stone
    Initial 382
    Recurrent 383
    Calcium Oxalate 384
    Struvite 385
    Uric Acid 386
Uremia 387
Urine, Red 388

CHAPTER 8

Neurology

Alzheimer's Disease
    Diagnosis 391
    Management 393
Amyotrophic Lateral
    Sclerosis (ALS), Diagnosis 394
Brain Mass
    History of Primary Extracranial
        Malignancy 395
    No Known Extracranial
        Malignancy 396
Carotid Stenosis, Asymptomatic .. 397
Cervical Bruit, Asymptomatic 398
Cervical Spondylosis with
    Myelopathy 399

Cranial Neuropathy,
  Immunocompromised
  Patient 400
Diplopia 401
Dizziness, Nonvertiginous 402
Episodic Loss of Consciousness,
  Seizure Versus Syncope 403
Facial Weakness 405
Gait Disorders 406
Headache
  Acute 407
  Chronic Recurrent 408
  Migraine 409
  Post-traumatic 410
Imaging Abnormality
  Hydrocephalus 411
  Hygroma 412
  Subdural, Asymptomatic 413
  Unidentified Bright
    Objects (UBOs) 414
Lyme Disease, Possible Cause of
  Neurologic Findings 415
Memory Loss 416
Mental Status Change
  Acute or Subacute 417
  Chronic Dementia 419
  Immunocompromised
    Patient 421
Multiple Sclerosis
  Diagnosis 422
  Management 423
Myasthenia Gravis, Diagnosis 424
Myopathic Weakness 425
Neuropathy, Peripheral 426
Paresthesias
  Feet 427
  Hands 428

Parkinsonian Syndrome,
  Atypical 429
Parkinson's Disease 430
Postconcussion Syndrome 431
Ptosis 432
Radiculopathy
  Cervical 433
  Thoracic 434
Seizures
  Generalized 435
  New Onset, in Adults 436
  Partial 438
Speech Disorder 439
Spells, Transient Ischemic
  Attack Versus Seizure 440
Swallowing Disorder 441
Tics 442
Transient Ischemic Attacks
  (TIAs) 443
Tremor 445
Vertigo 446
Visual Loss, Monocular 447
Weakness, Generalized 448

CHAPTER 9

Oncology

Adenopathy, Supraclavicular 451
Back Pain, History of Cancer 452
Bone Lesion, Lytic 453
Breast Mass 454
Breast Cancer
  Family History of 455
  History of 456
Head and Neck Irradiation,
  Childhood 457

CONTENTS

Lung Cancer
    Small Cell, History of 458
    Squamous Cell, History of 459
Lymphoma, History of 460
Mammogram, Suspicious 461
Mass, Extremity 462
Melanoma, History of 463
Prostate Cancer, History of 464
Renal Cell Cancer, History of 465
Sarcoma, History of 466
Testicular Cancer, History of 467
Thyroid Cancer
    History of 468
    Medullary, Family History of .. 469

CHAPTER 10
Pulmonary

Adenopathy, Hilar, Bilateral 473
Alpha-1-Antitrypsin Deficiency ... 474
Asbestos Lung Disease 475
Asthma 476
    Cold- and Exercise-Induced .. 478
    During Pregnancy 479
    In the Elderly 480
    Occupational 481
Atelectasis 482
Cavitary Lung Lesion 483
Chronic Obstructive Pulmonary
    Disease (COPD) 484
Chronic Obstructive Pulmonary
    Disease (COPD),
    Premature 486
Cor Pulmonale 487
Cough, Chronic 488
Cystic Fibrosis 489

Disability Evaluation,
    Lung Disease 490
Dyspnea
    Chronic 491
    Episodic 492
    Nocturnal 493
Hemoptysis 494
Inhalation, Toxic 496
Lung Cancer, Non-Small
    Cell 497
Lung Disease
    Air Travel with 498
    Handicapped License
        Plates with 499
    Occupational 500
    Scuba Diving Clearance
        with 501
Pleural Effusion 502
Pneumonia
    Immunocompromised Host ... 503
    Lobar 504
    Poorly Resolving 505
Pneumothorax, Recurrent 506
Preoperative Pulmonary
    Assessment 507
Pulmonary Consolidation 508
Pulmonary Fibrosis, Interstitial ... 509
Pulmonary Hypertension,
    Primary 510
Pulmonary Infiltrate with
    Eosinophilia 511
Pulmonary Nodules
    Multiple 512
    Solitary, Central 513
    Solitary, Peripheral 514
Reactive Airway Dysfunction
    Syndrome 515

Sarcoidosis 516
Sleep Apnea/Snoring 517
Smoking Cessation 518

CHAPTER 11
Rheumatology

Ankylosing Spondylitis 521
Antinuclear Antibody (ANA),
   Positive 523
Arthritis
   Rheumatoid, Diagnosis 524
   Rheumatoid, Management 526
   With Fever 527
   With Subcutaneous
      Nodules 528
Bursitis: Shoulder, Elbow, Hip ... 529
Carpal Tunnel Syndrome 530
Dermatomyositis 531
Discoid/Cutaneous Lupus
   Diagnosis 532
   Management 533
Fasciitis, Plantar 534
Fibrositis/Fibromyalgia 535
Giant Cell/Temporal Arteritis 536
Gout 537
Pain, Chronic Soft Tissue 538
Pain in a Few Joints
   Less Than or Equal to 4
      Joints 539
   Greater Than or Equal
      to 5 Joints 541

Painful
   Ankle, Foot, or Toe 543
   Elbow 545
   Hip 547
   Knee 549
   Lower Back/Lumbosacral
      Spine 551
   Neck 553
   Shoulder 555
   Upper Back/Thoracic
      Spine 557
   Wrist and/or Hand 559
Polymyalgia Rheumatica 561
Polymyositis 562
Pseudogout 563
Raynaud's Phenomenon 564
Reiter's Syndrome 565
Rheumatic Fever 566
Sarcoidosis with Joint
   Involvement 567
Scleroderma 568
Sicca Complex, Diagnosis 569
Sjögren's Syndrome, Diagnosis ... 570
Systemic Lupus Erythematosus (SLE)
   Diagnosis 572
   Management 574
   With Nephritis 575
   With Neurologic Involvement. . 576
Tendonitis 578
Tendonitis, Achilles 579

Index 581

How to Use This Book

The Consultation Guide is designed to support specialty consultation by primary care physicians in the ambulatory environment. Its recommendations are most relevant to decisions about the first consultative visit.

Does this patient's problem require consultation? And if so, when and by whom?

What test results should the primary care physician obtain in advance because they will be valuable to the consultant at the first visit?

And which tests are seldom, if ever, appropriate before consultation?

Some primary care physicians will also find it useful to review what further tests or other interventions their consultant may need to perform. It can crystallize their own thinking about a patient's problem, and help them prepare their patient for what the consultant may recommend. Finally, *The Consultation Guide* indicates what duration and intensity of follow up the consultant may require.

Finding the Clinical Problem

The most pertinent recommendations for a given clinical problem can be located in one of three places: the Table of Contents, the Problem Lists that precede each specialty section, or the Index. When a clinical problem overlaps more than one specialty, it has been primarily assigned to the specialty with which it is most closely associated, e.g., chest pain with Cardiology and dyspnea with Pulmonary. Finally, the recommendations for many problems include a See Also list, which directs the reader to related clinical problems covered by the Guide.

Understanding the Categories of Recommendations

Indications and Timing for Referral provide recommendations to support the primary care physician's decisions before referring the patient to the consultant.

Indications fall into several categories: 1) problem or disease-related factors, such as severity, chronicity, and lack of response to conventional therapy; 2) patient-related factors, such as age, co-morbidities, and familial predispositions; and 3) physician-related factors, such as diagnostic uncertainty and needing assistance with management. This final category of indication arising from the knowledge, skills, experience, and confidence of the primary care physician deserves special explanation. For many clinical problems, such as knee pain or anemia, their severity or duration actually matters less than whether the primary care physician knows why the problem is occurring, what else it means for the patient's health, and what to do about it. Consequently, the best referral indications cannot always be pegged to a specific characteristic of a symptom, sign, or lab abnormality. Finally, patient anxiety is an additional obvious and common referral indication that is implicit and not repeatedly listed.

HOW TO USE THIS BOOK

Timing for Referral is specified for each indication based on the problem's severity, duration, progression, or potential pathophysiological implications. The categories of optimal timing for consultation are: Urgent, which has been defined as within 24 hours in the ambulatory environment; Expedited, within one week; and Routine, which will vary among consultants and health systems, but hopefully occur within four weeks.

The **Advice for Referral** section offers a varied set of key clinical insights for the referring physician. While the Guide is not designed to elaborate diagnostic algorithms, this section often highlights pivotal steps in clinical assessment. When problems might be referred to more than one specialty (e.g., Should the patient with sinusitis be referred to the allergist, infectious disease specialist, or otolaryngologist?), this section lists clinical factors that may favor one consultant over the other. In some cases, this section also defines critical information from the medical history and past test results that must be passed along to the consultant.

For any clinical problem, there is typically a relatively large domain of tests and procedures that could be done to evaluate the patient. *The Consultation Guide* does not attempt to enumerate or categorize them all—that is why patients need the clinical wisdom of generalists and specialists. But the Guide does define important subsets from among all of these potential diagnostic procedures.

Tests to Prepare for Consult list those laboratory, imaging, and other test procedures that will yield important results for the consultant to consider at the time of the first consultative visit. Put another way, these are the tests that the consultant will otherwise order in nine out of ten cases if the results are not already available. Often these are the tests yielding key findings that direct the clinician at a critical juncture in differential diagnosis. Sometimes they are simply safe and relatively inexpensive tests that rule out certain possibilities. Not seeing a test included in this category does not mean that primary care physicians should not or cannot order it themselves in appropriate patients. It simply means that the consultant will not need the test result in many patients with that clinical problem.

Tests Not Useful Before Consult identifies tests and procedures that the Guide's contributors did not consider appropriate to order before the consultant personally evaluates the patient. Tests fell into this category for several reasons: they were often diagnostically inaccurate, outdated, or potentially dangerous or particularly expensive for their diagnostic yield. Some were included because their quality and safety was significantly better when performed or requested by the consultants themselves. Panelists and reviewers were reminded that they had to exercise the highest standard to recommend excluding a test before consultation.

Tests Consultant May Need to Do offers guidance about the additional studies that a consultant might consider appropriate after reviewing the patient's clinical findings and available test results at the initial consultative visit. This list is comprehensive, including virtually all tests that might prove appropriate to confirm or exclude diagnostic possibilities. Seldom would all or most of these tests be required in one patient's case. The aim is to empower the consultant to promptly provide the advice that the primary care physician and the patient are seeking. Tests in this category can also be ordered by primary care physicians who are confident about their diagnostic approach. While this set of recommendations is driven by the logic of diagnostic decision-making, it is obvious that an additional filter may have to be installed to control precisely when and where high-cost testing will be performed in many health systems. A glossary of test abbreviations used in *The Consultation Guide* begins on page xxvii.

Follow-Up Visits Generally Required enumerates how many follow-up visits would typically be required by the consultant: none, one, two, or long-term co-management. This number does not include the initial consultative visit.

Suggested Readings and Selected Guidelines direct physicians to primary sources of current information about the evaluation and management of the clinical problems.

Your Feedback to The Consultation Guide

At every stage in development of *The Consultation Guide,* thoughtful clinicians have made wise suggestions to improve it. The Editor and Contributors hope that readers of this book will participate in that process. Please send us your thoughts, either by e-mail at www.consultguide.com, or by post to 3908 North Charles Street, Suite 300, Baltimore, Maryland 21218.

Abbreviations

5'-HIAA	5-aminoacridine hydrochloride	ECG	electrocardiogram
		EEG	electroencephalogram
ACE	angiotensin converting enzyme	ELISA	enzyme-linked immunosorbent assay
ACTH	adrenocorticotropic hormone (stimulation test)	EMG	electromyogram
		ERCP	endoscopic retrograde cholangiopancreatography
AFB	acid-fast bacillus	ESR	erythrocyte sedimentation rate
AFP	α-fetoprotein		
ALT	alanine aminotransferase		
ANA	antinuclear antibody	FEV_1	forced expiratory volume, in 1 second
ANCA	antineutrophil cytoplasmic antibody	FSH	follicle-stimulating hormone
APC	antigen presenting cells	FTA-ABS	fluorescent treponemal antibody absorption
ASLO titer	Anti-streptolysin O		
AST	aspartate aminotransferase		
		G6PD	glucose-6-phosphate dehydrogenase
BP	blood pressure		
BUN	blood urea nitrogen	GBM	glomerular basement membrane
C&S	culture and sensitivity	GH	growth hormone
CA19-9	cancer antigen 19-9	GHRH	GH-releasing hormone
CA-125	cancer antigen 125 test		
CBC	complete blood count	Hb	hemoglobin
CEA	carcinoembryonic antigen	HB_cAb	hepatitis B core antibody
CMV	cytomegalovirus	HB_sAb	hepatitis B surface antibody
CPK	creatine phosphokinase	HB_sAg	hepatitis B surface antigen
Cr	creatinine	HCG	human chorionic gonadotropin
CRH	corticotropin releasing hormone (stimulation test)	HDL	high density lipoprotein
CSF	cerebrospinal fluid	HIV	human immunodeficiency virus
CT	computed tomography		
		HLA	human lymphocyte antigen
DLCO	diffusing capacity for CO	HSV	herpes simplex virus
DSA	digital subtraction angiography	HTLV-I	human T-cell lymphotropic virus, type 1
DTPA	diethylenetriamine pentaacetic acid	^{131}I	Iodine-131
		IEP	immunoelectrophoresis
EBV	Epstein-Barr virus	Ig	immunoglobulin

ABBREVIATIONS

IGF	insulin growth factor	RDW	red cell distribution width
IVP	intravenous pyelogram	RET	*RET* proto-oncogene
		RF	rheumatoid factor
KOH	potassium hydroxide	RNP	ribonucleoprotein
KUB	kidneys, ureters, bladders	RPR test	rapid plasma reagin test
CHANGED TO: Plain film, abdomen		RVVT	Russell viper venom time
LAC	lupus anticoagulant	SPECT	single photon emission computed tomography
LDH	lactate dehydrogenase		
LDL	low density lipoprotein		
LH	luteinizing hormone	T_3	triiodothyronine
LKM anti-body	liver-kidney-microsomal antibody	T_4	thyroxine
		TB	tuberculosis
MR	magnetic resonance	TIBC	total iron binding capacity
MRI	magnetic resonance imaging	TG	triglycerides
		TRH	thyrotropin-releasing hormone
OPG	oculoplethysmography	TSH	thyroid-stimulating hormone
PA	posterior-anterior (radiograph)	TSI	thyroid-stimulating immunoglobulin
PCP	*Pneumocystis carinii* pneumonia		
PCR	polymerase chain reaction	UA	urine analysis
PET scan	positron emission tomography scan	UGIS	upper gastrointestinal series
PPD	purified protein derivative of tuberculin	VDRL test	Venereal Disease Research Laboratories test
PSA	prostate-specific antigen	VIP	vasoactive intestinal polypeptide
PTH	parathyroid hormone		
PTT	partial thromboplastin time	VLCFA	very long chain fatty acids
		V/Q scan	perfusion ventilation scan
RAST	radioallergosorbent test		
RBC	red blood cell	WBC	white blood cell

CHAPTER 1

Allergy and Immunology

Allergen Disease, Environmental Controls for	2
Anaphylaxis or Anaphylactoid Reactions, History of	3
Beesting Allergy	4
Common Variable Hypogammaglobulinemia	5
Dermatitis	
Atopic	6
Contact	7
Occupational Contact	8
Drug Reactions	
Allergic	9
Assistance with Desensitization	10
Idiosyncratic	11
Eosinophilia	261
Food and Additive Reactions	
Allergic	12
Nonallergic	13
Immunoglobulin A Deficiency	14
Insect Sting Allergy	15
Latex Sensitivity	16
Mast Cell Disorders	17
Multiple Chemical Sensitivity Syndrome	18
Nasal Polyposis	19
Pneumonitis, Hypersensitivity, Episodic	20
Postnasal Drainage, Perennial	21
Pruritus	22
Pulmonary Infections, Recurrent	23
Rhinitis	
Seasonal	24
Perennial	25
Rhinorrhea, Refractory	26
Urticaria and Angioedema	
Acute Episodes	27
Chronic	28
Vasculitis with Cutaneous Lesions	29

Allergen Disease, Environmental Controls for

Indications and Timing for Referral

- Identification of responsible allergen
- Assistance with management

Timing: Routine (less than 4 weeks)

Advice for Referral

- Careful patient diary of environmental exposures before and during symptomatic periods is helpful.

Tests to Prepare for Consult

- None

Tests Not Useful Before Consult

- Immediate hypersensitivity skin testing
- RAST

Tests Consultant May Need to Do

- Immediate hypersensitivity skin testing
- RAST

Follow-up Visits Generally Required

- One

Suggested Readings

Fernandez-Caldas E, Trudeau WL, Ledford DK. Environmental control of indoor biologic agents. [Review]. J Allergy Clin Immunol 1994;94:404–412.

Fernandez-Caldas E, Fox RW. Environmental control of indoor air pollution. [Review]. Med Clin North Am 1992;76:935–952.

Klein GL, Ziering RW. Environmental control of the home. [Review]. Clin Rev Allergy 1988;6:3–22.

Novey HS. Environmental control of the workplace. [Review]. Clin Rev Allergy 1988;6:45–60.

Selected Guidelines

Allergen skin testing. Board of Directors. American Academy of Allergy and Immunology. J Allergy Clin Immunol 1993;92:636–637.

Allergy testing. American College of Physicians [see comments]. Ann Intern Med 1989;110:317–320.

Anaphylaxis or Anaphylactoid Reactions, History of

Indications and Timing for Referral
- Refer all patients except those with a clearly defined provocative agent that can be avoided.
- If assistance with management is needed and/or patient education regarding future exposure

Timing: Expedited (less than 1 week)

Advice for Referral
- Emergent care required if airway obstruction or hypotension are present.
- Obtain serum at time of acute episode if diagnosis of anaphylaxis is not clear-cut. (Store serum in freezer for serum tryptase levels done in several laboratories in the United States.)

Tests to Prepare for Consult
- None

Tests Not Useful Before Consult
- Histamine level
- Immediate hypersensitivity skin testing
- RAST

Tests Consultant May Need to Do
- Immediate hypersensitivity skin testing
- RAST
- Provocative food/drug testing
- 5'-HIAA, 24-hour urine
- Tryptase, in acute reactions
- Skin biopsy

Follow-up Visits Generally Required
- One

Suggested Readings
Atkinson TP, Kaliner MA. Anaphylaxis. [Review]. Med Clin North Am 1992;76:841–855.

Bochner BS, Lichtenstein LM. Anaphylaxis [see comments]. [Review]. N Engl J Med 1991;324:1785–1790.

Wiggins CA, Dykewicz MS, Patterson R. Idiopathic anaphylaxis: a review. [Review]. Ann Allergy 1989;62:1–4.

Austen KF. Diseases of immediate type sensitivity. In: Fauci AS, Braunwald E, Isselbacher KJ, et al., eds. Harrison's Principles of Internal Medicine. 14th ed. New York: McGraw Hill, 1998:1860–1869.

Selected Guidelines
Allergen skin testing. Board of Directors. American Academy of Allergy and Immunology. J Allergy Clin Immunol 1993;92:636–637.

Allergy testing. American College of Physicians [see comments]. Ann Intern Med 1989;110:317–320.

See Also
- Urticaria and angioedema, acute episodes
- Urticaria and angioedema, chronic

THE CONSULTATION GUIDE

Beesting Allergy

Indications and Timing for Referral

- Acute systemic reaction after sting
- Assistance with management regarding future sting avoidance and self-medication
- Syndrome consistent with serum sickness, especially after multiple stings

Timing: Expedited (less than 1 week)

Advice for Referral

- Positive identification of stinging insect is valuable if available.
- Evaluation should precede next potential exposure. (Seasonal timing increases risk of next exposure.)
- Definitive skin testing is more informative if performed more than 4 weeks after the sting when false-negatives are less likely.

Tests to Prepare for Consult

- None

Tests Not Useful Before Consult

- Immediate hypersensitivity skin testing
- RAST

Tests Consultant May Need to Do

- Immediate hypersensitivity skin testing
- ESR
- Creatinine
- Urinalysis with microscopic
- Complement factors (C3, C4)
- Venom IgG levels
- Venom IgE levels

Follow-up Visits Generally Required

- One

Suggested Readings

Freeman TM. Insect and fire ant hypersensitivity: what the primary care physician needs to know. Compr Ther 1997;23:38–43.

Reisman RE. Insect stings [see comments]. [Review]. N Engl J Med 1994;331:523–527.

Reisman RE. Stinging insect allergy. [Review]. Med Clin North Am 1992;76:883–894.

Valentine MD. Allergy to stinging insects [published erratum appears in Ann Allergy 1993;71:96]. [Review]. Ann Allergy 1993;70:427–432.

See Also

- Insect sting allergy

4

ALLERGY AND IMMUNOLOGY

Common Variable Hypogammaglobulinemia

Indications and Timing for Referral
- Assistance with management

Timing: Routine (less than 4 weeks)

Advice for Referral
- This condition often requires co-management with an allergist/immunologist.

Tests to Prepare for Consult
- CBC with differential
- Immunoglobulins, quantitative
- Albumin, total protein

Tests Not Useful Before Consult
- Globulin (total)

Tests Consultant May Need to Do
- Functional antibody response to immunization
- ANA
- IEP
  - Serum
  - Urine
- B-lymphocyte quantitative count
- Delayed hypersensitivity skin tests

Follow-up Visits Generally Required
- Co-management, see *Advice for Referral*

Suggested Readings
Rosen FS, Cooper MD, Wedgwood RJ. The primary immunodeficiencies. N Engl J Med 1995;333:431–440.

Eisenstein EM, Sneller MC. Common variable immunodeficiency: diagnosis and management. [Review]. Ann Allergy 1994;73:285–292.

Sneller MC, Strober W, Eisenstein E, et al. NIH conference. New insights into common variable immunodeficiency [see comments]. [Review]. Ann Intern Med 1993;118:720–730.

Sweinberg SK, Wodell RA, Grodofsky MP, et al. Retrospective analysis of the incidence of pulmonary disease in hypogammaglobulinemia. J Allergy Clin Immunol 1991;88:96–104.

Cooper MD, Lawson AR. Primary immune deficiency diseases. In: Fauci AS, Braunwald E, Isselbacher KJ, et al., eds. Harrison's Principles of Internal Medicine. 14th ed. New York: McGraw Hill, 1998:1783–1791.

See Also
- IgA deficiency
- Pulmonary infections, recurrent

Dermatitis, Atopic

Indications and Timing for Referral
- Diagnostic uncertainty
- Assistance with management
- Recurrent cutaneous infections

Timing: Routine (less than 4 weeks)

Tests to Prepare for Consult
- None

Tests Not Useful Before Consult
- Immediate hypersensitivity skin testing
- RAST

Tests Consultant May Need to Do
- CBC with differential
- Platelet count
- IgE, quantitative
- Skin testing for food and aeroallergens
- RAST
- Challenge tests

Follow-up Visits Generally Required
- One

Suggested Readings
Rothe MJ, Grant-Kels JM. Diagnostic criteria for atopic dermatitis [see comments]. Lancet 1996;348:769–0:

Friedmann PS, Tan BB, Musaba E, Strickland I. Pathogenesis and management of atopic dermatitis. Clin Exp Allergy 1995;25:799–806.

Morren MA, Przybilla B, Bamelis M, et al. Atopic dermatitis: triggering factors. [Review]. J Am Acad Dermatol 1994;31:467–473.

Whitmore SE. Should atopic individuals be patch tested?. [Review]. Dermatol Clin 1994;12:491–499.

Cooper KD. New therapeutic approaches in atopic dermatitis. [Review]. Clin Rev Allergy 1993;11:543–559.

Selected Guidelines
Guidelines of care for atopic dermatitis. American Academy of Dermatology. J Am Acad Dermatol 1992;26:485–488.

Allergen skin testing. Board of Directors. American Academy of Allergy and Immunology. J Allergy Clin Immunol 1993;92:636–637.

Allergy testing. American College of Physicians [see comments]. Ann Intern Med 1989;110:317–320.

See Also
- Dermatitis, contact
- Dermatitis, occupational contact

ALLERGY AND IMMUNOLOGY

Dermatitis, Contact

Indications and Timing for Referral

- Diagnostic uncertainty
- Assistance with management

Timing: Routine (less than 4 weeks)

Advice for Referral

- History of exposures at work and home are important.

Tests to Prepare for Consult

- None

Tests Not Useful Before Consult

- Immediate hypersensitivity skin testing
- RAST
- Skin biopsy

Tests Consultant May Need to Do

- CBC with differential
- Eosinophil count, total
- IgE, quantitative
- Patch tests

Follow-up Visits Generally Required

- One

Suggested Readings

Dooms-Goossens A. Cosmetics as causes of allergic contact dermatitis. [Review]. Cutis 1993;52:316–320.

Whitmore E. Common problems of the skin. In: Barker LR, Burton JR, Zieve PD, eds. Principles of Ambulatory Medicine. 4th ed. Baltimore: Williams & Wilkins, 1995: 1439–1479.

Williford PM, Sheretz EF. Poison ivy dermatitis. Nuances in treatment. [Review]. Arch Fam Med 1994;3:184–188.

Selected Guidelines

Allergen skin testing. Board of Directors. American Academy of Allergy and Immunology. J Allergy Clin Immunol 1993;92:636–637.

Allergy testing. American College of Physicians [see comments]. Ann Intern Med 1989;110: 317–320.

Guidelines of care for atopic dermatitis. American Academy of Dermatology. J Am Acad Dermatol 1992;26:485–488.

See Also

- Dermatitis, atopic
- Dermatitis, occupational contact

Dermatitis, Occupational Contact

Indications and Timing for Referral
- Diagnostic uncertainty
- Assistance with management

Timing: Routine (less than 4 weeks)

Tests to Prepare for Consult
- None

Tests Not Useful Before Consult
- Immediate hypersensitivity skin testing
- RAST

Tests Consultant May Need to Do
- Patch tests

Follow-up Visits Generally Required
- One

Suggested Readings

Rietschel RL. Occupational contact dermatitis. [Review] [18 refs]. Lancet 1997;349:1093–1095.

Marrakchi S, Maibach HI. What is occupational contact dermatitis? An operational definition. [Review]. Dermatol Clin 1994;12:477–484.

Turjanmaa K. Update on occupational natural rubber latex allergy. [Review]. Dermatol Clin 1994;12:561–567.

Epstein WL. Occupational poison ivy and oak dermatitis. [Review]. Dermatol Clin 1994;12:511–516.

Fisher AA. Allergic contact reactions in health personnel. [Review]. J Allergy Clin Immunol 1992;90:729–738.

Selected Guidelines

Guidelines of care for atopic dermatitis. American Academy of Dermatology. J Am Acad Dermatol 1992;26:485–488.

Allergen skin testing. Board of Directors. American Academy of Allergy and Immunology. J Allergy Clin Immunol 1993;92:636–637.

Allergy testing. American College of Physicians [see comments]. Ann Intern Med 1989;110:317–320.

See Also
- Latex sensitivity
- Dermatitis, contact
- Dermatitis, atopic

ALLERGY AND IMMUNOLOGY

Drug Reactions, Allergic

Indications and Timing for Referral
- Diagnostic uncertainty
- Drug is potentially or actually needed despite reaction
- Unusually prolonged or severe clinical manifestation after initial reaction

Timing: Routine (less than 4 weeks)

Advice for Referral
- Complete concurrent medication history is critical.
- Consult before next critical use.

Tests to Prepare for Consult
- None

Tests Not Useful Before Consult
- Immediate hypersensitivity skin testing
- RAST

Tests Consultant May Need to Do
- CBC with differential
- ESR
- Creatinine
- ALT, AST, alkaline phosphatase
- Urinalysis with microscopic
- Immediate hypersensitivity skin testing
- RAST
- Provocative testing for relevant drugs

Follow-up Visits Generally Required
- One

Suggested Readings
Roujeau JC, Stern RS. Severe adverse cutaneous reactions to drugs. [Review]. N Engl J Med 1994;331:1272–1285.

Weiss ME. Drug allergy. [Review]. Med Clin North Am 1992;76:857–882.

Anderson JA. Allergic reactions to drugs and biological agents. [Review]. JAMA 1992;268:2844–2857.

Coopman SA, Stern RS. Cutaneous drug reactions in human immunodeficiency virus infection [editorial; comment]. [Review]. Arch Dermatol 1991;127:714–717.

See Also
- Drug reactions, idiosyncratic
- Drug reactions, assistance with desensitization

Drug Reactions, Assistance with Desensitization

Indications and Timing for Referral

- Assistance with management
- Drug is potentially or actually needed despite reaction

Timing: Routine (less than 4 weeks)

Advice for Referral

- Complete concurrent medication history is critical.

Tests to Prepare for Consult

- None

Tests Not Useful Before Consult

- Immediate hypersensitivity skin testing
- RAST
- Provocative testing for relevant drugs

Tests Consultant May Need to Do

- Desensitization procedures
- Immediate hypersensitivity skin testing
- RAST
- Provocative testing for relevant drugs

Follow-up Visits Generally Required

- Two

Suggested Readings

Patterson R, DeSwarte RD, Greenberger PA, et al. Drug allergy and protocols for management of drug allergies. [Review]. Allergy Proc 1994;15:239–264.

Wintroub BU, Stern RS. Cutaneous drug reactions. In: Fauci AS, Braunwald E, Isselbacher KJ, et al., eds. Harrison's Principles of Internal Medicine. 14th ed. New York: McGraw Hill, 1998: 249–255.

See Also

- Drug reactions, idiosyncratic
- Drug reactions, allergic

ALLERGY AND IMMUNOLOGY

Drug Reactions, Idiosyncratic

Indications and Timing for Referral
- Diagnostic uncertainty
- Drug is potentially or actually needed despite reaction
- Unusually prolonged or severe clinical manifestation after initial reaction

Timing: Routine (less than 4 weeks)

Advice for Referral
- Complete concurrent medication history is critical.
- Consult before next critical use.

Tests to Prepare for Consult
- None

Tests Not Useful Before Consult
- Immediate hypersensitivity skin testing
- RAST

Tests Consultant May Need to Do
- CBC with differential
- ESR
- Creatinine
- ALT, AST, alkaline phosphatase
- Urinalysis with microscopic
- Immediate hypersensitivity skin testing
- RAST
- Provocative testing for relevant drugs

Follow-up Visits Generally Required
- One

Suggested Readings
Rieder MJ. Mechanisms of unpredictable adverse drug reactions. [Review]. Drug Saf 1994;11:196–212.

Bonnetblanc JM. Drug hypersensitivity syndrome. [Review]. Dermatology 1993;187:84–85.

Roujeau JC, Stern RS. Severe adverse cutaneous reactions to drugs. [Review]. N Engl J Med 1994;331:1272–1285.

See Also
- Drug reactions, allergic
- Drug reactions, assistance with desensitization

THE CONSULTATION GUIDE

Food and Additive Reactions, Allergic

Indications and Timing for Referral

- Assistance with management
- Diagnostic uncertainty
- History of anaphylactic reaction or significant angioedema to any food

Timing: Routine (less than 4 weeks)

Advice for Referral

- Careful patient diary critical

Tests to Prepare for Consult

- None

Tests Not Useful Before Consult

- IgE, quantitative
- Immediate hypersensitivity skin testing
- RAST

Tests Consultant May Need to Do

- Immediate hypersensitivity skin testing
- RAST
- Provocative food/drug testing
- Spirometry

Follow-up Visits Generally Required

- One

Suggested Readings

Bahna SL, Kanuga J. Food hypersensitivity. [Review]. Rheum Dis Clin North Am 1991;17:243–249.

Sampson HA, Metcalfe DD. Food allergies. [Review]. JAMA 1992;268:2840–2844.

Pearl ER. Food allergy. [Review] [38 refs]. Lippincotts Prim Care Pract 1997;1:154–167.

Weber RW. Food additives and allergy. [Review]. Ann Allergy 1993;70:183–190.

Daul CB, Morgan JE, Lehrer SB. Hypersensitivity reactions to crustacea and mollusks. [Review]. Clin Rev Allergy 1993;11:201–222.

O'Neil C, Helbling AA, Lehrer SB. Allergic reactions to fish. [Review]. Clin Rev Allergy 1993;11:183–200.

Pearson DJ. Pseudo-food allergy. [Review]. Rheum Dis Clin North Am 1991;17:343–349.

Zeiger RS. Prevention of food allergy and atopic disease. [Review] [90 refs]. J R Soc Med 1997;90(Suppl 30):21–33.

See Also

- Food and additive reactions, nonallergic

ALLERGY AND IMMUNOLOGY

Food and Additive Reactions, Nonallergic

Indications and Timing for Referral

- Assistance with management
- Diagnostic uncertainty

Timing: Routine (less than 4 weeks)

Advice for Referral

- Careful patient diary critical

Tests to Prepare for Consult

- None

Tests Not Useful Before Consult

- Immediate hypersensitivity skin testing
- RAST

Tests Consultant May Need to Do

- Provocative food/drug testing
- Spirometry

Follow-up Visits Generally Required

- One

Suggested Readings

Simon RA. Adverse reactions to food and drug additives [review]. Immunol Allergy Clin North Am 1996;16:137.

Sampson HA, Metcalfe DD. Food allergies. [Review]. JAMA 1992;268:2840–2844.

Pearl ER. Food allergy. [Review] [38 refs]. Lippincotts Prim Care Pract 1997;1:154–167.

Vaughan TR. The role of food in the pathogenesis of migraine headache. [Review]. Clin Rev Allergy 1994;12:167–180.

See Also

Food and additive reactions, allergic

Immunoglobulin A Deficiency

Indications and Timing for Referral

- Uncertainty regarding significance and implications

Timing: Routine (less than 4 weeks)

Tests to Prepare for Consult

- Immunoglobulins, quantitative

Tests Not Useful Before Consult

- IEP, serum

Tests Consultant May Need to Do

- Functional antibody response to immunization
- SPEP with immunofixation

Follow-up Visits Generally Required

- Two

Suggested Readings

Itescu S. Adult immunodeficiency and rheumatic disease. Rheum Dis Clin North Am 1996;22:53–73.

Johnson ML, Keeton LG, Zhu ZB, et al. Age-related changes in serum immunoglobulins in patients with familial IgA deficiency and common variable immunodeficiency (CVID). Clin Exp Immunol 1997;108:477–483.

Sethi DS, Winkelstein JA, Lederman H, Loury MC. Immunologic defects in patients with chronic recurrent sinusitis: diagnosis and management. Otolaryngol Head Neck Surg 1995;112:242–247.

Rosen FS, Cooper MD, Wedgwood RJ. The primary immunodeficiencies. N Engl J Med 1995;333:431–440.

Cooper MD, Lawson AR. Primary immune deficiency diseases. In: Fauci AS, Braunwald E, Isselbacher KJ, et al., eds. Harrison's Principles of Internal Medicine. 14th ed. New York: McGraw Hill, 1998:1783–1791.

Insect Sting Allergy

Indications and Timing for Referral
- Acute systemic reaction after sting
- Assistance with management regarding future sting avoidance and self-medication
- Syndrome consistent with serum sickness, especially after multiple stings

Timing: Expedited (less than 1 week)

Advice for Referral
- Positive identification of stinging insect is valuable if available.
- Evaluation should precede next potential exposure (seasonal timing increases risk of next exposure).
- Definitive testing is more accurate if performed more than 4 weeks after the sting.

Tests to Prepare for Consult
- None

Tests Not Useful Before Consult
- Immediate hypersensitivity skin testing
- RAST

Tests Consultant May Need to Do
- Immediate hypersensitivity skin testing
- RAST
- Creatinine
- Urinalysis with microscopic
- Complement factors (C3, C4)

Follow-up Visits Generally Required
- One

Suggested Readings
Freeman TM. Insect and fire ant hypersensitivity: what the primary care physician needs to know. Compr Ther 1997;23:38–43.

Reisman RE. Insect stings [see comments]. [Review]. N Engl J Med 1994;331:523–527.

Reisman RE. Stinging insect allergy. [Review]. Med Clin North Am 1992;76:883–894.

Valentine MD. Allergy to stinging insects [published erratum appears in Ann Allergy 1993;71:96]. [Review]. Ann Allergy 1993;70:427–432.

See Also
- Beesting allergy

THE CONSULTATION GUIDE

Latex Sensitivity

Indications and Timing for Referral

- Diagnostic uncertainty
- Assistance with management

Timing: Routine (less than 4 weeks)

Advice for Referral

- Skin and RAST testing for latex sensitivity is not generally advisable due to the lack of any standard commercial test material available. Also, difficulty in interpreting test results may occur.

Tests to Prepare for Consult

- None

Tests Not Useful Before Consult

- Immediate hypersensitivity skin testing
- Latex skin testing
- RAST

Tests Consultant May Need to Do

- RAST
- Patch tests
- Latex skin testing, epicutaneous

Follow-up Visits Generally Required

- One

Suggested Readings

Fisher AA. The diagnosis and management of health personnel allergic to natural rubber latex gloves. Part II. [Review] [17 refs]. Cutis 1997;59:168–170.

Sussman GL, Beezhold DH. Allergy to latex rubber. [Review]. Ann Intern Med 1995;122:43–46.

Slater JE. Latex allergy. [Review]. J Allergy Clinical Immunol 1994;94:139–149.

Yassin MS, Lierl MB, Fischer TJ, et al. Latex allergy in hospital employees. Ann Allergy 1994;72:245–249.

Selected Guidelines

Task Force on Allergic Reactions to Latex. American Academy of Allergy and Immunology. Committee report. J Allergy Clin Immunol 1993;92:16–18.

Guidelines of care for atopic dermatitis. American Academy of Dermatology. J Am Acad Dermatol 1992;26:485–488.

Allergen skin testing. Board of Directors. American Academy of Allergy and Immunology. J Allergy Clin Immunol 1993;92:636–637.

Allergy testing. American College of Physicians [see comments]. Ann Intern Med 1989;110:317–320.

See Also

- Dermatitis, occupational contact

ALLERGY AND IMMUNOLOGY

Mast Cell Disorders

Indications and Timing for Referral

- Diagnostic uncertainty
- Assistance with management

Timing: Routine (less than 4 weeks)

Advice for Referral

- Histologic documentation of diagnosis if available

Tests to Prepare for Consult

- CBC
- ALT, AST, alkaline phosphatase
- Bilirubin

Tests Not Useful Before Consult

- None

Tests Consultant May Need to Do

- Tryptase
- 24-hour urine histamine
- Skin biopsy
- Bone marrow biopsy

Follow-up Visits Generally Required

- Two

Suggested Readings

Longley J, Duffy TP, Kohn S. The mast cell and mast cell disease. [Review]. J Am Acad Dermatology 1995;32:545–561.

Horan RF, Schneider LC, Sheffer AL. Allergic skin disorders and mastocytosis. [Review]. JAMA 1992;268:2858–2868.

Metcalfe DD. Mastocytosis. In: Bennett JC, Plum F, eds. Cecil Textbook of Medicine. 20th ed. Philadelphia: WB Saunders, 1996:1435–1437.

See Also

- Flushing

THE CONSULTATION GUIDE

Multiple Chemical Sensitivity Syndrome

Indications and Timing for Referral

- Diagnostic uncertainty
- Assistance with management
- Disability assessment

Timing: Routine (less than 4 weeks)

Tests to Prepare for Consult

- CBC
- Creatinine
- Glucose
- Electrolytes (Na, K, Cl, CO_2)
- Calcium
- ALT, AST, alkaline phosphatase
- TSH (assay sensitivity <0.1 mU/L)
- Urinalysis with microscopic

Tests Not Useful Before Consult

- Immediate hypersensitivity skin testing
- RAST
- Environmental chemical analyses
  - Serum
  - Tissue
- Lymphocyte phenotyping profiles
- Environmental allergen serologies

Tests Consultant May Need to Do

- Immediate hypersensitivity skin testing
- RAST
- Double-blind challenge tests

Follow-up Visits Generally Required

- One

Suggested Readings

Weaver VM. Medical management of the multiple chemical sensitivity patient. Regul Toxicol Pharmacol 1996;24:S111–S115.

Hahn M, Bonkovsky HL. Multiple chemical sensitivity syndrome and porphyria. A note of caution and concern. [Review] [35 refs]. Arch Intern Med 1997;157:281–285.

Menzies D, Bourbeau J. Current concepts: building-related illnesses. N Engl J Med 1997;337(21):1524–1531.

McCampbell A. Controversy over multiple chemical sensitivities [letter; comment]. Ann Intern Med 1994;120:250–251.

Selected Guidelines

Allergy testing. American College of Physicians [see comments]. Ann Intern Med 1989;110:317–320.

Allergen skin testing. Board of Directors. American Academy of Allergy and Immunology. J Allergy Clin Immunol 1993;92:636–637.

ALLERGY AND IMMUNOLOGY

Nasal Polyposis

Indications and Timing for Referral
- Patient has coexisting persistent asthma
- Unresponsive or intolerant to conventional therapies
- Associated recurrences of sinusitis
- Need for either multiple or prolonged bursts of systemic glucocorticoids
- Associated with anosmia
- Associated with aspirin hypersensitivity

Timing: Routine (less than 4 weeks)

Advice for Referral
- Co-management with an allergist may be useful to evaluate allergic basis and determine management plan.
- Sinus CT, focused series is a limited series of appropriate regional cuts to include coronal images of the osteomeatal complex.
- Imaging should not be obtained during or within 2 weeks of an acute episode of sinusitis or other respiratory tract infection.
- History of aspirin intolerance or signs of cystic fibrosis are important.

Tests to Prepare for Consult
- CT, sinuses, focused series (see *Advice for Referral*)

Tests Not Useful Before Consult
- None

Tests Consultant May Need to Do
- Immediate hypersensitivity skin testing
- RAST
- Nasal cytology
- Fiberoptic rhinolaryngoscopy

Follow-up Visits Generally Required
- Co-management, see *Advice for Referral*

Suggested Readings
Hosemann W, Gode U, Wagner W. Epidemiology, pathophysiology of nasal polyposis, and spectrum of endonasal sinus surgery. [Review]. Am J Otolaryngol 1994;15:85–98.

King VV. Upper respiratory disease, sinusitis, and polyposis. [Review]. Clin Rev Allergy 1991;9:143–157.

Mygind N, Lildholdt T. Nasal polyps treatment: medical management. Allergy Asthma Proc 1996;17:275–282.

Holmberg K, Karlsson G. Nasal polyps: medical or surgical management? Clin Exp Allergy 1996;26:275–282.

Bernstein JM, Gorfien J, Noble B. Role of allergy in nasal polyposis: a review. Otolaryngol Head Neck Surg 1995;113:724–732.

See Also
- Rhinitis, perennial
- Rhinitis, refractory

Pneumonitis, Hypersensitivity, Episodic

Indications and Timing for Referral

- Etiology unclear
- Assistance with management

Timing: Routine (less than 4 weeks)

Advice for Referral

- Histories of potential occupational or recreational exposure, and of related medication ingestion are important.

Tests to Prepare for Consult

- CBC with differential
- Chest radiograph

Tests Not Useful Before Consult

- Immediate hypersensitivity skin testing
- RAST

Tests Consultant May Need to Do

- Precipitin tests
- Spirometry, before and after bronchodilator
- Diffusing capacity for CO (DLCO)
- Lung volumes
- *Aspergillus* skin test

Follow-up Visits Generally Required

- Two

Suggested Readings

Schuyler MR. Hypersensitivity pneumonitis. In: Fishman AP, Elias JA, Fishman JA, et al., eds. Fishman's Pulmonary Diseases and Disorders. 3rd ed. New York: McGraw Hill, 1998:1085–1097.

Craig TJ, Richerson HB. Update on hypersensitivity pneumonitis. [Review] [24 refs]. Compr Ther 1996;22:559–564.

Krasnick J, Meuwissen HJ, Nakao MA, et al. Hypersensitivity pneumonitis—problems in diagnosis. J Allergy Clin Immunol 1996;97:1027–1030.

Schuyler M, Cormier Y. The diagnosis of hypersensitivity pneumonitis [editorial; comment]. Chest 1997;111:534–536.

See Also

- Asthma
- Dyspnea, episodic
- Cough, chronic

ALLERGY AND IMMUNOLOGY

Postnasal Drainage, Perennial

Indications and Timing for Referral

- Patient has co-existing persistent asthma
- Unresponsive or intolerant to conventional therapies
- Associated recurrences of sinusitis
- Need for either multiple or prolonged courses of systemic glucocorticoids

Timing: Routine (less than 4 weeks)

Advice for Referral

- Sinus CT, focused series is a limited series of appropriate cuts to include coronal images of the osteomeatal complex.

Tests to Prepare for Consult

- None

Tests Not Useful Before Consult

- IgE, quantitative
- Immediate hypersensitivity skin testing
- RAST
- Sinus radiographs
- CT scan, sinuses

Tests Consultant May Need to Do

- Immediate hypersensitivity skin testing
- RAST
- Sinus radiographs
- CT, sinuses, focused series (see *Advice for Referral*)
- Fiberoptic rhinolaryngoscopy
- Nasal smear

Follow-up Visits Generally Required

- One

Suggested Readings

Badhwar AK, Druce HM. Allergic rhinitis. [Review]. Med Clin North Am 1992;76:789–803.

Naclerio RM. Allergic rhinitis [see comments]. [Review]. N Engl J Med 1991;325:860–869.

Curley FJ, Irwin RS, Pratter MR, et al. Cough and the common cold. Am Rev Respir Dis 1988;138:305–311.

Suonpaa J. Treatment of allergic rhinitis. Ann Med 1996;28:17–22.

DeShazo RD. Allergic rhinitis. In: Bennett JC, Plum F, eds. Cecil Textbook of Medicine. 20th ed. Philadelphia: WB Saunders, 1996:1413–1417.

Selected Guidelines

Allergy testing. American College of Physicians [see comments]. Ann Intern Med 1989;110:317–320.

See Also

- Nasal polyposis
- Rhinitis, seasonal
- Rhinitis, perennial
- Rhinorrhea, refractory

Pruritus

Indications and Timing for Referral

- Symptoms are persistent, unexplained and generalized

Timing: Routine (less than 4 weeks)

Tests to Prepare for Consult

- Glucose
- CBC with differential
- BUN, Creatinine
- TSH (assay sensitivity <0.1 mU/L)
- Bilirubin
- ALT, AST, alkaline phosphatase
- Calcium

Tests Consultant May Need to Do

- Eosinophil count, total
- Immediate hypersensitivity skin testing
- RAST
- IEP
  - Serum
  - Urine
- Radiograph, chest
- ALT, AST, alkaline phosphatase
- Bilirubin
- Glucose
  - Fasting
  - Postprandial
- Skin biopsy

Follow-up Visits Generally Required

- One

Suggested Readings

Greaves MW, Wall PD. Pathophysiology of itching [see comments]. [Review] [30 refs]. Lancet 1996;348:938–940.

Klecz RJ, Schwartz RA. Pruritus. [Review]. Am Fam Physician 1992;45:2681–2686.

Lober CW. Pruritus and malignancy. [Review]. Clin Dermatol 1993;11:125–128.

Fried RG. Evaluation and treatment of "psychogenic" pruritus and self-excoriation. [Review]. J Am Acad Dermatol 1994;30:993–999.

Berger TG. Evaluation and treatment of pruritus in the HIV-infected patient. [Review]. AIDS Clin Rev 1989:205–220.

ALLERGY AND IMMUNOLOGY

Pulmonary Infections, Recurrent

Indications and Timing for Referral

- Uncertain etiology
- Nonsmoker with more than three episodes per year without obvious underlying factors and requiring treatment with antibiotics
- Patient with suspected associated host defense deficiency or asthma

Timing: Routine (less than 4 weeks)

Advice for Referral

- Sinus CT, focused series is a limited series of appropriate regional cuts to include coronal images of the osteomeatal complex.
- Functional antibody response is measured by detecting an antibody to an immunogen (e.g., diptheria, tetanus).

Tests to Prepare for Consult

- CBC with differential
- Immunoglobulins, quantitative
- Radiograph, chest

Tests Not Useful Before Consult

- None

Tests Consultant May Need to Do

- IgG subclasses
- Immediate hypersensitivity skin testing
- Functional antibody response to immunization
- CH50
- Human immunodeficiency virus (HIV) antibody testing
- IEP
  - Serum
  - Urine
- CT, sinuses, focused series (see *Advice for Referral*)
- CT scan, thorax

Follow-up Visits Generally Required

- Two

Suggested Readings

Geppert EF. Chronic and recurrent pneumonia. [Review]. Sem Respir Infect 1992;7:282–288.

Gross TJ, Chavis AD, Lynch JP 3d. Noninfectious pulmonary diseases masquerading as community-acquired pneumonia. [Review]. Clin Chest Med 1991;12:363–393.

See Also

- Common variable hypogammaglobulinemia

THE CONSULTATION GUIDE

Rhinitis, Seasonal

Indications and Timing for Referral

- Patient has co-existing persistent asthma
- Associated recurrences of sinusitis or otitis media
- Unresponsive or intolerant to conventional therapies
- Need for either multiple or prolonged courses of systemic glucocorticoids

Timing: Routine (less than 4 weeks)

Advice for Referral

- Careful medication history vital, e.g., chronicle of medications taken and responses to them.
- Patient should be off usual antihistamines 3 to 4 days before referral. Astemizole (Hismanal) may interfere with skin testing for up to 14 weeks.
- RAST testing infrequently required.

Tests to Prepare for Consult

- None

Tests Not Useful Before Consult

- IgE, quantitative
- Immediate hypersensitivity skin testing
- RAST
- Sinus radiographs
- CT scan, sinuses

Tests Consultant May Need to Do

- Skin testing for relevant aeroallergens
- RAST
- Nasal cytology

Follow-up Visits Generally Required

- One

Suggested Readings

Badhwar AK, Druce HM. Allergic rhinitis. [Review]. Med Clin North Am 1992;76:789–803.

Naclerio RM. Allergic rhinitis [see comments]. [Review]. N Engl J Med 1991;325:860–869.

Lund VJ. Seasonal allergic rhinitis – a review of current therapy. Allergy 1996;51(Suppl 28):5–7.

Suonpaa J. Treatment of allergic rhinitis. Ann Med 1996;28:17–22.

Selected Guidelines

Allergen skin testing. Board of Directors. American Academy of Allergy and Immunology. J Allergy Clin Immunol 1993;92:636–637.

Allergy testing. American College of Physicians [see comments]. Ann Intern Med 1989;110:317–320.

See Also

- Rhinitis, perennial
- Rhinorrhea, refractory
- Postnasal drainage, perennial

ALLERGY AND IMMUNOLOGY

Rhinitis, Perennial

Indications and Timing for Referral

- Patient snores or has anosmia
- Patient has co-existing persistent asthma
- Unresponsive or intolerant to conventional therapies
- Associated recurrences of sinusitis
- Need for either multiple or prolonged courses of systemic glucocorticoids

Timing: Routine (less than 4 weeks)

Advice for Referral

- Sinus CT, focused series is a limited series of appropriate regional cuts to include coronal images of the osteomeatal complex.
- History of medications that may induce nasal congestion (e.g., antihypertensive drugs), and chronic decongestant use is important.

Tests to Prepare for Consult

- None

Tests Not Useful Before Consult

- IgE, quantitative
- Immediate hypersensitivity skin testing
- RAST

Tests Consultant May Need to Do

- CBC with differential
- Skin testing for relevant aeroallergens
- RAST
- Sinus radiographs
- CT, sinuses, focused series (see *Advice for Referral*)
- Fiberoptic rhinolaryngoscopy
- Nasal cytology
- TSH

Follow-up Visits Generally Required

- One

Suggested Readings

Badhwar AK, Druce HM. Allergic rhinitis. [Review]. Med Clin North Am 1992;76:789–803.

Naclerio RM. Allergic rhinitis [see comments]. [Review]. N Engl J Med 1991;325:860–869.

Suonpaa J. Treatment of allergic rhinitis. Ann Med 1996;28:17–22.

Selected Guidelines

Allergen skin testing. Board of Directors. American Academy of Allergy and Immunology. J Allergy Clin Immunol 1993;92:636–637.

Allergy testing. American College of Physicians [see comments]. Ann Intern Med 1989;110:317–320.

See Also

- Postnasal drainage, perennial
- Rhinorrhea, refractory
- Rhinitis, seasonal
- Nasal polyposis

Rhinorrhea, Refractory

Indications and Timing for Referral

- Unresponsive to conventional therapy

Timing: Routine (less than 4 weeks)

Advice for Referral

- Careful medication history is vital, including a chronicle of medications taken and responses to them.
- Sinus CT, focused series is a limited series of appropriate regional cuts to include coronal images of the osteomeatal complex.
- If there is a history of recent head trauma, obtain radiographic views for cribriform plate fracture.

Tests to Prepare for Consult

- None

Tests Not Useful Before Consult

- IgE, quantitative
- Immediate hypersensitivity skin testing
- RAST
- Sinus radiographs
- CT scan, sinuses

Tests Consultant May Need to Do

- Immediate hypersensitivity skin testing
- RAST
- Sinus radiographs
- CT, sinuses, focused series (see *Advice for Referral*)
- Fiberoptic rhinolaryngoscopy
- Glucose nasal secretions
- Nasal smear

Follow-up Visits Generally Required

- Two

Suggested Readings

Badhwar AK, Druce HM. Allergic rhinitis. [Review]. Med Clin North Am 1992;76:789–803.

Naclerio RM. Allergic rhinitis [see comments]. [Review]. N Engl J Med 1991;325:860–869.

Evans KL. Diagnosis and management of sinusitis. [Review]. Br Med J 1994;309:1415–1422.

Druce HM. Diagnosis of sinusitis in adults: history, physical examination, nasal cytology, echo, and rhinoscope. [Review]. J Allergy Clin Immunol 1992;90:436–441.

Daley CL, Sande M. The runny nose. Infection of the paranasal sinuses. [Review]. Infectious Dis Clin North Am 1988;2:131–147.

Suonpaa J. Treatment of allergic rhinitis. Ann Med 1996;28:17–22.

Selected Guidelines

Allergy testing. American College of Physicians [see comments]. Ann Intern Med 1989;110:317–320.

See Also

- Rhinitis, seasonal
- Rhinitis, perennial
- Postnasal drainage, perennial
- Nasal polyposis

ALLERGY AND IMMUNOLOGY

Urticaria and Angioedema, Acute Episodes

Indications and Timing for Referral
- Previous episode involving upper airway
- Multiple, unexplained or uncontrolled episodes

Timing: Expedited (less than 1 week)

Advice for Referral
- Careful patient diary of events and meals within 4 hours of symptom onset is helpful.

Tests to Prepare for Consult
- CBC with differential
- ALT, AST, alkaline phosphatase

Tests Not Useful Before Consult
- Immediate hypersensitivity skin testing
- RAST

Tests Consultant May Need to Do
- ESR
- C1 inhibitor
- Complement factors (C3, C4)
- Immediate hypersensitivity skin testing
- RAST
- Skin biopsy

Follow-up Visits Generally Required
- One

Suggested Readings
Charlesworth EN. Urticaria and angioedema: a clinical spectrum. [Review] [90 refs]. Ann Allergy Asthma Immunol 1996;76:484–495.

Casale TB, Sampson HA, Hanifin J, et al. Guide to physical urticarias [see comments]. J Allergy Clin Immunol 1988;82:758–763.

Mahmood T. Urticaria. [Review]. Am Fam Physician 1995;51:811–816.

Harvell J, Bason M, Maibach HI. Contact urticaria (immediate reaction syndrome). [Review]. Clin Rev Allergy 1992;10:303–323.

Stafford CT. Urticaria as a sign of systemic disease. [Review]. Ann Allergy 1990;64:264–270.

Selected Guidelines
Allergen skin testing. Board of Directors. American Academy of Allergy and Immunology. J Allergy Clin Immunol 1993;92:636–637.

Allergy testing. American College of Physicians [see comments]. Ann Intern Med 1989;110:317–320.

See Also
- Anaphylaxis or anaphylactoid reactions, history of
- Urticaria and angioedema, chronic

Urticaria and Angioedema, Chronic

Indications and Timing for Referral

- Persistent for longer than 6 weeks
- Assistance with management

Timing: Routine (less than 4 weeks)

Tests to Prepare for Consult

- CBC with differential
- ESR
- BUN, Creatinine
- ALT
- Bilirubin

Tests Not Useful Before Consult

- Immediate hypersensitivity skin testing
- RAST

Tests Consultant May Need to Do

- Immediate hypersensitivity skin testing
- RAST
- TSH (assay sensitivity <0.1 mU/L)
- ANA
- C1 inhibitor
- Complement factors (C3, C4)
- Hepatitis
    - A antibody
    - B surface antigen
    - B core antibody
    - C antibody
    - E antigen
- Stool O&P
- Amebic serology
- Skin biopsy

Follow-up Visits Generally Required

- Two

Suggested Readings

Cicardi M, Agostoni A. Hereditary angioedema. N Engl J Med 1996;334:1666–1667.

Charlesworth EN. Urticaria and angioedema: a clinical spectrum. [Review] [90 refs]. Ann Allergy Asthma Immunol 1996;76:484–495.

Huston DP, Bressler RB. Urticaria and angioedema. [Review]. Med Clin North Am 1992;76:805–840.

Casale TB, Sampson HA, Hanifin J, et al. Guide to physical urticarias [see comments]. J Allergy Clin Immunol 1988;82:758–763.

Mahmood T. Urticaria. [Review]. Am Fam Physician 1995;51:811–816.

Stafford CT. Urticaria as a sign of systemic disease. [Review]. Ann Allergy 1990;64:264–270.

Armenaka M, Lehach J, Rosenstreich DL. Successful management of chronic urticaria. Clin Rev Allergy 1992;10:371–390.

Selected Guidelines

Allergen skin testing. Board of Directors. American Academy of Allergy and Immunology. J Allergy Clin Immunol 1993;92:636–637.

Allergy testing. American College of Physicians [see comments]. Ann Intern Med 1989;110:317–320.

See Also

- Urticaria and angioedema, acute episodes
- Anaphylaxis or anaphylactoid reactions, history of

ALLERGY AND IMMUNOLOGY

Vasculitis with Cutaneous Lesions

Indications and Timing for Referral

- Assistance with management

Timing: Expedited (less than 1 week)

Tests to Prepare for Consult

- CBC with differential
- ESR
- BUN, Creatinine
- ALT, AST, alkaline phosphatase
- Urinalysis with microscopic

Tests Not Useful Before Consult

- RAST

Tests Consultant May Need to Do

- CBC with differential
- Creatinine
- Urinalysis with microscopic
- 24-hour urine protein
- Cryoglobulins
- CH50
- Complement factors (C3, C4)
- Rheumatoid factor
- Hepatitis B surface antigen
- Skin biopsy

Follow-up Visits Generally Required

- Two

Suggested Readings

Allen NB, Bressler PB. Diagnosis and treatment of the systemic and cutaneous necrotizing vasculitis syndromes. [Review] [39 refs]. Med Clin North Am 1997;81:243–259.

Gibson LE. Cutaneous vasculitis: approach to diagnosis and systemic associations. [Review]. Mayo Clin Proc 1990;65:221–229.

Roujeau JC, Stern RS. Severe adverse cutaneous reactions to drugs. [Review]. N Engl J Med 1994;331:1272–1285.

Dumler JS, Walker DH. Diagnostic tests for Rocky Mountain spotted fever and other rickettsial diseases. [Review]. Dermatol Clin 1994;12:25–36.

CHAPTER 2

Cardiology

Aneurysm, Ventricular 33
Aortic Valve, Bicuspid/Calcified 35
Atrial Fibrillation 36
Atrial Flutter 38
Bradycardia 39
Cardiomyopathy 40
Cerebrovascular Accident (CVA) or Transient Ischemic
   Attack (TIA), Possible Cardiac Source of Embolus 42
Chest Discomfort
   Anginal 43
   Non-Anginal 45
   Possible Angina 47
Conduction Defect
   Left Bundle Branch Block 49
   Right Bundle Branch Block 50
   Left Anterior Fascicular Block 51
Coronary Artery Disease, History of Previous Coronary
   Bypass Grafting, or Percutaneous Transluminal Coronary
   Angioplasty 52
Coronary Bypass Grafting or Percutaneous Transluminal Coronary
   Angioplasty—Second Opinion 54
Dyspnea
   Chronic 56
   Episodic 57
   Nocturnal 58
Edema, Dependent 59
Electrocardiogram
   Abnormal 60
   Abnormal Stress 62
Fenfluramine/Dexfenfluramine Use, History of 64
Heart Block
   First-Degree Atrioventricular 65
   Second-Degree Atrioventricular, Mobitz 1 66
   Second-Degree Atrioventricular, Mobitz 2 67
   Third-Degree Atrioventricular 68

(continued)

THE CONSULTATION GUIDE

Cardiology (continued)

Heart Failure
    Etiology Uncertain, New Onset 70
    Management 72
Heart Murmur
    Aortic 74
    Diastolic 75
    Mitral 77
Hypotension, Orthostatic 79
Lightheadedness/Near Syncope 80
Mitral Annulus Calcification 82
Mitral Valve Prolapse
    Click-Murmur/Suspected 83
    Echocardiographically Confirmed 84
Myocardial Infarction (MI)
    Recent, Uncomplicated 85
    Silent/Electrocardiographic Evidence of 87
Palpitations 89
Pericardial Effusion 90
Pericarditis 91
Premature Ventricular Complexes (PVCs) 92
Preoperative Evaluation 93
Q-T Interval Abnormality 94
Syncope 95
Tachycardia
    Supraventricular 97
    Ventricular, Nonsustained 99
Valve Replacement, Postoperative Management 101
Wolff-Parkinson-White (WPW) Syndrome 102

CARDIOLOGY

Aneurysm, Ventricular

Indications and Timing for Referral
- Serious consideration should be given to having all such patients seen in consultation by a cardiologist

Timing: Routine (less than 4 weeks)

- Presence of congestive heart failure, arrhythmias, or recent embolic event

Timing: Expedited (less than 1 week)

  Appropriate timing of referral may be Immediate or Urgent (less than 24 hours) depending upon the severity, duration, frequency, or progression of symptoms

Advice for Referral
- In general, electrocardiographic stress testing is appropriate if the resting ECG is normal, whereas stress imaging procedures are preferred when the resting ECG is abnormal.
- The need for cardiac catheterization may be apparent at the initial consultative visit. Actual procedures for preliminary discussion with primary care physician, authorization, and scheduling will depend upon the practice setting. If cardiac catheterization is performed, an additional follow-up visit is appropriate.

Tests to Prepare for Consult
- Radiograph, chest
- ECG
- Echocardiogram

Tests Not Useful Before Consult
- None

Tests Consultant May Need to Do
- Stress ECG
- Stress radionuclide imaging
- Stress echocardiography
- Cardiac catheterization (see *Advice for Referral*)

Follow-up Visits Generally Required
- See *Advice for Referral*

Suggested Readings
Brown SL, Gropler RJ, Harris KM. Distinguishing left ventricular aneurysm from pseudoaneurysm. A review of the literature. [Review] [44 refs]. Chest 1997;111:1403–1409.

Hamer DH, Lindsay J Jr. Redefining true ventricular aneurysm. [Review]. Am J Cardiol 1989;64:1192–1194.

Gersh BJ, Braunwald E, Rutherford JD. Chronic coronary artery disease: left ventricular aneurysm. In: Braunwald E, ed. Heart Disease: a Textbook of Cardiovascular Medicine. Philadelphia: WB Saunders, 1997;1347–1348.

Aneurysm, Ventricular (continued)

Selected Guidelines

Ritchie JL, Bateman TM, Bonow RO, et al. Guidelines for clinical use of cardiac radionuclide imaging. Report of the American College of Cardiology/American Heart Association Task Force on Assessment of Diagnostic and Therapeutic Cardiovascular Procedures (Committee on Radionuclide Imaging), developed in collaboration with the American Society of Nuclear Cardiology. J Am Coll Cardiol 1995;25:521–547.

Efficacy of exercise thallium-201 scintigraphy in the diagnosis and prognosis of coronary artery disease. American College of Physicians. Ann Intern Med 1990;113:703–704.

See Also

- Myocardial infarction, silent/ECG evidence of
- Myocardial infarction, recent, uncomplicated

CARDIOLOGY

Aortic Valve, Bicuspid/Calcified

Indications and Timing for Referral

- Fever or other signs of infection, potentially caused by endocarditis

Timing: Urgent (less than 24 hours)
- Associated, progressive cardiac symptoms present (e.g., angina, CHF, syncope)
- Assistance in determining clinical significance

Timing: Routine (less than 4 weeks)

Appropriate timing of referral may be Immediate or Urgent (under 24 hours) depending upon the severity, duration, frequency, or progression of symptoms

Advice for Referral

- Reports of all previous cardiac studies are vital.
- The need for cardiac catheterization may be apparent at the initial consultative visit. Actual procedures for preliminary discussion with primary care physician, authorization, and scheduling will depend upon the practice setting. If cardiac catheterization is performed an additional follow-up visit is appropriate.

Tests to Prepare for Consult

- Radiograph, chest
- ECG
- Echocardiogram with Doppler studies

Tests Not Useful Before Consult

- Stress ECG

Tests Consultant May Need to Do

- CBC
- Blood culture
- ESR
- Echocardiogram with Doppler studies
- Cardiac catheterization (see *Advice for Referral*)

Follow-up Visits Generally Required

- One

Suggested Readings

Stewart BF, Pearlman AS. Aortic stenosis or aortic sclerosis [review]. Cardiology in the Elderly 1995;3:259–264.

Baxley WA. Aortic valve disease. [Review]. Curr Opin Cardiol 1994;9:152–157.

Roger VL, Tajik AJ, Reeder GS, et al. Effect of doppler echocardiography on utilization of hemodynamic cardiac catheterization in the preoperative evaluation of aortic stenosis. Mayo Clin Proc 1996;71:141–149.

Selected Guidelines

Ewy GA. ACC/AHA Guidelines for the clinical application of echocardiography. JACC 1990;17:1505–1528.

Dajani AS, Bisno AL, Chung KJ, et al. Prevention of bacterial endocarditis. Recommendations by the American Heart Association. JAMA 1990;264:2919–2922.

See Also

- Heart murmur, aortic

Atrial Fibrillation

Indications and Timing for Referral

- Patient symptomatic (e.g., angina, heart failure, or change in mental status)

Timing: Urgent (less than 24 hours)

- Assistance with management (e.g., rate control, anticoagulant therapy)

Timing: Expedited (less than 1 week)

- Determine underlying cause

Timing: Routine (less than 4 weeks)

Appropriate timing of referral may be Immediate or Urgent (under 24 hours) depending upon the severity, duration, frequency, or progression of symptoms

Advice for Referral

- Complete history of medication, alcohol, and caffeine intake is vital.
- Echocardiogram most helpful if it includes evaluation of structural abnormalities (left atrial size, presence or absence of mitral annulus calcification), thrombus, left ventricular function with ejection fraction, and the pericardium.
- Serious consideration should be given to having all such patients seen in consultation with a cardiologist.

Tests to Prepare for Consult

- CBC
- Prothrombin time
- Platelet count
- TSH (assay sensitivity <0.1 mU/L)
- ECG
- Echocardiogram

Tests Not Useful Before Consult

- None

Tests Consultant May Need to Do

- ECG
- Radiograph, chest
- Ambulatory ECG (Holter)
- Echocardiogram with Doppler studies
- Transesophageal echocardiography

Follow-up Visits Generally Required

- See *Advice for Referral*

CARDIOLOGY

Atrial Fibrillation (continued)

Suggested Readings

Golzari H, Cebul RD, Bahler RC. Atrial fibrillation: restoration and maintenance of sinus rhythm and indications for anticoagulation therapy. [Review] [205 refs]. Ann Intern Med 1996;125:311–323.

Pritchett EL. Management of atrial fibrillation [see comments]. [Review]. N Engl J Med 1992;326:1264–1271.

Blackshear JL, Kopecky SL, Litin SC, et al. Management of atrial fibrillation in adults: Prevention of thromboembolism and symptomatic treatment. Mayo Clin Proc 1996;71:150–160.

Falk RH. Current management of atrial fibrillation. [Review]. Curr Opin Cardiol 1994;9:30–39.

Havranek EP. The management of atrial fibrillation: current perspectives [see comments]. [Review]. Am Fam Physician 1994;50:959–968.

Selected Guidelines

Knoebel SB, Williams SV, Achord JL, et al. Clinical competence in ambulatory electrocardiography. A statement for physicians from the AHA/ACC/ACP Task Force on Clinical Privileges in Cardiology. Circulation 1993;88:337–341.

See Also

- PVCs
- Ventricular tachycardia, nonsustained
- Supraventricular tachycardia
- Atrial flutter
- Palpitations

Atrial Flutter

Indications and Timing for Referral

- Patient symptomatic (e.g., angina, heart failure, or change in mental status)

Timing: Urgent (less than 24 hours)

- Determine underlying cause
- Assistance with management (e.g., rate control, anticoagulation therapy)

Timing: Expedited (less than 1 week)

Appropriate timing of referral may be Immediate or Urgent (under 24 hours) depending upon the severity, duration, frequency, or progression of symptoms

Advice for Referral

- Complete history of medication, alcohol, and caffeine intake is vital.
- Echocardiogram most helpful if it includes evaluation of structural abnormalities (e.g., left atrial size, presence or absence of mitral annulus calcification), thrombus, left ventricular function with ejection fraction, and the pericardium.
- Serious consideration should be given to having all such patients seen in consultation with a cardiologist.
- Co-management with a cardiologist is indicated until sinus rhythm is restored.

Tests to Prepare for Consult

- CBC
- Prothrombin time
- Platelet count
- TSH (assay sensitivity <0.1 mU/L)
- ECG
- Echocardiogram

Tests Not Useful Before Consult

- None

Tests Consultant May Need to Do

- ECG
- Radiograph, chest
- Ambulatory ECG (Holter)
- Echocardiogram with Doppler studies
- Transesophageal echocardiography

Follow-up Visits Generally Required

- See *Advice for Referral*

Suggested Readings

Lesh MD, Kalman JM, Olgin JE. New approaches to treatment of atrial flutter and tachycardia. J Cardiovasc Electrophysiol 1996;7:368–381.

Waldo AL. Clinical evaluation in therapy of patients with atrial fibrillation or flutter. [Review]. Cardiol Clin 1990;8:479–490.

Saoudi N, Nair M, Poty H, et al. Catheter ablation for the common type of atrial flutter—where do we stand. J Intervention Cardiol 1996;9:35–44.

Fitzgerald DM, Hawthorne HR, Crossley GH, et al. Effects of atrial fibrillation and atrial flutter on the signal-averaged electrocardiogram. Am J Cardiol 1996;77:205–209.

Selected Guidelines

Knoebel SB, Williams SV, Achord JL, et al. Clinical competence in ambulatory electrocardiography. A statement for physicians from the AHA/ACC/ACP Task Force on Clinical Privileges in Cardiology. Circulation 1993;88:337–341.

See Also

- Palpitations
- Atrial fibrillation
- Supraventricular tachycardia
- PVCs
- Ventricular tachycardia, nonsustained

CARDIOLOGY

Bradycardia

Indications and Timing for Referral
- Potentially associated neurologic or constitutional symptoms

Timing: Expedited (less than 1 week)

- Assistance with management of patients on contributory cardiac medications with heart rate less than 50/minute
- Consultation may be particularly appropriate for patients over 60 years old with a heart rate of less than 50/minute

Timing: Routine (less than 4 weeks)

Advice for Referral
- A complete medication history is vital, including all levels of cardioactive drugs, e.g., digitalis, quinidine, procainamide.
- Asymptomatic persons under 60 years old with otherwise normal ECGs generally do not require consultation.

Tests to Prepare for Consult
- TSH
- ECG
- Ambulatory ECG (Holter)

Tests Not Useful Before Consult
- Echocardiogram

Tests Consultant May Need to Do
- ECG
- Radiograph, chest
- Event monitor
- Loop monitor
- Drug levels

Follow-up Visits Generally Required
- None

Suggested Readings
Maloney JD, Jaeger FJ, Rizo-Patron C, Zhu DW. The role of pacing for the management of neurally mediated syncope: carotid sinus syndrome and vasovagal syncope. [Review]. Am Heart J 1994;127:1030–1037.

Wellens HJ, Gorgels AP, Smeets JL, den Dulk K. Ambulatory electrocardiography evaluation of supraventricular tachyarrhythmias and bradyarrhythmias. [Review]. Cardiol Clin 1992;10:361–70.

DiMarco JP, Philbrick JT. Use of ambulatory electrocardiographic (Holter) monitoring. Ann Intern Med 1990;113:53–68.

Kapoor WN, Smith MA, Miller NL. Upright tilt testing in evaluating syncope: a comprehensive literature review. [Review]. Am J Med 1994;97:78–88.

Selected Guidelines
Ambulatory electrocardiographic (Holter) monitoring. American College of Physicians [comment]. Ann Intern Med 1990;113:77–79.

See Also
- Orthostatic hypotension
- Hypothyroidism

THE CONSULTATION GUIDE

Cardiomyopathy

Indications and Timing for Referral

- Diagnostic uncertainty
- Assistance with management when refractory to conventional treatment
- Consideration of a cardiac transplant
- Presence of uncontrolled arrhythmias

Timing: Expedited (less than 1 week)

Appropriate timing of referral may be Immediate or Urgent (less than 24 hours) depending upon the severity, duration, frequency, or progression of symptoms

Advice for Referral

- Complete medication and alcohol intake histories are vital.
- In general, ECG stress testing is appropriate if the resting ECG is normal, whereas stress imaging procedures are preferred when the resting ECG is abnormal.
- The need for cardiac catheterization and biopsy may be apparent at the initial consultative visit. Actual procedures for preliminary discussion with primary care physician, authorization, and scheduling will depend upon the practice setting. If cardiac catheterization and biopsy are performed an additional follow-up visit is appropriate.
- Serious consideration should be given to having all such patients seen in consultation with a cardiologist.

Tests to Prepare for Consult

- CBC
- Sodium
- Potassium
- Albumin, total protein
- BUN, Creatinine
- Radiograph, chest
- ECG with prolonged rhythm strip
- Echocardiogram

Tests Not Useful Before Consult

- Ambulatory ECG (Holter)

Tests Consultant May Need to Do

- CPK
- ESR
- TSH (assay sensitivity <0.1 mU/L)
- 24-hour urine metanephrines
- Echocardiogram
- Ambulatory ECG (Holter)
- Stress ECG
- Stress radionuclide imaging
- Stress echocardiography
- Cardiac catheterization (see *Advice for Referral*)
- Myocardial biopsy (see *Advice for Referral*)

Follow-up Visits Generally Required

- See *Advice for Referral*

Cardiomyopathy (continued)

Suggested Readings

Kushwaha SS, Fallon JT, Fuster V. Restrictive cardiomyopathy. [Review] [136 refs]. N Engl J Med 1997;336:267–276.

Spirito P, Seidman CE, McKenna WJ, Maron BJ. The management of hypertrophic cardiomyopathy. [Review] [151 refs]. N Engl J Med 1997;336:775–785.

Borggrefe M, Block M, Breithardt G. Identification and management of the high risk patient with dilated cardiomyopathy. [Review]. Br Heart J 1995;72(Suppl):S42–S45.

Posma JL, van der Wall EE, Blanksma PK, et al. New diagnostic options in hypertrophic cardiomyopathy. [Review] [148 refs]. Am Heart J 1996;132:1031–1041.

Selected Guidelines

Konstam M, Dracup K, Baker D. [Anonymous] Heart failure: evaluation and care of patients with left-ventricular systolic dysfunction. Clinical Practice Guideline No.11. 1994; AHCPR Publication No. 94–0612. Agency for Health Care Policy and Research, Public Health Service. 50940038.

Ritchie JL, Bateman TM, Bonow RO, et al. Guidelines for clinical use of cardiac radionuclide imaging. Report of the American College of Cardiology/American Heart Association Task Force on Assessment of Diagnostic and Therapeutic Cardiovascular Procedures (Committee on Radionuclide Imaging), developed in collaboration with the American Society of Nuclear Cardiology. J Am Coll Cardiol 1995;25:521–547.

See Also

- Heart failure, management
- Heart failure, etiology uncertain, new onset

THE CONSULTATION GUIDE

Cerebrovascular Accident (CVA) or Transient Ischemic Attack (TIA), Possible Cardiac Source of Embolus

Indications and Timing for Referral

- Diagnostic uncertainty
- Clinical or test evidence of heart disease

Timing: Urgent (less than 24 hours)

Tests to Prepare for Consult

- ECG
- Echocardiogram with contrast

Tests Consultant May Need to Do

- CBC
- Prothrombin time
- PTT
- Platelet count
- Ambulatory ECG (Holter)
- Transesophageal echocardiography
- Carotid duplex study

Follow-up Visits Generally Required

- One

Suggested Readings

Streifler JY, Katz M. Cardiogenic cerebral emboli: diagnosis and treatment. [Review]. Curr Opin Neurol 1995;8:45–54.

Hart RG. Cardiogenic embolism to the brain [see comments]. [Review]. Lancet 1992;339:589–594.

Sherman DG. Cardiac embolism: the neurologist's perspective. [Review]. Am J Cardiol 1990;65:32C–37C.

Cardiogenic brain embolism. The second report of the Cerebral Embolism Task Force [published erratum appears in Arch Neurol 1989;46:1079] [see comments]. [Review]. Arch Neurol 1989;46:727–743.

Suggested Guidelines

Ewy GA. ACC/AHA Guidelines for the clinical application of echocardiography. JACC 1990;17:1505–1528.

See Also

- Episodic loss of consciousness, seizure versus syncope
- Vertigo
- Facial weakness
- Ptosis
- Diplopia
- Visual loss, monocular
- Swallowing disorder
- Speech disorder
- Carotid stenosis, asymptomatic
- Spells, TIA versus seizure
- Cervical bruit, asymptomatic

CARDIOLOGY

Chest Discomfort, Anginal

Indications and Timing for Referral

- Diagnostic uncertainty
- Assistance with risk stratification and management

Timing: Urgent (less than 24 hours)

Appropriate timing of referral may be Immediate or Urgent (less than 24 hours) depending upon the severity, duration, frequency, or progression of symptoms

Advice for Referral

- Stress testing may be associated with increased risk of cardiac events when there is a pattern of unstable angina.
- In general, ECG stress testing is appropriate if the resting ECG is normal, whereas stress imaging procedures are preferred when the resting ECG is abnormal.
- The need for coronary angiography may be apparent at the initial consultative visit. Actual procedures for preliminary discussion with primary care physician, authorization, and scheduling will depend upon the practice setting. If coronary angiography is performed an additional follow-up visit is appropriate.

Tests to Prepare for Consult

- Glucose, fasting
- Lipid profile (cholesterol, TG, HDL)
- ECG

Tests Not Useful Before Consult

- Ambulatory ECG (Holter)

Tests Consultant May Need to Do

- CBC
- ECG
- Stress ECG
- Stress radionuclide imaging
- Stress echocardiography
- Coronary angiography (see *Advice for Referral*)

Follow-up Visits Generally Required

- Two

Suggested Readings

Katz DA, Griffith JL, Beshansky JR, Selker HP. The use of empiric clinical data in the evaluation of practice guidelines for unstable angina [see comments]. JAMA 1996;276:1568–1574.

Catherwood E, O'Rourke DJ. Critical pathway management of unstable angina. [Review]. Prog Cardiovasc Dis 1994;37:121–148.

Shub C. Stable angina pectoris: 2. Cardiac evaluation and diagnostic testing. [Review]. Mayo Clin Proc 1990;65:243–255.

Mayo Clinic Cardiovascular Working Group on Stress Testing. Cardiovascular stress testing: a description of the various types of stress tests and indications for their use. Mayo Clin Proc 1996;71:43–52.

Bernstein SJ. Coronary angiography: a literature review and ratings of appropriateness and necessity. RAND 1992;JRA-03.

Hamm CW, Goldmann BU, Heeschen C, et al. Emergency room triage of patients with acute chest pain by means of rapid testing for cardiac troponin T or troponin I. N Engl J Med 1997;337:1648–1653.

Goldman L, Cook EF, Johnson PA, et al. Prediction of the need for intensive care in patients who come to emergency departments with acute chest pain. N Engl J Med 1996;334:1498–1504.

THE CONSULTATION GUIDE

Chest Discomfort, Anginal (continued)

Selected Guidelines

Diagnosing and managing unstable angina. Unstable Angina Guideline Panel. Agency for Health Care Policy and Research. Am Fam Physician 1994;49:1459–1462, 1465–1468, 1473–1475.

Pina IL, Balady GJ, Hanson P, et al. Guidelines for clinical exercise testing laboratories. A statement for healthcare professionals from the Committee on Exercise and Cardiac Rehabilitation, American Heart Association. Circulation 1995;91:912–921.

Ritchie JL, Bateman TM, Bonow RO, et al. Guidelines for clinical use of cardiac radionuclide imaging. Report of the American College of Cardiology/American Heart Association Task Force on Assessment of Diagnostic and Therapeutic Cardiovascular Procedures (Committee on Radionuclide Imaging), developed in collaboration with the American Society of Nuclear Cardiology. J Am Coll Cardiol 1995;25:521–547.

Kirklin JW. Guidelines and indications for coronary artery bypass graft surgery. ACC/AHA Task Force Report. JACC 1991;17:543–589.

See Also

- Chest discomfort, nonanginal
- Chest discomfort, possible angina
- Pre-CABG or PTCA second opinion

CARDIOLOGY

Chest Discomfort, Non-Anginal

Indications and Timing for Referral

- Diagnostic uncertainty
- Multiple risk factors for coronary artery disease (CAD)
- High requirement to exclude CAD (e.g., occupational concerns for airline pilot)

Timing: Routine (less than 4 weeks)

Appropriate timing of referral may be Immediate or Urgent (less than 24 hours) depending upon the severity, duration, frequency, or progression of symptoms

Advice for Referral

- ECG tracing during pain is extremely helpful whenever possible.
- In general, ECG stress testing is appropriate if the resting ECG is normal, whereas stress imaging procedures are preferred when the resting ECG is abnormal.
- Echocardiography is generally uninformative in the absence of other specific clinical findings indicating cardiac disease.
- Transient appearance of paradoxical splitting of S2 during pain is highly suggestive of cardiac origin.
- Exclude chest wall tenderness, but do not dismiss if some discomfort can be provoked by exertion.

Tests to Prepare for Consult

- Glucose, fasting
- Lipid profile (cholesterol, TG, HDL)
- ECG
- Radiograph, chest

Tests Not Useful Before Consult

- Ambulatory ECG (Holter)

Tests Consultant May Need to Do

- ECG
- Stress ECG
- Stress radionuclide imaging
- Stress echocardiography

Follow-up Visits Generally Required

- One

Suggested Readings

Pryor DB. Value of the history and physical in identifying patients at increased risk for coronary artery disease. Ann Intern Med 1993;118:81–90.

Richter JE. Overview of diagnostic testing for chest pain of unknown origin. [Review]. Am J Med 1992;92(5A):41S–45S.

Hackshaw BT. Excluding heart disease in the patient with chest pain. [Review]. Am J Med 1992;92(5A):46S–51S.

Rao SS, Gregersen H, Hayek B, et al. Unexplained chest pain: the hypersensitive, hyperreactive, and poorly compliant esophagus [comment] [see comments]. Ann Intern Med 1996;124:950–958.

Disla E, Rhim HR, Reddy A, et al. Costochondritis. A prospective analysis in an emergency department setting. Arch Intern Med 1994;154:2466–2469.

Fleet RP, Beitman BD. Unexplained chest pain: when is it panic disorder?. [Review] [68 refs]. Clin Cardiol 1997;20:187–194.

Chest Discomfort, Nonanginal (*continued*)

Selected Guidelines

Ritchie JL, Bateman TM, Bonow RO, et al. Guidelines for clinical use of cardiac radionuclide imaging. Report of the American College of Cardiology/American Heart Association Task Force on Assessment of Diagnostic and Therapeutic Cardiovascular Procedures (Committee on Radionuclide Imaging), developed in collaboration with the American Society of Nuclear Cardiology. J Am Coll Cardiol 1995;25:521–547.

Pina IL, Balady GJ, Hanson P, et al. Guidelines for clinical exercise testing laboratories. A statement for healthcare professionals from the Committee on Exercise and Cardiac Rehabilitation, American Heart Association. Circulation 1995;91:912–921.

Browning TH. Diagnosis of chest pain of esophageal origin. A guideline of the Patient Care Committee of the American Gastroenterological Association. Dig Dis Sci 1990;35:289–293.

See Also

- Chest discomfort, possible angina
- Chest discomfort, anginal

CARDIOLOGY

Chest Discomfort, Possible Angina

Indications and Timing for Referral

- Diagnostic uncertainty
- Multiple risk factors for coronary artery disease (CAD)
- High requirement to exclude CAD (e.g., occupational concerns for airline pilot)

Timing: Routine (less than 4 weeks)

Appropriate timing of referral may be Immediate or Urgent (less than 24 hours) depending upon the severity, duration, frequency, or progression of symptoms

Advice for Referral

- ECG tracing during pain is extremely helpful whenever possible.
- Stress testing may be associated with increased risk of cardiac events when there is a pattern of unstable angina.
- In general, ECG stress testing is appropriate if the resting ECG is normal, whereas stress imaging procedures are preferred when the resting ECG is abnormal.
- The need for coronary angiography may be apparent at the initial consultative visit. Actual procedures for preliminary discussion with primary care physician, authorization, and scheduling will depend upon the practice setting. If coronary angiography is performed an additional follow-up visit is appropriate.

Tests to Prepare for Consult

- Glucose, fasting
- Lipid profile (cholesterol, TG, HDL)
- ECG

Tests Not Useful Before Consult

- Ambulatory ECG (Holter)

Tests Consultant May Need to Do

- ECG
- TSH (assay sensitivity <0.1 mU/L)
- CBC
- Stress ECG
- Stress radionuclide imaging
- Stress echocardiography
- Coronary angiography (see *Advice for Referral*)

Follow-up Visits Generally Required

- Two

Suggested Readings

Pryor DB. Value of the history and physical in identifying patients at increased risk for coronary artery disease. Ann Intern Med 1993;118:81–90.

Zucker DR, Griffith JL, Beshansky JR, Selker HP. Presentations of acute myocardial infarction in men and women (see comments). J Gen Intern Med 1997;12:79–87.

Hackshaw BT. Excluding heart disease in the patient with chest pain. [Review]. Am J Med 1992;92(5A):46S–51S.

Bernstein SJ. Coronary angiography: a literature review and ratings of appropriateness and necessity. RAND 1992;JRA-03

Fam AG. Approach to musculoskeletal chest wall pain. [Review]. Primary Care; Clin Office Pract 1988;15:767–782.

Goldman L, Cook EF, Johnson PA, et al. Prediction of the need for intensive care in patients who come to emergency departments with acute chest pain. N Engl J Med 1996;334:1498–1504.

Hamm CW, Goldmann BU, Heeschen C, et al. Emergency room triage of patients with acute chest pain by means of rapid testing for cardiac troponin T or troponin I. N Engl J Med 1997;337:1648–1653.

THE CONSULTATION GUIDE

Chest Discomfort, Possible Angina (*continued*)

Selected Guidelines

Braunwald E, Jones RH, Mark DB, et al. Diagnosing and managing unstable angina. Agency for Health Care Policy and Research. Circulation 1994;90:613–622.

Ritchie JL, Bateman TM, Bonow RO, et al. Guidelines for clinical use of cardiac radionuclide imaging. Report of the American College of Cardiology/American Heart Association Task Force on Assessment of Diagnostic and Therapeutic Cardiovascular Procedures (Committee on Radionuclide Imaging), developed in collaboration with the American Society of Nuclear Cardiology. J Am Coll Cardiol 1995;25:521–547.

Browning TH. Diagnosis of chest pain of esophageal origin. A guideline of the Patient Care Committee of the American Gastroenterological Association. Dig Dis Sci 1990;35:289–293.

See Also

- Chest discomfort, nonanginal
- Chest discomfort, anginal

CARDIOLOGY

Conduction Defect, Left Bundle Branch Block

Indications and Timing for Referral

- Associated signs or symptoms of cardiac disease
- Risk factors for cardiac disease present
- Unexplained finding
- Pre-procedure evaluation

Timing: Routine (less than 4 weeks)

Appropriate timing of referral may be Immediate or Urgent (less than 24 hours) depending upon associated findings

Advice for Referral

- Old ECG tracings important

Tests to Prepare for Consult

- ECG

Tests Not Useful Before Consult

- Stress ECG

Tests Consultant May Need to Do

- Echocardiogram with Doppler studies
- MUGA scan
- Stress radionuclide imaging
- Stress echocardiography
- Ambulatory ECG (Holter)

Follow-up Visits Generally Required

- One

Suggested Readings

Sgarbossa EB, Pinski SL, Barbagelata A, et al. Electrocardiographic diagnosis of evolving acute myocardial infarction in the presence of left bundle-branch block. N Engl J Med 1996;334:481–487.

Fisher JD, Aronson RS. Rate-dependent bundle branch block: occurrence, causes and clinical correlations. [Review]. J Am Coll Cardiol 1990;16:240–243.

Fisch C. Electrocardiography: intraventricular conduction defects. In: Braunwald E, ed. Heart disease: a textbook of cardiovascular medicine. 5th ed. Philadelphia: WB Saunders, 1997;119–123.

Suggested Guidelines

Knoebel SB, Williams SV, Achord JL, et al. Clinical competence in ambulatory electrocardiography. A statement for physicians from the AHA/ACC/ACP Task Force on Clinical Privileges in Cardiology. Circulation 1993;88:337–341.

See Also

- Left anterior fascicular block
- Right bundle branch block
- Heart block, third-degree AV
- Heart block, second-degree AV, Mobitz 2
- Heart block, first-degree AV
- Heart block, second-degree AV, Mobitz 1

THE CONSULTATION GUIDE

Conduction Defect, Right Bundle Branch Block

Indications and Timing for Referral

- Associated signs or symptoms of cardiac disease
- Risk factors for cardiac disease present
- Unexplained finding
- Pre-procedure evaluation

Timing: Routine (less than 4 weeks)

Appropriate timing of referral may be Immediate or Urgent (less than 24 hours) depending upon associated findings

Advice for Referral

- Old ECG tracings are important.
- In general, ECG stress testing is appropriate if the resting ECG is normal, whereas stress imaging procedures are preferred when the resting ECG is abnormal.

Tests to Prepare for Consult

- ECG

Tests Not Useful Before Consult

- None

Tests Consultant May Need to Do

- Echocardiogram with Doppler studies
- MUGA scan
- Stress ECG
- Stress radionuclide imaging
- Stress echocardiography

Follow-up Visits Generally Required

- One

Suggested Readings

Fisher JD, Aronson RS. Rate-dependent bundle branch block: occurrence, causes and clinical correlations. [Review]. J Am Coll Cardiol 1990;16:240–243.

Hancock EW. Chest pain and a change in right bundle branch block. Hosp Pract (Off Ed) 1996;31:53–54.

Suggested Guidelines

Knoebel SB, Williams SV, Achord JL, et al. Clinical competence in ambulatory electrocardiography. A statement for physicians from the AHA/ACC/ACP Task Force on Clinical Privileges in Cardiology. Circulation 1993;88:337–341.

See Also

- Heart block, first-degree AV
- Heart block, second-degree AV, Mobitz 1
- Heart block, second-degree AV, Mobitz 2
- Heart block, third-degree AV
- Conduction defect, left bundle branch block
- Left anterior fascicular block

CARDIOLOGY

Conduction Defect, Left Anterior Fascicular Block

Indications and Timing for Referral

- Associated signs or symptoms of cardiac disease
- Risk factors for cardiac disease present
- Pre-procedure evaluation

Timing: Routine (less than 4 weeks)

Advice for Referral

- Old ECG tracings important
- In general, ECG stress testing is appropriate if the resting ECG is normal, whereas stress imaging procedures are preferred when the resting ECG is abnormal.

Tests to Prepare for Consult

- ECG

Tests Not Useful Before Consult

- None

Tests Consultant May Need to Do

- Echocardiogram with Doppler studies
- MUGA scan
- Stress ECG
- Stress radionuclide imaging
- Stress echocardiography

Follow-up Visits Generally Required

- One

Suggested Readings

Fisch C. Electrocardiography: intraventricular conduction defects. In: Braunwald E, ed. Heart Disease: a Textbook of Cardiovascular Medicine. 5th ed. Philadelphia: WB Saunders, 1997; 119–123.

See Also

- Heart block, third-degree AV
- Conduction defect, left bundle branch block
- Conduction defect, right bundle branch block
- Heart block, second-degree AV, Mobitz 1
- Heart block, first-degree AV
- Heart block, second-degree AV, Mobitz 2

Coronary Artery Disease, History of Previous Coronary Bypass Grafting, or Percutaneous Transluminal Coronary Angioplasty

Indications and Timing for Referral
- Assistance with evaluation of future risk of cardiac events
- Assistance with evaluation of clinical or ECG findings suggesting recurrent cardiac ischemia

Timing: Routine (less than 4 weeks)

Appropriate timing of referral may be Immediate or Urgent (less than 24 hours) depending upon the severity, duration, frequency, or progression of symptoms

Advice for Referral
- Records of all previous cardiac catheterization, operative/procedure, and stress test reports are vital.
- In general, ECG stress testing is appropriate if the resting ECG is normal, whereas stress imaging procedures are preferred when the resting ECG is abnormal.
- Stress testing may be associated with increased risk of cardiac events when there is a pattern of unstable angina.
- The need for coronary angiography may be apparent at the initial consultative visit. Actual procedures for preliminary discussion with primary care physician, authorization, and scheduling will depend upon the practice setting. If coronary angiography is performed an additional follow-up visit is appropriate.
- Co-management with a cardiologist may be appropriate if recurrent ischemia or a high-risk profile is present

Tests to Prepare for Consult
- Glucose, fasting
- Lipid profile (cholesterol, TG, HDL)
- ECG

Tests Not Useful Before Consult
- Ambulatory ECG (Holter)

Tests Consultant May Need to Do
- ECG
- Echocardiogram with Doppler studies
- MUGA scan
- Stress ECG
- Stress radionuclide imaging
- Stress echocardiography
- Coronary angiography (see *Advice for Referral*)

Follow-up Visits Generally Required
- See *Advice for Referral*

Suggested Readings
Campeau L. Coronary risk factors and the postbypass patient. [Review]. Cardiovasc Clin 1991;21:123–133.

Stark RM. Review of the major intervention trials of lowering coronary artery disease risk through cholesterol reduction. [Review] [27 refs]. Am J Cardiol 1996;78:13–19.

Deedwania PC, Carbajal EV. Can ambulatory monitoring identify high-risk patients with stable coronary artery disease? [letter]. JAMA 1997;277:1760–1761.

Kadel C, Vallbracht C, Buss F, et al. Long-term follow-up after percutaneous transluminal coronary angioplasty in patients with single-vessel disease [published erratum appears in Am Heart J 1993;12:1818] [see comments]. [Review]. Am Heart J 1992;124:1159–1169.

CARDIOLOGY

Coronary Artery Disease, History of Previous Coronary Bypass Grafting, or Percutaneous Transluminal Coronary Angioplasty (*continued*)

Selected Guidelines

Pearson T, Rapaport E, Criqui M, et al. Optimal risk factor management in the patient after coronary revascularization. A statement for healthcare professionals from an American Heart Association Writing Group. Circulation 1994;90:3125–3133.

Ritchie JL, Bateman TM, Bonow RO, et al. Guidelines for clinical use of cardiac radionuclide imaging. Report of the American College of Cardiology/American Heart Association Task Force on Assessment of Diagnostic and Therapeutic Cardiovascular Procedures (Committee on Radionuclide Imaging), developed in collaboration with the American Society of Nuclear Cardiology. J Am Coll Cardiol 1995;25:521–547.

Triglyceride, high density lipoprotein, and coronary heart disease. NIH Consensus Statement 1992;10:1–28.

See Also

- Chest discomfort, anginal
- Chest discomfort, possible angina

THE CONSULTATION GUIDE

Coronary Bypass Grafting or Percutaneous Transluminal Coronary Angioplasty—Second Opinion

Indications and Timing for Referral

- Physician or patient uncertainty about appropriateness of recommended procedure

Timing: Expedited (less than 1 week)

Appropriate timing of referral may be Immediate or Urgent (less than 24 hours) depending upon the severity, duration, frequency, or progression of symptoms

Advice for Referral

- All records on which the recommendation was based are vital (e.g., cines, images, and tracings).
- If appropriate tests have not yet been performed or are of insufficient quality, they may need to be done or repeated.
- In general, ECG stress testing is appropriate if the resting ECG is normal, whereas stress imaging procedures are preferred when the resting ECG is abnormal.
- Stress testing may be associated with increased risk of cardiac events when there is a pattern of unstable angina.

Tests to Prepare for Consult

- None

Tests Not Useful Before Consult

- None

Tests Consultant May Need to Do

- ECG
- Stress ECG
- Stress echocardiography
- Rest and reperfusion radionuclide imaging
- Dobutamine echocardiography
- PET scan, myocardial

Follow-up Visits Generally Required

- One

Suggested Readings

Five-year clinical and functional outcome comparing bypass surgery and angioplasty in patients with multivessel coronary disease. A multicenter randomized trial. Writing Group for the Bypass Angioplasty Revascularization Investigation (BARI) Investigators. JAMA 1997;277:715–721.

Comparison of coronary bypass surgery with angioplasty in patients with multivessel disease. The Bypass Angioplasty Revascularization Investigation (BARI) Investigators [see comments] [published erratum appears in N Engl J Med 1997;336:147]. N Engl J Med 1996;335:217–225.

Bernstein SJ. Coronary angiography: a literature review and ratings of appropriateness and necessity. RAND 1992;JRA-03

Hilborne LH. Percutaneous transluminal coronary angioplasty: a review and ratings of appropriateness and necessity. RAND 1991;JRA-01

Hecht HS. Radionuclide techniques in the selection of patients for PTCA and in post-PTCA evaluation. [Review]. Cardiol Clin 1994;12:373–383.

Landau C, Lange RA, Hillis LD. Percutaneous transluminal coronary angioplasty. [Review]. N Engl J Med 1994;330:981–993.

CARDIOLOGY

Coronary Bypass Grafting or Percutaneous Transluminal Coronary Angioplasty—Second Opinion (*continued*)

Suggested Guidelines

Kirklin JW. Guidelines and indications for coronary artery bypass graft surgery. ACC/AHA Task Force Report. JACC 1991;17:543–589.

Braunwald E, Mark DB, Jones RH. [Anonymous] Unstable angina: diagnosis and management. 1994; AHCPR Publication No. 94–0602. Agency for Health Care Policy and Research and the National Heart, Lung, and Blood Institute, Public Health Service. 50940032.

Ritchie JL, Bateman TM, Bonow RO, et al. Guidelines for clinical use of cardiac radionuclide imaging. Report of the American College of Cardiology/American Heart Association Task Force on Assessment of Diagnostic and Therapeutic Cardiovascular Procedures (Committee on Radionuclide Imaging), developed in collaboration with the American Society of Nuclear Cardiology. J Am Coll Cardiol 1995;25:521–547.

See Also

- Chest discomfort, anginal
- Chest discomfort, possible angina

Dyspnea, Chronic

Indications and Timing for Referral

- Diagnostic uncertainty

Timing: Routine (less than 4 weeks)

Appropriate timing of referral may be Immediate or Urgent (less than 24 hours) depending upon the severity, duration, frequency, or progression of symptoms

Advice for Referral

- In general, ECG stress testing is appropriate if the resting ECG is normal, whereas stress imaging procedures are preferred when the resting ECG is abnormal.

Tests to Prepare for Consult

- CBC
- Radiograph, chest
- ECG
- Echocardiogram

Tests Not Useful Before Consult

- None

Tests Consultant May Need to Do

- ECG
- Oxygen saturation or arterial blood gas
- MUGA scan
- Transesophageal echocardiography
- Stress ECG
- Stress radionuclide imaging
- Stress echocardiography
- V/Q scan
- Metabolic stress test

Follow-up Visits Generally Required

- One

Suggested Readings

Pryor DB. Value of the history and physical in identifying patients at increased risk for coronary artery disease. Ann Intern Med 1993;118:81–90.

Silvestri GA, Mahler DA. Evaluation of dyspnea in the elderly patient. [Review]. Clin Chest Med 1993;14:393–404.

Suggested Guidelines

Konstam M, Dracup K, Baker D. Heart failure: evaluation and care of patients with left-ventricular systolic dysfunction. Clinical Practice Guideline No.11. 1994; AHCPR Publication No. 94-0612. Agency for Health Care Policy and Research, Public Health Service. 50940038.

Pina IL, Balady GJ, Hanson P, et al. Guidelines for clinical exercise testing laboratories. A statement for healthcare professionals from the Committee on Exercise and Cardiac Rehabilitation, American Heart Association. Circulation 1995;91:912–921.

Efficacy of exercise thallium-201 scintigraphy in the diagnosis and prognosis of coronary artery disease. American College of Physicians. Ann Intern Med 1990;113:703–704.

See Also

- Asthma
- Chronic obstructive pulmonary disease (COPD)

CARDIOLOGY

Dyspnea, Episodic

Indications and Timing for Referral

- Diagnostic uncertainty

Timing: Routine (less than 4 weeks)

Appropriate timing of referral may be Immediate or Urgent (less than 24 hours) depending upon the severity, duration, frequency, or progression of symptoms

Advice for Referral

- In general, ECG stress testing is appropriate if the resting ECG is normal, whereas stress imaging procedures are preferred when the resting ECG is abnormal.

Tests to Prepare for Consult

- CBC
- Radiograph, chest
- ECG with prolonged rhythm strip
- Echocardiogram

Tests Not Useful Before Consult

- None

Tests Consultant May Need to Do

- ECG
- Oxygen saturation
- MUGA scan
- Transesophageal echocardiography
- Stress ECG
- Stress radionuclide imaging
- Stress echocardiography
- V/Q scan
- Ambulatory ECG (Holter)
- Lower extremity venous Doppler study

Follow-up Visits Generally Required

- One

Suggested Readings

Gillespie ND, McNeill G, Pringle T, et al. Cross sectional study of contribution of clinical assessment and simple cardiac investigations to diagnosis of left ventricular systolic dysfunction in patients admitted with acute dyspnoea. Br Med J 1997;314:936–940.

Mahler DA, Horowitz MB. Clinical evaluation of exertional dyspnea. [Review]. Clin Chest Med 1994;15:259–269.

Silvestri GA, Mahler DA. Evaluation of dyspnea in the elderly patient. [Review]. Clin Chest Med 1993;14(3):393–404.

Suggested Guidelines

Pina IL, Balady GJ, Hanson P, et al. Guidelines for clinical exercise testing laboratories. A statement for healthcare professionals from the Committee on Exercise and Cardiac Rehabilitation, American Heart Association. Circulation 1995;91:912–921.

Kotler TS, Diamond GA. Exercise thallium-201 scintigraphy in the diagnosis and prognosis of coronary artery disease. Ann Intern Med 1990;113:684–702.

See Also

- Asthma
- Chronic obstructive pulmonary disease (COPD)

Dyspnea, Nocturnal

Indications and Timing for Referral

- Diagnostic uncertainty

Timing: Routine (less than 4 weeks)

Appropriate timing of referral may be Immediate or Urgent (less than 24 hours) depending upon the severity, duration, frequency, or progression of symptoms

Advice for Referral

- In general, ECG stress testing is appropriate if the resting ECG is normal, whereas stress imaging procedures are preferred when the resting ECG is abnormal.

Tests to Prepare for Consult

- CBC
- Radiograph, chest
- ECG with prolonged rhythm strip
- Echocardiogram

Tests Not Useful Before Consult

- None

Tests Consultant May Need to Do

- Oxygen saturation
- MUGA scan
- Transesophageal echocardiography
- Stress ECG
- Stress radionuclide imaging
- Stress echocardiography

Follow-up Visits Generally Required

- One

Suggested Readings

Gillespie ND, McNeill G, Pringle T, et al. Cross sectional study of contribution of clinical assessment and simple cardiac investigations to diagnosis of left ventricular systolic dysfunction in patients admitted with acute dyspnoea. Br Med J 1997;314:936–940.

Pryor DB. Value of the history and physical in identifying patients at increased risk for coronary artery disease. Ann Intern Med 1993;118:81–90.

Suggested Guidelines

Konstam M, Dracup K, Baker D. Heart failure: evaluation and care of patients with left-ventricular systolic dysfunction. Clinical Practice Guideline No.11. 1994; AHCPR Publication No. 94-0612. Agency for Health Care Policy and Research, Public Health Service. 50940038.

Ritchie JL, Bateman TM, Bonow RO, et al. Guidelines for clinical use of cardiac radionuclide imaging. Report of the American College of Cardiology/American Heart Association Task Force on Assessment of Diagnostic and Therapeutic Cardiovascular Procedures (Committee on Radionuclide Imaging), developed in collaboration with the American Society of Nuclear Cardiology. J Am Coll Cardiol 1995;25:521–547.

See Also

- Sleep apnea/snoring

CARDIOLOGY

Edema, Dependent

Indications and Timing for Referral

- Suspected cardiac etiology

Timing: Routine (less than 4 weeks)

Advice for Referral

- A complete medication history vital.

Tests to Prepare for Consult

- CBC
- BUN, Creatinine
- Albumin, total protein
- TSH (assay sensitivity <0.1 mU/L)
- Urinalysis with microscopic
- Radiograph, chest
- ECG

Tests Not Useful Before Consult

- None

Tests Consultant May Need to Do

- Echocardiogram with Doppler studies
- Noninvasive venous flow studies

Follow-up Visits Generally Required

- One

Suggested Readings

Morrison RT. Edema and principles of diuretic use. [Review] [55 refs]. Med Clin North Am 1997;81:689–704.

Powell AA, Armstrong MA. Peripheral edema. [Review] [20 refs]. Am Fam Physician 1997;55:1721–1726.

MacGregor GA, de Wardener HE. Idiopathic edema. In: Schrier RW, Gottschalk CW, eds. Diseases of the kidney. 5th ed. Boston: Little, Brown, and Company, 1993;2493–2502.

Pryor DB. Value of the history and physical in identifying patients at increased risk for coronary artery disease. Ann Intern Med 1993;118:81–90.

Braunwald E. Edema. In: Fauci AS, Braunwald E, Isselbacher KJ, eds. Harrison's Principles of Internal Medicine. 14th ed. New York: McGraw Hill, 1998:210–214.

THE CONSULTATION GUIDE

Electrocardiogram (ECG), Abnormal

Indications and Timing for Referral

- Associated cardiac symptoms or signs that are not understood or controlled.
- Risk factors for cardiac disease present
- Unexplained electrocardiographic finding
- Preprocedure evaluation

Timing: Routine (less than 4 weeks)

- ECG changes are consistent with acute ischemia
- Ventricular tachycardia
- Rapid supraventricular tachycardia
- Significant conduction abnormalities such as Mobitz II or third-degree Heart Block (see these specific topics)
- Patient is clinically unstable

Timing: Urgent (less than 24 hours) or Immediate

Advice for Referral

- Old ECG tracings are important.
- Complete medication history is vital, including all levels of cardioactive drugs, e.g., digitalis, quinidine, procainamide.
- In general, ECG stress testing is appropriate if the resting ECG is normal, whereas stress imaging procedures are preferred when the resting ECG is abnormal.
- Recognition of simple technical errors such as lead reversal and reduced voltage scale may obviate need for some consultations.

Tests to Prepare for Consult

- ECG
- Electrolytes (Na, K, Cl, CO_2)

Tests Not Useful Before Consult

- None

Tests Consultant May Need to Do

- Calcium
- TSH
- Lipid profile (cholesterol, TG, HDL)
- Radiograph, chest
- Echocardiogram with Doppler studies
- Ambulatory ECG (Holter)
- Stress radionuclide imaging
- Stress echocardiography
- Stress ECG
- MUGA scan

Follow-up Visits Generally Required

- None

CARDIOLOGY

Electrocardiogram (ECG), Abnormal (continued)

Suggested Readings

Hurst JW. The rise, fall, and rise again of the ECG as a diagnostic tool. Chest 1997;111:800–801

Cohen JD. Abnormal electrocardiograms and cardiovascular risk: role of silent myocardial ischemia. Evidence from MRFIT. Am J Cardiol 1992;70:14F–18F.

Mayo Clinic Cardiovascular Working Group on Stress Testing. Cardiovascular stress testing: a description of the various types of stress tests and indications for their use. Mayo Clin Proc 1996;71:43–52.

Suggested Guidelines

Knoebel SB, Williams SV, Achord JL, et al. Clinical competence in ambulatory electrocardiography. A statement for physicians from the AHA/ACC/ACP Task Force on Clinical Privileges in Cardiology. Circulation 1993;88:337–341.

Pina IL, Balady GJ, Hanson P, et al. Guidelines for clinical exercise testing laboratories. A statement for healthcare professionals from the Committee on Exercise and Cardiac Rehabilitation, American Heart Association. Circulation 1995;91:912–921.

See Also

- Left anterior fascicular block
- Q-T interval abnormality
- Conduction defect, left bundle branch block
- Conduction defect, right bundle branch block
- Heart block, third-degree AV
- Heart block, second-degree AV, Mobitz 2
- Heart block, second-degree AV, Mobitz 1
- Heart block, first-degree AV
- Electrocardiogram, abnormal stress

Electrocardiogram (ECG), Abnormal Stress

Indications and Timing for Referral

- Ventricular tachyarrhythmia present
- Markedly positive ECG changes or drop in blood pressure with exercise compatible with ischemia
- Clinical instability
- Patient at high risk for cardiac event

Timing: Urgent (less than 24 hours)

- High patient anxiety

Timing: Expedited (less than 1 week)

- Assistance with interpretation of clinical significance
- Assistance with risk stratification

Timing: Routine (less than 4 weeks)

Advice for Referral

- Appropriate timing of referral may be best determined after preliminary discussion with the consulting cardiologist.
- Record of medications being taken when test was administered is vital.
- In general, ECG stress testing is appropriate if the resting ECG is normal, whereas stress imaging procedures are preferred when the resting ECG is abnormal.
- The need for coronary angiography may be apparent at the initial consultative visit. Actual procedures for preliminary discussion with primary care physician, authorization, and scheduling will depend upon the practice setting. If coronary angiography is performed an additional follow-up visit is appropriate.

Tests to Prepare for Consult

- ECG

Tests Not Useful Before Consult

- None

Tests Consultant May Need to Do

- Glucose
- Lipid profile (cholesterol, TG, HDL)
- ECG
- Echocardiogram with Doppler studies
- Stress ECG
- Stress radionuclide imaging
- Stress echocardiography
- Coronary angiography (see *Advice for Referral*)

Follow-up Visits Generally Required

- One

CARDIOLOGY

Electrocardiogram (ECG), Abnormal Stress (*continued*)

Suggested Readings

Mayo Clinic Cardiovascular Working Group on Stress Testing. Cardiovascular stress testing: a description of the various types of stress tests and indications for their use. Mayo Clin Proc 1996;71:43–52.

Okin PM, Kligfield P. Heart rate adjustment of ST segment depression and performance of the exercise electrocardiogram: a critical evaluation. [Review]. J Am Coll Cardiol 1995;25:1726–1735.

Mickelson JK, Bates ER, Hartigan P, et al. Is computer interpretation of the exercise electrocardiogram a reasonable surrogate for visual reading? Veterans Affairs ACME Investigators. Clin Cardiol 1997;20:391–397.

Gianrossi R, Detrano R, Mulvihill D, et al. Exercise-induced ST depression in the diagnosis of coronary artery disease. A meta-analysis. [Review]. Circulation 1989;80:87–98.

Suggested Guidelines

Pina IL, Balady GJ, Hanson P, et al. Guidelines for clinical exercise testing laboratories. A statement for healthcare professionals from the Committee on Exercise and Cardiac Rehabilitation, American Heart Association. Circulation 1995;91:912–921.

Ritchie JL, Bateman TM, Bonow RO, et al. Guidelines for clinical use of cardiac radionuclide imaging. Report of the American College of Cardiology/American Heart Association Task Force on Assessment of Diagnostic and Therapeutic Cardiovascular Procedures (Committee on Radionuclide Imaging), developed in collaboration with the American Society of Nuclear Cardiology. J Am Coll Cardiol 1995;25:521–547.

See Also

- Chest discomfort, nonanginal
- Chest discomfort, possible angina
- Chest discomfort, anginal
- ECG, abnormal

THE CONSULTATION GUIDE

Fenfluramine/Dexfenfluramine Use, History of

Indications and Timing for Referral

- Clinical findings suggesting valvular heart disease
- Echocardiographically confirmed valvular abnormality

Timing: Routine (less than 4 weeks)

Appropriate timing of referral may be Immediate or Urgent (less than 24 hours) depending upon the severity, duration, frequency, or progression of symptoms

Advice for Referral

- Patients without symptoms and/or murmurs on initial examination should undergo repeat clinical examination in 6 to 8 months to rule out progression of valvular heart disease.
- Echocardiography is only recommended when symptoms or cardiac murmur present, when body type or size prevents adequate auscultation of murmur, or when patient is undergoing an invasive procedure for which antibiotic prophylaxis is recommended to prevent bacterial endocarditis.
- Although the need for cardiac catheterization may be apparent at the initial consultative visit, appropriate procedures for preliminary discussion with primary care physician, authorization, and scheduling will depend upon the practice setting. If cardiac catheterization is performed an additional follow-up visit is appropriate.

Tests to Prepare for Consult

- None

Tests Not Useful Before Consult

- None

Tests Consultant May Need to Do

- ECG
- Echocardiogram with Doppler studies
- Cardiac catheterization (see *Advice for Referral*)

Follow-up Visits Generally Required

- One

Suggested Readings

Connolly HM, Crary JL, McGoon MD, et al. Valvular heart disease associated with fenfluramine-phentermine. N Engl J Med 1997;337:581–588.

From the Centers for Disease Control and Prevention. Cardiac valvulopathy associated with exposure to fenfluramine or dexfenfluramine: US Department of Health and Human Services interim public health recommendations, November 1997. JAMA 1997;278:1729–1731.

Centers for Disease Control and Prevention. Cardiac valvulopathy associated with exposure to fenfluramine or dexfenfluramine: U. S. Department of Health and Human Services interim public health recommendations, November 1997. MMWR 1997;46:1061–1066.

Roldan CA, Shively BK, Crawford MH. Value of the cardiovascular physical examination for detecting valvular heart disease in asymptomatic subjects. Am J Cardiol 1996;77:1327–1331.

Suggested Guidelines

Ewy GA. ACC/AHA Guidelines for the clinical application of echocardiography. JACC 1990;17:1505–1528.

CARDIOLOGY

Heart Block, First-Degree Atrioventricular

Indications and Timing for Referral

- Symptoms suggesting a more serious cardiac abnormality

Timing: Routine (less than 4 weeks)

Advice for Referral

- Complete medication history and old ECG tracings vital.

Tests to Prepare for Consult

- ECG

Tests Not Useful Before Consult

- Echocardiogram

Tests Consultant May Need to Do

- ECG
- Drug levels
- ESR
- Ambulatory ECG (Holter)

Follow-up Visits Generally Required

- None

Suggested Readings

Narula OS. Wenckebach type I and type II atrioventricular block (revisited). Cardiovasc Clin 1974;6:137–167.

Zipes DP. Specific arrhythmias; diagnosis and treatment: heart block. In: Braunwald E, ed. Heart Disease: a Textbook of Cardiovascular Medicine. 5th ed. Philadelphia: WB Saunders, 1997;887–893.

Suggested Guidelines

Knoebel SB, Williams SV, Achord JL, et al. Clinical competence in ambulatory electrocardiography. A statement for physicians from the AHA/ACC/ACP Task Force on Clinical Privileges in Cardiology. Circulation 1993;88:337–341.

See Also

- Right bundle branch block
- Conduction defect, left bundle branch block
- Conduction defect, left anterior fascicular block
- Heart block, second-degree AV, Mobitz 2
- Heart block, second-degree AV, Mobitz 1
- Heart block, third-degree AV

THE CONSULTATION GUIDE

Heart Block, Second-Degree Atrioventricular, Mobitz 1

Indications and Timing for Referral

- Symptoms suggesting more serious cardiac abnormalities

Timing: Routine (less than 4 weeks)

Advice for Referral

- Can be physiologic in well-trained athletes.
- Complete medication history is vital.
- Echocardiography is generally uninformative in the absence of other specific clinical findings indicating cardiac disease.
- Old ECG tracings are helpful.

Tests to Prepare for Consult

- ECG with prolonged rhythm strip

Tests Not Useful Before Consult

- Echocardiogram

Tests Consultant May Need to Do

- ECG
- Ambulatory ECG (Holter)
- Drug levels

Follow-up Visits Generally Required

- One

Suggested Readings

Connelly DT, Steinhaus DM. Mobitz type 1 atrioventricular block—an indication for permanent pacing. Pacing Clinical Electrophysiol 1996;19:261–264.

DiMarco JP, Philbrick JT. Use of ambulatory electrocardiographic (Holter) monitoring. Ann Intern Med 1990;113:53–68.

Zipes DP. Specific arrhythmias; diagnosis and treatment: heart block. In: Braunwald E, ed. Heart disease: a textbook of cardiovascular medicine. 5th ed. Philadelphia: WB Saunders, 1997;887–893.

Suggested Guidelines

Ambulatory electrocardiographic (Holter) monitoring. American College of Physicians [comment]. Ann Intern Med 1990;113:77–79.

See Also

- Heart block, first-degree AV
- Heart block, second-degree AV, Mobitz 2
- Heart block, third-degree AV
- Conduction defect, right bundle branch block
- Conduction defect, left bundle branch block
- Conduction defect, left anterior fascicular block

CARDIOLOGY

Heart Block, Second-Degree Atrioventricular, Mobitz 2

Indications and Timing for Referral

- All patients presenting with this finding should be evaluated by a cardiologist.

Timing: Routine (less than 4 weeks)

Appropriate timing of referral may be Urgent (less than 24 hours) or Expedited (less than 1 week), depending upon the severity, duration, frequency, or progression of symptoms

Advice for Referral

- In general, ECG stress testing is appropriate if the resting ECG is normal, whereas stress imaging procedures are preferred when the resting ECG is abnormal.
- A complete medication history is vital.

Tests to Prepare for Consult

- ECG
- Ambulatory ECG (Holter)

Tests Not Useful Before Consult

- None

Tests Consultant May Need to Do

- Echocardiogram with Doppler studies
- Stress ECG
- Stress radionuclide imaging
- Stress echocardiography
- Drug levels
- Ambulatory ECG (Holter)
- Event monitor
- Loop monitor

Follow-up Visits Generally Required

- One

Suggested Readings

Aggarwal RK, Ray SG, Connelly DT, et al. Trends in pacemaker mode prescription 1984–1994—a single centre study of 3710 patients. Heart 1996;75:518–521.

Alagona P. New indications for permanent cardiac pacing. Curr Opin Cardiol 1996;11:9–15.

Zipes DP. Specific arrhythmias; diagnosis and treatment: heart block. In: Braunwald E, ed. Heart Disease: a Textbook of Cardiovascular Medicine. 5th ed. Philadelphia: WB Saunders, 1997;887–893.

Suggested Guidelines

Recommended guidelines for in-hospital cardiac monitoring of adults for detection of arrhythmia. Emergency Cardiac Care Committee members. J Am Coll Cardiol 1991;18:1431–1433.

See Also

- Heart block, first-degree AV
- Conduction defect, left anterior fascicular block
- Conduction defect, left bundle branch block
- Conduction defect, right bundle branch block
- Heart block, second-degree AV, Mobitz 1
- Heart block, third-degree AV

THE CONSULTATION GUIDE

Heart Block, Third-Degree Atrioventricular

Indications and Timing for Referral

- Patient symptomatic or heart rate less than 40/minute

Timing: Urgent (less than 24 hours)

- Patient asymptomatic

Timing: Expedited (less than 1 week)

Appropriate timing of referral may be Immediate or Urgent (less than 24 hours) depending upon the severity, duration, frequency, or progression of symptoms

Advice for Referral

- The need for temporary transvenous pacemaker may be apparent at the initial consultative visit. Actual procedures for preliminary discussion with primary care physician, authorization, and scheduling will depend upon the practice setting.
- Echocardiography is generally uninformative in the absence of other specific clinical findings indicating cardiac disease.
- A complete medication history is vital.
- Old ECG tracings are vital.
- Patient will benefit from co-management with a cardiologist.

Tests to Prepare for Consult

- ECG with prolonged rhythm strip

Tests Not Useful Before Consult

- None

Tests Consultant May Need to Do

- ECG
- Digoxin level
- TSH (assay sensitivity <0.1 mU/L)
- BUN, Creatinine
- Potassium
- Echocardiogram
- Ambulatory ECG (Holter)

Follow-up Visits Generally Required

- Co-management, see *Advice for Referral*

Suggested Readings

Aggarwal RK, Ray SG, Connelly DT, et al. Trends in pacemaker mode prescription 1984–1994—a single centre study of 3710 patients. Heart 1996;75:518–521.

Alagona P. New indications for permanent cardiac pacing. Curr Opin Cardiol 1996;11:9–15.

DiMarco JP, Philbrick JT. Use of ambulatory electrocardiographic (Holter) monitoring. Ann Intern Med 1990;113:53–68.

Zipes DP. Specific arrhythmias; diagnosis and treatment: heart block. In: Braunwald E, ed. Heart Disease: a Textbook of Cardiovascular Medicine. 5th ed. Philadelphia: WB Saunders, 1997;887–893.

CARDIOLOGY

Heart Block, Third-Degree Atrioventricular

Suggested Guidelines

Ambulatory electrocardiographic (Holter) monitoring. American College of Physicians [comment]. Ann Intern Med 1990;113:77–79.

Recommended guidelines for in-hospital cardiac monitoring of adults for detection of arrhythmia. Emergency Cardiac Care Committee members. J Am Coll Cardiol 1991;18:1431–1433.

See Also

- Conduction defect, right bundle branch block
- Conduction defect, left bundle branch block
- Conduction defect, left anterior fascicular block
- Heart block, first-degree AV
- Heart block, second-degree AV, Mobitz 1
- Heart block, second-degree AV, Mobitz 2

THE CONSULTATION GUIDE

Heart Failure, Etiology Uncertain, New Onset

Indications and Timing for Referral

- Diagnostic uncertainty

Timing: Expedited (less than 1 week)

Appropriate timing of referral may be Immediate or Urgent (less than 24 hours) depending upon the severity, duration, frequency, or progression of symptoms

Advice for Referral

- In general, ECG stress testing is appropriate if the resting ECG is normal, whereas stress imaging procedures are preferred when the resting ECG is abnormal.
- The need for cardiac catheterization and biopsy may be apparent at the initial consultative visit. Actual procedures for preliminary discussion with primary care physician, authorization, and scheduling will depend upon the practice setting. If cardiac catheterization and biopsy are performed an additional follow-up visit is appropriate.
- Serious consideration should be given to having all such patients seen in consultation with a cardiologist.

Tests to Prepare for Consult

- CBC
- Sodium
- Potassium
- Albumin, total protein
- BUN, Creatinine
- Radiograph, chest
- ECG with prolonged rhythm strip
- Echocardiogram

Tests Not Useful Before Consult

- Ambulatory ECG (Holter)

Tests Consultant May Need to Do

- CPK
- ESR
- TSH (assay sensitivity <0.1 mU/L)
- Echocardiogram
- Stress ECG
- Stress radionuclide imaging
- Stress echocardiography
- Cardiac catheterization (see *Advice for Referral*)
- Endomyocardial biopsy (see *Advice for Referral*)

Follow-up Visits Generally Required

- See *Advice for Referral*

CARDIOLOGY

Heart Failure, Etiology Uncertain, New Onset (*continued*)

Suggested Readings

Karon BL. Diagnosis and outpatient management of congestive heart failure. Mayo Clin Proc 1995;70:1080–1085.

Borggrefe M, Block M, Breithardt G. Identification and management of the high risk patient with dilated cardiomyopathy. [Review]. Br Heart J 1995;72(Suppl):S42–S45.

The effect of digoxin on mortality and morbidity in patients with heart failure. The Digitalis Investigation Group [see comments]. N Engl J Med 1997;336:525–533.

Rahko PS, Orie JE. The clinical presentation and laboratory evaluation of congestive and ischemic cardiomyopathies. [Review]. Cardiovasc Clin 1988;19:75–119.

Suggested Guidelines

Heart failure: management of patients with left-ventricular systolic dysfunction. Agency for Health Care Policy and Research. Clin Pract Guidel Quick Ref Guide Clin 1994; 11:1–25.

Konstam M, Dracup K, Baker D. [Anonymous] Heart failure: evaluation and care of patients with left-ventricular systolic dysfunction. Clinical Practice Guideline No.11. 1994; AHCPR Publication No. 94-0612. Agency for Health Care Policy and Research, Public Health Service. 50940038. Anonymous

See Also

- Heart failure, management
- Cardiomyopathy

THE CONSULTATION GUIDE

Heart Failure, Management

Indications and Timing for Referral

- Change in pattern of signs and/or symptoms
- Refractory to conventional therapy
- Consideration of cardiac transplant
- Assistance with management

Timing: Routine (less than 4 weeks)

Advice for Referral

- A record of the patient's serial weights can be extremely valuable.
- A complete medication history is vital, including levels of all cardioactive drugs.
- Patients with a confirmed diagnosis of heart failure may benefit from co-management with a cardiologist.
- In general, ECG stress testing is appropriate if the resting ECG is normal, whereas stress imaging procedures are preferred when the resting ECG is abnormal.
- The need for cardiac catheterization may be apparent at the initial consultative visit. Actual procedures for preliminary discussion with primary care physician, authorization, and scheduling will depend upon the practice setting. If cardiac catheterization is performed an additional follow-up visit is appropriate.

Tests to Prepare for Consult

- CBC
- BUN, Creatinine
- Electrolytes (Na, K, Cl, CO_2)
- Albumin, total protein
- Radiograph, chest
- ECG with prolonged rhythm strip
- Echocardiogram or MUGA scan
- Weight

Tests Not Useful Before Consult

- None

Tests Consultant May Need to Do

- TSH (assay sensitivity <0.1 mU/L)
- Stress ECG
- Stress radionuclide imaging
- Stress echocardiography
- Metabolic stress test
- Cardiac catheterization (see *Advice for Referral*)
- Drug levels

Follow-up Visits Generally Required

- Co-management, see *Advice for Referral*

CARDIOLOGY

Heart Failure, Management (*continued*)

Suggested Readings

Karon BL. Diagnosis and outpatient management of congestive heart failure. Mayo Clin Proc 1995;70:1080–1085.

Eichhorn EJ, Bristow MR. Medical therapy can improve the biological properties of the chronically failing heart. A new era in the treatment of heart failure. [Review] [156 refs]. Circulation 1996;94:2285–2296.

Adams KF, Ellis ML, Williamson KM, Patterson JH. The AHCPR clinical practice guideline for heart failure revisited. Ann Pharmacother 1997;31:1197–1204.

Aranow WS. Treatment for congestive heart failure in older persons. J Am Geriatr Soc 1997;45:1252–1258.

The effect of digoxin on mortality and morbidity in patients with heart failure. The Digitalis Investigation Group [see comments]. N Engl J Med 1997;336:525–533.

Suggested Guidelines

Konstam M, Dracup K, Baker D. [Anonymous] Heart failure: evaluation and care of patients with left-ventricular systolic dysfunction. Clinical Practice Guideline No.11. 1994; AHCPR Publication No. 94–0612. Agency for Health Care Policy and Research, Public Health Service. 50940038.

ASHP therapeutic guidelines on angiotensin-converting-enzyme inhibitors in patients with left ventricular dysfunction. This official ASHP practice standard was developed through the ASHP Commission on Therapeutics and approved by the ASHP Board of Directors on November 16, 1996 [see comments]. [Review] [109 refs]. Am J Health Syst Pharm 1997;54:299–313.

See Also

- Heart failure, etiology uncertain, new onset
- Cardiomyopathy

Heart Murmur, Aortic

Indications and Timing for Referral

- Fever or other signs of infection, potentially because of endocarditis

Timing: Urgent (less than 24 hours)

- Associated, progressive cardiac symptoms present (e.g., angina, CHF, syncope)
- Assistance in determining clinical significance

Timing: Routine (less than 4 weeks)

Appropriate timing of referral may be Immediate or Urgent (less than 24 hours) depending upon the severity, duration, frequency, or progression of symptoms

Advice for Referral

- Reports of all previous cardiac studies vital.
- The need for cardiac catheterization may be apparent at the initial consultative visit. Actual procedures for preliminary discussion with primary care physician, authorization, and scheduling will depend upon the practice setting. If cardiac catheterization is performed an additional follow-up visit is appropriate.

Tests to Prepare for Consult

- Radiograph, chest
- ECG
- Echocardiogram with Doppler studies

Tests Not Useful Before Consult

- Stress ECG

Tests Consultant May Need to Do

- Echocardiogram with Doppler studies
- Cardiac catheterization (see *Advice for Referral*)
- Radiograph, spine

Follow-up Visits Generally Required

- One

Suggested Readings

Baxley WA. Aortic valve disease. [Review]. Curr Opin Cardiol 1994;9:152–157.

Stewart BF, Pearlman AS. Aortic stenosis or aortic sclerosis [review]. Cardiology in the Elderly 1995;3:259–264.

Lembo NJ, Dell'Italia LJ, Crawford MH, O'Rourke RA. Bedside diagnosis of systolic murmurs. N Engl J Med 1988;318:1572–1578.

Shaver JA. Cardiac auscultation: a cost-effective diagnostic skill. Curr Probl Cardiol 1995;20:441–530.

Dajani AS, Bisno AL, Chung KJ, et al. Prevention of bacterial endocarditis. Recommendations by the American Heart Association. JAMA 1990;264:2919–2922.

See Also

- Aortic valve, bicuspid/calcified valve
- Heart murmur, mitral

CARDIOLOGY

Heart Murmur, Diastolic

Indications and Timing for Referral

- Fever or other signs of infection, potentially because of endocarditis

Timing: Urgent (less than 24 hours)

- Associated, progressive cardiac symptoms present (e.g., angina, CHF, syncope)
- Assistance in determining clinical significance

Timing: Routine (less than 4 weeks)

Appropriate timing of referral may be Immediate or Urgent (less than 24 hours) depending upon the severity, duration, frequency, or progression of symptoms

Advice for Referral

- Reports of all previous cardiac studies is vital.
- In general, ECG stress testing is appropriate if the resting ECG is normal, whereas stress imaging procedures are preferred when the resting ECG is abnormal.
- The need for cardiac catheterization may be apparent at the initial consultative visit. Actual procedures for preliminary discussion with primary care physician, authorization, and scheduling will depend upon the practice setting. If cardiac catheterization is performed an additional follow-up visit is appropriate.
- Serious consideration should be given to having all such patients seen in consultation with a cardiologist.

Tests to Prepare for Consult

- Radiograph, chest
- ECG
- Echocardiogram

Tests Not Useful Before Consult

- None

Tests Consultant May Need to Do

- CBC
- Blood culture
- ESR
- VDRL test
- Echocardiogram with Doppler studies
- Stress ECG
- Stress radionuclide imaging
- Stress echocardiography
- Cardiac catheterization (see *Advice for Referral*)
- 5′-HIAA, 24-hour urine

Follow-up Visits Generally Required

- See *Advice for Referral*

Suggested Readings

Desjardins VA, Enriquezsarano M, Tajik AJ, et al. Intensity of murmurs correlates with severity of valvular regurgitation. Am J Med 1996;100:149–156.

Braunwald E. Valvular heart disease: mitral stenosis and mitral regurgitation. In: Braunwald E, ed. Heart Disease: a Textbook of Cardiovascular Medicine. Philadelphia: WB Saunders, 1997;1007–1035.

O'Rourke RA, Braunwald E. Physical examination of the cardiovascular system. In: Fauci AS, Braunwald E, Isselbacher KJ, et al., eds. Harrison's Principles of Internal Medicine. 14th ed. New York: McGraw Hill, 1998;1231–1237.

Shaver JA. Cardiac auscultation: a cost-effective diagnostic skill. Curr Probl Cardiol 1995;20:441–530.

Heart Murmur, Diastolic (*continued*)

Suggested Guidelines

Dajani AS, Bisno AL, Chung KJ, et al. Prevention of bacterial endocarditis. Recommendations by the American Heart Association. JAMA 1990;264:2919–2922.

Ritchie JL, Bateman TM, Bonow RO, et al. Guidelines for clinical use of cardiac radionuclide imaging. Report of the American College of Cardiology/American Heart Association Task Force on Assessment of Diagnostic and Therapeutic Cardiovascular Procedures (Committee on Radionuclide Imaging), developed in collaboration with the American Society of Nuclear Cardiology. J Am Coll Cardiol 1995;25:521–547.

See Also

- Heart murmur, mitral
- Mitral valve prolapse, click-murmur/suspected
- Mitral valve prolapse, echocardiographically confirmed
- Mitral annulus calcification

CARDIOLOGY

Heart Murmur, Mitral

Indications and Timing for Referral

- Fever or other signs of infection, potentially because of endocarditis

Timing: Urgent (less than 24 hours)

- Associated, progressive cardiac symptoms present (e.g., angina, dyspnea, CHF, hemoptysis, syncope)
- Assistance in determining clinical significance

Timing: Routine (less than 4 weeks)

Appropriate timing of referral may be Immediate or Urgent (less than 24 hours) depending upon the severity, duration, frequency, or progression of symptoms

Advice for Referral

- Reports of all previous cardiac studies are vital.
- In general, ECG stress testing is appropriate if the resting ECG is normal, whereas stress imaging procedures are preferred when the resting ECG is abnormal.
- The need for cardiac catheterization may be apparent at the initial consultative visit. Actual procedures for preliminary discussion with primary care physician, authorization, and scheduling will depend upon the practice setting. If cardiac catheterization is performed an additional follow-up visit is appropriate.

Tests to Prepare for Consult

- Radiograph, chest
- ECG with prolonged rhythm strip
- Echocardiogram with Doppler studies

Tests Not Useful Before Consult

- None

Tests Consultant May Need to Do

- CBC
- Blood culture
- ESR
- Echocardiogram with Doppler studies
- Stress ECG
- Stress radionuclide imaging
- Stress echocardiography
- Cardiac catheterization (see *Advice for Referral*)

Follow-up Visits Generally Required

- One

Heart Murmur, Mitral (continued)

Suggested Readings

Desjardins VA, Enriquezsarano M, Tajik AJ, et al. Intensity of murmurs correlates with severity of valvular regurgitation. Am J Med 1996;100:149–156.

Wisenbaugh T. Mitral valve disease. [Review]. Curr Opin Cardiol 1994;9:146–151.

Lembo NJ, Dell'Italia LJ, Crawford MH, O'Rourke RA. Bedside diagnosis of systolic murmurs. N Engl J Med 1988;318:1572–1578.

Shaver JA. Cardiac auscultation: a cost-effective diagnostic skill. Curr Probl Cardiol 1995;20:441–530.

Braunwald E. Valvular heart disease: mitral stenosis and mitral regurgitation. In: Braunwald E, ed. Heart Disease: a Textbook of Cardiovascular Medicine. Philadelphia: WB Saunders, 1997;1007–1035.

O'Rourke RA, Braunwald E. Physical examination of the cardiovascular system. In: Fauci AS, Braunwald E, Isselbacher KJ, et al., eds. Harrison's Principles of Internal Medicine. 14th ed. New York: McGraw Hill, 1998;1231–1237.

Suggested Guidelines

Ewy GA. ACC/AHA Guidelines for the clinical application of echocardiography. JACC 1990;17:1505–1528.

Dajani AS, Bisno AL, Chung KJ, et al. Prevention of bacterial endocarditis. Recommendations by the American Heart Association. JAMA 1990;264:2919–2922.

See Also

- Heart murmur, aortic
- Heart murmur, diastolic
- Mitral valve prolapse, click-murmur/suspected
- Mitral valve prolapse, echocardiographically confirmed

CARDIOLOGY

Hypotension, Orthostatic

Indications and Timing for Referral

- Assistance with management of medications

Timing: Routine (less than 4 weeks)

Advice for Referral

- Complete medication history vital.
- Records documenting postural blood pressure readings and pulse rates are vital.

Tests to Prepare for Consult

- CBC
- Glucose
- Sodium
- Potassium
- BUN, Creatinine

Tests Not Useful Before Consult

- None

Tests Consultant May Need to Do

- ECG
- ACTH stimulation test, 1 hour
- Tilt table test

Follow-up Visits Generally Required

- One

Suggested Readings

Consensus statement on the definition of orthostatic hypotension, pure autonomic failure, and multiple system atrophy. [Review] [0 refs]. J Neurol Sci 1996;144:218–219.

Lipsitz LA. Orthostatic hypotension in the elderly. [Review]. N Engl J Med 1989;321:952–957.

Mader SL. Orthostatic hypotension. [Review]. Med Clin North Am 1989;73:1337–1349.

Susman J. Orthostatic hypotension. [Review]. Am Fam Physician 1988;37:115–118.

See Also

- Lightheadedness/near syncope
- Bradycardia
- Syncope
- Episodic loss of consciousness, seizure versus syncope

Lightheadedness/Near Syncope

Indications and Timing for Referral

- Diagnostic uncertainty
- Assistance with management

Timing: Routine (less than 4 weeks)

Appropriate timing of referral may be Immediate or Urgent (less than 24 hours) depending upon the severity, duration, frequency, or progression of symptoms

Advice for Referral

- Evaluation of orthostatic blood pressures are vital before consultation.
- Complete medication history is vital, including all levels of cardioactive drugs, e.g., digitalis, quinidine, procainamide.
- The need for electrophysiologic study may be apparent at the initial consultative visit. Actual procedures for preliminary discussion with primary care physician, authorization, and scheduling will depend upon the practice setting. If electrophysiologic study is performed an additional follow-up visit is appropriate.
- In general, ECG stress testing is appropriate if the resting ECG is normal, whereas stress imaging procedures are preferred when the resting ECG is abnormal.
- Factors favoring referral to a cardiologist include:
  - Evidence of cardiac abnormalities or rhythm disturbances
- Factors favoring referral to a neurologist include:
  - Abnormal neurological findings persisting after event
  - History of TIAs or seizures

Tests to Prepare for Consult

- CBC
- Glucose, fasting
- Calcium
- Sodium
- Potassium
- BUN, creatinine
- ECG with prolonged rhythm strip

Tests Not Useful Before Consult

- None

Tests Consultant May Need to Do

- TSH (assay sensitivity <0.1 mU/L)
- ECG
- Echocardiogram with Doppler studies
- Ambulatory ECG (Holter)
- Event monitor
- Loop monitor
- Stress ECG
- Stress radionuclide imaging
- Stress echocardiography
- Tilt table test
- Electrophysiologic study (see *Advice for Referral*)

CARDIOLOGY

Lightheadedness/Near Syncope (continued)

Follow-up Visits Generally Required

- One

Suggested Readings

Benditt DG, Remole S, Milstein S, Bailin S. Syncope: causes, clinical evaluation, and current therapy. [Review]. Annu Rev Med 1992;43:283–300.

Cohen NL. The dizzy patient. Update on vestibular disorders. [Review]. Med Clin North Am 1991;75:1251–1260.

Kapoor WN. Evaluation and management of the patient with syncope. [Review]. JAMA 1992;268:2553–2560.

Smith DB. Dizziness. A clinical perspective. [Review]. Neurol Clin 1990;8:199–207.

DiMarco JP, Philbrick JT. Use of ambulatory electrocardiographic (Holter) monitoring. Ann Intern Med 1990;113:53–68.

Suggested Guidelines

Linzer M, Yang EH, Estes NA 3rd, et al. Diagnosing syncope. Part 1: Value of history, physical examination, and electrocardiography. Clinical Efficacy Assessment Project of the American College of Physicians. [Review] [34 refs]. Ann Intern Med 1997;126:989–996.

Ambulatory electrocardiographic (Holter) monitoring. American College of Physicians [comment]. Ann Intern Med 1990;113:77–99.

See Also

- Syncope
- Hypotension, orthostatic
- Episodic loss of consciousness, seizure versus syncope

Mitral Annulus Calcification

Indications and Timing for Referral

- Patient has associated cardiac symptoms or signs

Timing: Routine (less than 4 weeks)

Tests to Prepare for Consult

- ECG
- Echocardiogram

Tests Not Useful Before Consult

- None

Tests Consultant May Need to Do

- None

Follow-up Visits Generally Required

- None

Suggested Readings

Benjamin EJ, Plehn JF, D'Agostino RB, et al. Mitral annular calcification and the risk of stroke in an elderly cohort [see comments]. N Engl J Med 1992;327:374–379.

Rubin DC, Hawke MW, Plotnick GD. Relation between mitral annular calcium and complex intra-aortic debris. Am J Cardiol 1993;71:1251–1252.

Suggested Guidelines

Ewy GA. ACC/AHA Guidelines for the clinical application of echocardiography. JACC 1990;17:1505–1528.

See Also

- Heart murmur, diastolic

CARDIOLOGY

Mitral Valve Prolapse, Click-Murmur/Suspected

Indications and Timing for Referral

- Assistance with management of symptoms and/or assessment of potential complications, e.g., decision-making about antibiotic prophylaxis and/or management of arrhythmias

Timing: Routine (less than 4 weeks)

Advice for Referral

- Echocardiogram may need to be repeated if previous study is inadequate to establish diagnosis.
- Reports of all previous cardiac studies are vital.

Tests to Prepare for Consult

- ECG with prolonged rhythm strip
- Echocardiogram with Doppler studies

Tests Not Useful Before Consult

- None

Tests Consultant May Need to Do

- Ambulatory ECG (Holter)
- Echocardiogram with Doppler studies

Follow-up Visits Generally Required

- One

Suggested Readings

Desjardins VA, Enriquezsarano M, Tajik AJ, et al. Intensity of murmurs correlates with severity of valvular regurgitation. Am J Med 1996;100:149–156.

Wisenbaugh T. Mitral valve disease. [Review]. Curr Opin Cardiol 1994;9:146–151.

Roldan CA, Shively BK, Crawford MH. Value of the cardiovascular physical examination for detecting valvular heart disease in asymptomatic subjects. Am J Cardiol 1996;77:1327–1331.

Braunwald E. Valvular heart disease: mitral valve prolapse. In: Braunwald E, ed. Heart Disease: a Textbook of Cardiovascular Medicine. Philadelphia: WB Saunders, 1997;1029–1035.

O'Rourke RA, Braunwald E. Physical examination of the cardiovascular system. In: Fauci AS, Braunwald E, Isselbacher KJ, et al., eds. Harrison's Principles of Internal Medicine. 14th ed. New York: McGraw Hill, 1998:1231–1237.

Suggested Guidelines

Dajani AS, Bisno AL, Chung KJ, et al. Prevention of bacterial endocarditis. Recommendations by the American Heart Association. JAMA 1990;264:2919–2922.

Ewy GA. ACC/AHA Guidelines for the clinical application of echocardiography. JACC 1990;17:1505–1528.

See Also

- Mitral valve prolapse, echocardiographically confirmed
- Heart murmur, mitral
- Heart murmur, diastolic

Mitral Valve Prolapse, Echocardiographically Confirmed

Indications and Timing for Referral

- Assistance with management of symptoms and/or assessment of potential complications, e.g., decision-making about antibiotic prophylaxis, and/or management of arrhythmias

Timing: Routine (less than 4 weeks)

Advice for Referral

- In general, ECG stress testing is appropriate if the resting ECG is normal, whereas stress imaging procedures are preferred when the resting ECG is abnormal.

Tests to Prepare for Consult

- ECG with prolonged rhythm strip

Tests Not Useful Before Consult

- None

Tests Consultant May Need to Do

- Ambulatory ECG (Holter)
- Stress ECG
- Stress radionuclide imaging
- Stress echocardiography

Follow-up Visits Generally Required

- One

Suggested Readings

Desjardins VA, Enriquezsarano M, Tajik AJ, et al. Intensity of murmurs correlates with severity of valvular regurgitation. Am J Med 1996;100:149–156.

Coghlan HC. Mitral valve prolapse: is echocardiography yielding too little or too much to the practicing physician? Am J Med 1989;87:367–370.

Wisenbaugh T. Mitral valve disease. [Review]. Curr Opin Cardiol 1994;9:146–151.

Suggested Guidelines

Ewy GA. ACC/AHA Guidelines for the clinical application of echocardiography. JACC 1990;17:1505–1528.

See Also

- Heart murmur, mitral
- Mitral valve prolapse, click-murmur/suspected
- Heart murmur, diastolic

CARDIOLOGY

Myocardial Infarction (MI), Recent, Uncomplicated

Indications and Timing for Referral

- Assistance with evaluation of future risk of cardiac events
- Assistance with management

Timing: Routine (less than 4 weeks)

Advice for Referral

- All records related to acute event are vital.
- In general, ECG stress testing is appropriate if the resting ECG is normal, whereas stress imaging procedures are preferred when the resting ECG is abnormal.
- The need for coronary angiography may be apparent at the initial consultative visit. Actual procedures for preliminary discussion with primary care physician, authorization, and scheduling will depend upon the practice setting. If coronary angiography is performed an additional follow-up visit is appropriate.

Tests to Prepare for Consult

- Glucose, fasting
- Lipid profile (cholesterol, TG, HDL)
- ECG
- Echocardiogram or MUGA scan

Tests Not Useful Before Consult

- None

Tests Consultant May Need to Do

- Radiograph, chest
- Echocardiogram with Doppler studies
- Stress ECG
- Stress radionuclide imaging
- Stress echocardiography
- Ambulatory ECG (Holter)
- Coronary angiography (see *Advice for Referral*)

Follow-up Visits Generally Required

- One

Suggested Readings

Peterson ED, Shaw LJ, Califf RM. Risk stratification after myocardial infarction. [Review] [280 refs]. Ann Intern Med 1997;126:561–582.

Stevenson WG, Ridker PM. Should survivors of myocardial infarction with low ejection fraction be routinely referred to arrhythmia specialists? [see comments]. JAMA 1996;276:481–485.

Loh E, Sutton MS, Wun CC, et al. Ventricular dysfunction and the risk of stroke after myocardial infarction. N Engl J Med 1997;336:251–257.

Sacks FM, Pfeffer MA, Moye LA, et al. The effect of pravastatin on coronary events after myocardial infarction in patients with average cholesterol levels. Cholesterol and Recurrent Events Trial investigators [see comments]. N Engl J Med 1996;335:1001–1009.

Kulick DL, Rahimtoola SH. Is noninvasive risk stratification sufficient, or should all patients undergo cardiac catheterization and angiography after a myocardial infarction? [Review]. Cardiovasc Clin 1990;21:3–25.

Myocardial Infarction (MI), Recent, Uncomplicated (continued)

Suggested Guidelines

Guidelines for risk stratification after myocardial infarction. American College of Physicians. Ann Intern Med 1997;126:556–560.

Ryan TJ, Anderson JL, Antman EM, et al. ACC/AHA Guidelines for the management of patients with acute myocardial infarction. A report of the American College of Cardiology/American Heart Association Task Force on Practice Guidelines (Committee on Management of Acute Myocardial Infarction). J Am Coll Cardiol 1996;28:1328–1428.

Triglyceride, high density lipoprotein, and coronary heart disease. NIH Consens Statement 1992;10:1–28.

See Also

- MI, silent/ECG evidence of

CARDIOLOGY

Myocardial Infarction (MI), Silent/Electrocardiographic Evidence of

Indications and Timing for Referral

- Patient asymptomatic
- Assistance with risk stratification and management
- Confirmation of clinical significance of ECG finding

Timing: Routine (less than 4 weeks)

Appropriate timing of referral may be Immediate or Urgent (less than 24 hours) depending upon the severity, duration, frequency, or progression of symptoms

Advice for Referral

- All old ECG tracings are vital.
- In general, ECG stress testing is appropriate if the resting ECG is normal, whereas stress imaging procedures are preferred when the resting ECG is abnormal.
- Stress testing may be associated with increased risk of cardiac events when recent MI is suspected.
- The need for coronary angiography may be apparent at the initial consultative visit. Actual procedures for preliminary discussion with primary care physician, authorization, and scheduling will depend upon the practice setting. If coronary angiography is performed an additional follow-up visit is appropriate.

Tests to Prepare for Consult

- Glucose, fasting
- Lipid profile (cholesterol, TG, HDL)
- ECG

Tests Not Useful Before Consult

- Ambulatory ECG (Holter)

Tests Consultant May Need to Do

- ECG
- Echocardiogram with Doppler studies
- Stress ECG
- Stress radionuclide imaging
- Stress echocardiography
- Coronary angiography (see *Advice for Referral*)

Follow-up Visits Generally Required

- One

Suggested Readings

Taylor GJ, Katholi RE, Womack K, et al. Increased incidence of silent ischemia after acute myocardial infarction. JAMA 1992;268:1448–1450.

Tzivoni D, Benhorin J, Stern S. Significance and management of silent myocardial ischemia. [Review]. Adv Cardiol 1990;37:312–319.

Gottlieb SO. Management strategies for high-risk patients with silent myocardial ischemia. [Review]. Adv Cardiol 1990;37:320–327.

Bernstein SJ. Coronary angiography: a literature review and ratings of appropriateness and necessity. RAND 1992;JRA-03

Myocardial Infarction (MI), Silent/Electrocardiographic Evidence of (*continued*)

Suggested Guidelines

Ritchie JL, Bateman TM, Bonow RO, et al. Guidelines for clinical use of cardiac radionuclide imaging. Report of the American College of Cardiology/American Heart Association Task Force on Assessment of Diagnostic and Therapeutic Cardiovascular Procedures (Committee on Radionuclide Imaging), developed in collaboration with the American Society of Nuclear Cardiology. J Am Coll Cardiol 1995;25:521–547.

Ewy GA. ACC/AHA Guidelines for the clinical application of echocardiography. JACC 1990;17:1505–1528.

Pina IL, Balady GJ, Hanson P, et al. Guidelines for clinical exercise testing laboratories. A statement for healthcare professionals from the Committee on Exercise and Cardiac Rehabilitation, American Heart Association. Circulation 1995;91:912–921.

See Also

- MI, recent, uncomplicated

CARDIOLOGY

Palpitations

Indications and Timing for Referral

- Diagnostic uncertainty
- High patient anxiety

Timing: Routine (less than 4 weeks)

Appropriate timing of referral may be Immediate or Urgent (less than 24 hours) depending upon associated findings

Advice for Referral

- Complete medication history is vital including alcohol and caffeine intake.

Tests to Prepare for Consult

- CBC
- ECG with prolonged rhythm strip

Tests Not Useful Before Consult

- None

Tests Consultant May Need to Do

- ECG
- TSH (assay sensitivity <0.1 mU/L)
- Ambulatory ECG (Holter)
- Event monitor
- Loop monitor
- Echocardiogram with Doppler studies
- Drug levels
- Electrolytes (Na, K, Cl, CO_2)

Follow-up Visits Generally Required

- One

Suggested Readings

Weber BE, Kapoor WN. Evaluation and outcomes of patients with palpitations. Am J Med 1996;100:138–148.

Weitz HH, Weinstock PJ. Approach to the patient with palpitations. [Review]. Med Clin North Am 1995;79:449–456.

Kinlay S, Leitch JW, Neil A, et al. Cardiac event recorders yield more diagnoses and are more cost-effective than 48-hour Holter monitoring in patients with palpitations—a controlled clinical trial. Ann Intern Med 1996;124:16–20.

DiMarco JP, Philbrick JT. Use of ambulatory electrocardiographic (Holter) monitoring. Ann Intern Med 1990;113:53–68.

Suggested Guidelines

Ambulatory electrocardiographic (Holter) monitoring. American College of Physicians [comment]. Ann Intern Med 1990;113:77–79.

See Also

- Atrial flutter
- Supraventricular tachycardia
- PVCs
- Tachycardia, ventricular, nonsustained
- Atrial fibrillation

Pericardial Effusion

Indications and Timing for Referral

- Acute pericardial effusion
- Recurrent or persistent pericardial effusion
- Etiology unclear

Timing: Expedited (less than 1 week)

- Chronic pericardial effusion
- Assistance with management

Timing: Routine (less than 4 weeks)

Advice for Referral

- Patient should be seen immediately if hemodynamic compromise is suspected.
- Serious consideration should be given to having all such patients be seen with a cardiologist unless known predisposing illness is present (e.g., systemic lupus erythematosus [SLE], renal failure, hypothyroidism).
- The need for pericardiocentesis may be apparent at the initial consultative visit. Actual procedures for preliminary discussion with primary care physician, authorization, and scheduling will depend upon the practice setting. If pericardiocentesis is performed an additional follow-up visit is appropriate.

Tests to Prepare for Consult

- CBC
- CPK
- Creatinine
- ESR
- TSH
- PPD
- Radiograph, chest
- ECG
- Echocardiogram

Tests Not Useful Before Consult

- None

Tests Consultant May Need to Do

- Radiograph, chest
- ECG
- Echocardiogram with Doppler studies
- Pericardiocentesis (see *Advice for Referral*)
- Pericardial biopsy

Follow-up Visits Generally Required

- See *Advice for Referral*

Suggested Readings

Hoit BD. Imaging the pericardium. [Review]. Cardiol Clin 1990;8:587–600.

Vaitkus PT, Herrmann HC, LeWinter MM. Treatment of malignant pericardial effusion. [Review]. JAMA 1994;272:59–64.

Lovell BH. Pericardial diseases: Acute pericarditis. In: Braunwald E, ed. Heart Disease: a Textbook of Cardiovascular Medicine. Philadelphia: WB Saunders, 1997; 1485–1495.

Suggested Guidelines

Ewy GA. ACC/AHA Guidelines for the clinical application of echocardiography. JACC 1990;17:1505–1528.

See Also

- Pericarditis

CARDIOLOGY

Pericarditis

Indications and Timing for Referral

- Acute pericarditis
- Recurrent or persistent pericarditis
- Etiology unclear

Timing: Expedited (less than 1 week)

- Chronic pericarditis

Timing: Routine (less than 4 weeks)

Advice for Referral

- Patient should be seen immediately if hemodynamic compromise or myocarditis is suspected.
- Serious consideration should be given to having all such patients be seen with a cardiologist unless known predisposing illness is present (e.g., SLE, renal failure).

Tests to Prepare for Consult

- CBC
- CPK
- Creatinine
- ESR
- PPD
- Radiograph, chest
- ECG
- Echocardiogram

Tests Consultant May Need to Do

- Radiograph, chest
- ECG
- Echocardiogram with Doppler studies

Follow-up Visits Generally Required

- See *Advice for Referral*

Suggested Readings

Hoit BD. Imaging the pericardium. [Review]. Cardiol Clin 1990;8:587–600.

Lovell BH. Pericardial diseases: acute pericarditis. In: Braunwald E, ed. Heart Disease: a Textbook of Cardiovascular Medicine. Philadelphia: WB Saunders, 1997;1481–1485.

Suggested Guidelines

Ewy GA. ACC/AHA Guidelines for the clinical application of echocardiography. JACC 1990;17:1505–1528.

See Also

- Pericardial effusion

THE CONSULTATION GUIDE

Premature Ventricular Complexes (PVCs)

Indications and Timing for Referral

- Associated symptoms or signs of cardiac disease
- Highly anxious patient

Timing: Expedited (less than 1 week)

- Risk factors for cardiac disease present
- Preprocedure evaluation

Timing: Routine (less than 4 weeks)

Appropriate timing of referral may be Immediate or Urgent (less than 24 hours) depending on the severity, duration, frequency or progression of symptoms

Advice for Referral

- In general, ECG stress testing is appropriate if the resting ECG is normal, whereas stress imaging procedures are preferred when the resting ECG is abnormal.
- Complete medication history is vital, including alcohol and caffeine intake.

Tests to Prepare for Consult

- Potassium
- Magnesium
- Creatinine
- CBC
- ECG with prolonged rhythm strip

Tests Not Useful Before Consult

- None

Tests Consultant May Need to Do

- Ambulatory ECG (Holter)
- Echocardiogram with Doppler studies
- Stress ECG
- Antiarrhythmic drug levels

Follow-up Visits Generally Required

- One

Suggested Readings

Wang K, Hodges M. The premature ventricular complex as a diagnostic aid. [Review]. Ann Intern Med 1992;117:766–770.

Messineo FC. Ventricular ectopic activity: prevalence and risk. [Review]. Am J Cardiol 1989;64:53J–56J.

Sung RJ, Fan W, Huycke EC. Ventricular arrhythmias in the absence of organic heart disease. [Review]. Cardiovasc Clin 1992;22:149–163.

Mitchell LB. Treatment of ventricular arrhythmias after recovery from myocardial infarction. [Review]. Annu Rev Med 1994;45:119–138.

DiMarco JP, Philbrick JT. Use of ambulatory electrocardiographic (Holter) monitoring. Ann Intern Med 1990;113:53–68.

Suggested Guidelines

Ambulatory electrocardiographic (Holter) monitoring. American College of Physicians [comment]. Ann Intern Med 1990;113:77–79.

Pina IL, Balady GJ, Hanson P, Labovitz AJ, et al. Guidelines for clinical exercise testing laboratories. A statement for healthcare professionals from the Committee on Exercise and Cardiac Rehabilitation, American Heart Association. Circulation 1995;91:912–921.

See Also

- Ventricular tachycardia, nonsustained
- Palpitations
- Atrial fibrillation
- Atrial flutter
- Supraventricular tachycardia

CARDIOLOGY

Preoperative Evaluation

Indications and Timing for Referral

- Clinical or test evidence of cardiac disease

Timing: Routine (less than 4 weeks)

Advice for Referral

- See specific cardiac condition for additional information
- In general, ECG stress testing is appropriate if the resting ECG is normal, whereas stress imaging procedures are preferred when the resting ECG is abnormal.

Tests to Prepare for Consult

- ECG

Tests Not Useful Before Consult

- None

Tests Consultant May Need to Do

- Echocardiogram with Doppler studies
- Stress ECG
- Stress radionuclide imaging
- Stress echocardiography

Follow-up Visits Generally Required

- None

Suggested Readings

Leppo JA. Preoperative cardiac risk assessment for noncardiac surgery. [Review]. Am J Cardiol 1995;75:42D–51D.

Freeman WK, Gibbons RJ, Shub C. Preoperative assessment of cardiac patients undergoing noncardiac surgical procedures. [Review]. Mayo Clin Proc 1989;64:1105–1117.

McCallion J, Krenis LJ. Preoperative cardiac evaluation. [Review]. Am Fam Physician 1992;45:1723–1732.

Pryor DB. Value of the history and physical in identifying patients at increased risk for coronary artery disease. Ann Intern Med 1993;118:81–90.

Mayo Clinic Cardiovascular Working Group on Stress Testing. Cardiovascular stress testing: a description of the various types of stress tests and indications for their use. Mayo Clin Proc 1996;71:43–52.

Goldman L. Assessment of perioperative cardiac risk. N Engl J Med 1994;330:707–709.

Mangano DT, Goldman L. Preoperative assessment of patients with known or suspected coronary disease. N Engl J Med 1995;333:1750–1756.

DeLisser HM, Grippi M. Perioperative respiratory considerations in the surgical patient. In: Fishman AP, Elias JA, Fishman JA, et al., eds. Fishman's Pulmonary Diseases and Disorders. 3rd ed. New York: McGraw Hill, 1998;619–629.

THE CONSULTATION GUIDE

Q-T Interval Abnormality

Indications and Timing for Referral

- Q-T interval prolonged and patient symptomatic (e.g., syncopal or ventricular arrhythmia present)

Timing: Urgent (less than 24 hours)

- Q-T interval prolonged and patient has family history of sudden death

Timing: Expedited (less than 1 week)

- Patient asymptomatic

Timing: Routine (less than 4 weeks)

Advice for Referral

- A complete family and medication history is vital.
- In general, ECG stress testing is appropriate if the resting ECG is normal, whereas stress imaging procedures are preferred when the resting ECG is abnormal.

Tests to Prepare for Consult

- Calcium
- Potassium
- ECG

Tests Not Useful Before Consult

- None

Tests Consultant May Need to Do

- ECG
- Ambulatory ECG (Holter)
- Event monitor
- Loop monitor
- Echocardiogram with Doppler studies
- Stress ECG
- Stress radionuclide imaging
- Stress echocardiography
- Drug levels

Follow-up Visits Generally Required

- One

Suggested Readings

Roden DM. A practical approach to torsade de pointes. Clin Cardiol 1997;20:285–290.

Fisch C. Electrocardiography: ST segment and T-wave changes. In: Braunwald E, ed. Heart Disease: a Textbook of Cardiovascular Medicine. 5th ed. Philadelphia: WB Saunders, 1997;136–143.

CARDIOLOGY

Syncope

Indications and Timing for Referral

- Diagnostic uncertainty, particularly in patients with known coronary artery disease, reduced ejection fraction (< 35%), hypertrophic or congestive cardiomyopathy, or a prolonged Q-T interval
- Assistance with management

Timing: Expedited (less than 1 week)

Appropriate timing of referral may be Immediate or Urgent (less than 24 hours) depending upon the severity, duration, frequency, or progression of symptoms

Advice for Referral

- Evaluation of orthostatic blood pressures are vital before consultation.
- Complete medication history is vital, including all levels of cardioactive drugs, e.g., digitalis, quinidine, procainamide.
- The need for electrophysiologic study may be apparent at the initial consultative visit. Actual procedures for preliminary discussion with primary care physician, authorization, and scheduling will depend upon the practice setting. If electrophysiologic study is performed, an additional follow-up visit is appropriate.
- In general, ECG stress testing is appropriate if the resting ECG is normal, whereas stress imaging procedures are preferred when the resting ECG is abnormal.

- Factors favoring referral to a cardiologist include:
    - Evidence of cardiac abnormalities or rhythm disturbances
- Factors favoring referral to a neurologist include:
    - Abnormal neurological findings persisting after event
    - History of TIAs or seizures

Tests to Prepare for Consult

- CBC
- Glucose, fasting
- Calcium
- Sodium
- Potassium
- BUN, Creatinine
- ECG with prolonged rhythm strip

Tests Not Useful Before Consult

- None

Tests Consultant May Need to Do

- TSH (assay sensitivity <0.1 mU/L)
- ECG
- Echocardiogram with Doppler studies
- Ambulatory ECG (Holter)
- Event monitor
- Loop monitor
- Tilt table test
- Stress ECG
- Stress radionuclide imaging
- Stress echocardiography
- Electrophysiologic study (see *Advice for Referral*)

Syncope (continued)

Follow-up Visits Generally Required

- One

Suggested Readings

Kapoor WN. Evaluation and management of the patient with syncope. [Review]. JAMA 1992;268:2553–2560.

Benditt DG, Ferguson DW, Grubb BP, et al. Tilt table testing for assessing syncope. American College of Cardiology. [Review] [97 refs]. J Am Coll Cardiol 1996;28:263–275.

Hart GT. Evaluation of syncope. [Review]. Am Fam Physician 1995;51:1941–1948.

Benditt DG, Remole S, Milstein S, Bailin S. Syncope: causes, clinical evaluation, and current therapy. [Review]. Annu Rev Med 1992;43:283–300.

Sra JS, Jazayeri MR, Dhala A, et al. Neurocardiogenic syncope. Diagnosis, mechanisms, and treatment. [Review]. Cardiol Clin 1993;11:183–191.

Suggested Guidelines

Linzer M, Yang EH, Estes NA 3rd, et al. Diagnosing syncope. Part 1: Value of history, physical examination, and electrocardiography. Clinical Efficacy Assessment Project of the American College of Physicians. [Review] [34 refs]. Ann Intern Med 1997;126:989–996.

Ambulatory electrocardiographic (Holter) monitoring. American College of Physicians [comment]. Ann Intern Med 1990;113:77–79.

See Also

- Lightheadedness/near syncope
- Hypotension, orthostatic
- Episodic loss of consciousness, seizure versus syncope

CARDIOLOGY

Tachycardia, Supraventricular

Indications and Timing for Referral

- Patient symptomatic (e.g., angina, heart failure, or change in mental status)
- Assistance with management

Timing: Urgent (less than 24 hours)

- Diagnostic uncertainty

Timing: Routine (less than 4 weeks)

Appropriate timing of referral may be Immediate or Urgent (less than 24 hours) depending upon the severity, duration, frequency, or progression of symptoms

Advice for Referral

- Complete history of medication, alcohol, and caffeine intake is vital.
- Echocardiogram most helpful if it includes evaluation of structural abnormalities (e.g., left atrial size, presence or absence of mitral annulus calcification), thrombus, and assessment of left ventricular function with ejection fraction.
- The need for electrophysiologic studies may be apparent at the initial consultative visit. Actual procedures for preliminary discussion with primary care physician, authorization, and scheduling will depend upon the practice setting. If electrophysiologic study is performed, additional follow-up visit may be appropriate.
- Serious consideration should be given to having all such patients seen in consultation with a cardiologist.

Tests to Prepare for Consult

- ECG with prolonged rhythm strip
- Ambulatory ECG (Holter)

Tests Not Useful Before Consult

- None

Tests Consultant May Need to Do

- TSH (assay sensitivity <0.1 mU/L)
- Drug levels
- Event monitor
- Loop monitor
- Echocardiogram with Doppler studies
- Electrophysiologic study (see *Advice for Referral*)

Follow-up Visits Generally Required

- See *Advice for Referral*

THE CONSULTATION GUIDE

Tachycardia, Supraventricular (continued)

Suggested Readings

Ganz LI, Friedman PL. Supraventricular tachycardia. [Review]. N Engl J Med 1995;332:162–173.

Lessmeier TJ, Gamperling D, Johnson-Liddon V, et al. Unrecognized paroxysmal supraventricular tachycardia. Potential for misdiagnosis as panic disorder. Arch Intern Med 1997;157:537–543.

Wathen MS, Klein GJ, Yee R, Natale A. Classification and terminology of supraventricular tachycardia. Diagnosis and management of the atrial tachycardias. [Review]. Cardiol Clin 1993;11:109–120.

Wellens HJ, Gorgels AP, Smeets JL, den Dulk K. Ambulatory electrocardiography evaluation of supraventricular tachyarrhythmias and bradyarrhythmias. [Review]. Cardiol Clin 1992;10:361–370.

Wanless RS, Anderson K, Joy M, Joseph SP. Multicenter comparative study of the efficacy and safety of sotalol in the prophylactic treatment of patients with paroxysmal supraventricular tachyarrhythmias. Am Heart J 1997;133:441–446.

Suggested Guidelines

Akhtar M, Williams SV, Achord JL, et al. Clinical competence in invasive cardiac electrophysiological studies. A statement for physicians from the ACP/ACC/AHA Task Force on Clinical Privileges in Cardiology. Circulation 1994;89:1917–1920.

Ambulatory electrocardiographic (Holter) monitoring. American College of Physicians [comment]. Ann Intern Med 1990;113:77–79.

See Also

- Palpitations
- PVCs
- Ventricular tachycardia, nonsustained
- Wolff-Parkinson-White (WPW) syndrome
- Atrial fibrillation
- Atrial flutter

CARDIOLOGY

Tachycardia, Ventricular, Nonsustained

Indications and Timing for Referral

- See *Advice for Referral*

Timing: Urgent or Immediate

- Assistance with rhythm control
- Assistance with assessing clinical significance
- Patient is symptomatic and/or highly anxious

Timing: Routine (less than 4 weeks)

Appropriate timing of referral may be Immediate or Urgent (less than 24 hours) depending upon the severity, duration, frequency, or progression of symptoms, e.g., recent history of MI, cardiomyopathy, or a prolonged Q-T interval

Advice for Referral

- Nonsustained ventricular tachycardia is defined as more than three consecutive beats of ventricular origin at a rate of greater than 120/minute.
- Complete history of medication, alcohol, and caffeine intake is vital.
- Echocardiogram most helpful if it includes evaluation of structural abnormalities (e.g., left atrial size, presence or absence of mitral annulus calcification) and assessment of left ventricular function with ejection fraction.
- In general, ECG stress testing is appropriate if the resting ECG is normal, whereas stress imaging procedures are preferred when the resting ECG is abnormal.
- Co-management with a cardiologist is indicated.

Tests to Prepare for Consult

- Potassium
- Magnesium
- ECG with prolonged rhythm strip

Tests Not Useful Before Consult

- None

Tests Consultant May Need to Do

- Ambulatory ECG (Holter)
- Echocardiogram
- Stress ECG
- Stress radionuclide imaging
- Stress echocardiography
- Antiarrhythmic drug levels

Follow-up Visits Generally Required

- Co-management

THE CONSULTATION GUIDE

Tachycardia, Ventricular, Nonsustained (*continued*)

Suggested Readings

Hsia HH, Buxton AE. Work-up and management of patients with sustained and nonsustained monomorphic ventricular tachycardias. [Review]. Cardiol Clin 1993;11:21–37.

Simons GR, Klein GJ, Natale A. Ventricular tachycardia: pathophysiology and radiofrequency catheter ablation. [Review] [126 refs]. Pacing Clin Electrophysiol 1997;20:534–551.

Pires LA, Huang SK. Nonsustained ventricular tachycardia: identification and management of high-risk patients. [Review]. Am Heart J 1993;126:189–200.

Mitchell LB. Treatment of ventricular arrhythmias after recovery from myocardial infarction. [Review]. Annu Rev Med 1994;45:119–138.

Reiter MJ. The ESVEM trial: impact on treatment of ventricular tachyarrhythmias. Electrophysiologic study versus electrocardiographic monitoring. [Review] [59 refs]. Pacing Clin Electrophysiol 1997;20:468–477.

Waldo AL, Henthorn RW, Carlson MD. A perspective on ventricular arrhythmias: patient assessment for therapy and outcome. [Review]. Am J Cardiol 1990;65:30B–35B.

Suggested Guidelines

Recommended guidelines for in-hospital cardiac monitoring of adults for detection of arrhythmia. Emergency Cardiac Care Committee members. J Am Coll Cardiol 1991;18:1431–1433.

Ambulatory electrocardiographic (Holter) monitoring. American College of Physicians [comment]. Ann Intern Med 1990;113:77–79.

See Also

- PVCs
- Supraventricular tachycardia
- Atrial flutter
- Palpitations
- Atrial fibrillation

CARDIOLOGY

Valve Replacement, Postoperative Management

Indications and Timing for Referral

- Assistance with management

Timing: Routine (less than 4 weeks)

Advice for Referral

- Patients with porcine valves may benefit from seeing a cardiologist on a yearly basis to reassess valve function.
- Patients with mechanical valves that have been recalled (i.e., the Shiley valve prone to strut fracture) should be evaluated by a cardiologist.
- Routine echocardiograms not usually required in absence of abnormal cardiac findings.
- Records of preoperative status, operative notes, and radiographs are important.

Tests to Prepare for Consult

- ECG

Tests Not Useful Before Consult

- None

Tests Consultant May Need to Do

- Prothrombin time
- Radiograph, chest
- Echocardiogram with Doppler studies

Follow-up Visits Generally Required

- See *Advice for Referral*

Suggested Readings

Cannegieter SC, Rosendaal FR, Briet E. Thromboembolic and bleeding complications in patients with mechanical heart valve prostheses. [Review]. Circulation 1994;89:635–641.

Grunkemeier GL, Rahimtoola SH. Artificial heart valves. [Review]. Annu Rev Med 1990;41:251–263.

Crumbley AJ 3d, Crawford FA Jr. Long-term results of aortic valve replacement. [Review]. Cardiol Clin 1991;9:353–380.

Heimberger TS, Duma RJ. Infections of prosthetic heart valves and cardiac pacemakers. [Review]. Infect Dis Clin North Am 1989;3:221–245.

Suggested Guidelines

Dajani AS, Bisno AL, Chung KJ, et al. Prevention of bacterial endocarditis. Recommendations by the American Heart Association. JAMA 1990;264:2919–2922.

THE CONSULTATION GUIDE

Wolff-Parkinson-White (WPW) Syndrome

Indications and Timing for Referral

- Patient symptomatic (e.g., angina, heart failure, syncope, or change in mental status)

Timing: Urgent (less than 24 hours)

- Confirmation of diagnosis
- Assistance with management of recurrent tachycardia

Timing: Routine (less than 4 weeks)

Appropriate timing of referral may be Immediate or Urgent (less than 24 hours) depending upon the severity, duration, frequency, or progression of symptoms

Advice for Referral

- The need for electrophysiologic studies may be apparent at the initial consultative visit. Actual procedures for preliminary discussion with primary care physician, authorization, and scheduling will depend upon the practice setting. If electrophysiologic study is performed, an additional follow-up visit is appropriate.
- Serious consideration should be given to having all such patients seen in consultation with a cardiologist.

Tests to Prepare for Consult

- ECG with prolonged rhythm strip
- Echocardiogram

Tests Not Useful Before Consult

- None

Tests Consultant May Need to Do

- Ambulatory ECG (Holter)
- Event monitor
- Loop monitor
- Electrophysiologic study (see *Advice for Referral*)

Follow-up Visits Generally Required

- See *Advice for Referral*

Suggested Readings

Miller JM. Therapy of Wolff-Parkinson-White syndrome and concealed bypass tracts. 1. J Cardiovascul Electrophysiol 1996;7:85–93.

Prystowsky EN, Packer DL, Schier JJ, Lowe JE. Nonpharmacologic treatment of the Wolff-Parkinson-White syndrome and other supraventricular tachycardias. [Review]. Annu Rev Med 1990;41:239–250.

Waldo AL, Akhtar M, Benditt DG, et al. Appropriate electrophysiologic study and treatment of patients with the Wolff-Parkinson-White syndrome. J Am Coll Cardiol 1988;11:1124–1129.

Suggested Guidelines

Knoebel SB, Williams SV, Achord JL, et al. Clinical competence in ambulatory electrocardiography. A statement for physicians from the AHA/ACC/ACP Task Force on Clinical Privileges in Cardiology. Circulation 1993;88:337–341.

See Also

- Supraventricular tachycardia

CHAPTER 3

Endocrinology and Metabolism

Acromegaly	105
Adrenal Insufficiency	106
Adrenal Mass, Radiologically Detected	108
Amenorrhea, Secondary	109
Anovulatory Syndrome, Chronic	110
Carcinoid Syndrome	111
Cushing's Syndrome	112
Delayed Puberty	
Female	114
Male	115
Diabetes Insipidus	116
Diabetes Mellitus, Glycemic Control	117
Diabetes, with Gastrointestinal Complications	119
Diabetic Nephropathy	120
Diabetic Neuropathy	122
Empty Sella Syndrome	123
Flushing	124
Galactorrhea	125
Glucocorticoid Taper	126
Goiter, Simple/Diffuse	127
Gynecomastia	128
High Density Lipoprotein (HDL) Cholesterol, Low	129
Hirsutism	130
Hyperaldosteronism, Primary	131
Hypercalcemia	132
Hypercalcemia, Low PTH	133
Hypercholesterolemia	134
Hyperparathyroidism	135
Hyperprolactinemia	137
Hypertension	138
Hyperthyroidism (see Thyrotoxicosis)	172
Hypertriglyceridemia	139
Hypoaldosteronism	140
Hypocalcemia	141
Hypocalcemia with Elevated PTH	142
Hypogonadism, Male	143

(continued)

Endocrinology and Metabolism (continued)

Hypoglycemia
    Fasting 144
    Reactive 145
Hypoparathyroidism 146
Hypopituitarism 147
Hypothyroidism 148
Impotence 149
Menopausal Hormone Replacement 150
Menopause, Premature 151
Multiple Endocrine Neoplasia I 152
Multiple Endocrine Neoplasia II 153
Obesity 154
Osteodystrophy, Renal 155
Osteomalacia 156
Osteopenia 157
Osteoporosis 158
Paget's Disease 160
Pheochromocytoma 161
Pituitary Tumor 163
Polycystic Ovaries 165
Sella Turcica, Enlarged 166
Thyroid Nodule 167
Thyroid Ophthalmopathy 168
Thyroid, Painful 169
Thyroid Function Tests, Abnormal 170
Thyroiditis, Subacute 171
Thyrotoxicosis 172

ENDOCRINOLOGY AND METABOLISM

Acromegaly

Indications and Timing for Referral
- Severe headache
- Change of vision

Timing: Urgent (less than 24 hours) or Expedited (less than 1 week)

- Diagnostic uncertainty
- Assistance with management

Timing: Routine (less than 4 weeks)

Advice for Referral
- Optimal long-term management includes screening for colonic polyposis.
- Serious consideration should be given to having such patients co-managed with an endocrinologist.

Tests to Prepare for Consult
- IGF-1
- Glucose

Tests Not Useful Before Consult
- Radiograph, skull
- Sellar tomograms

Tests Consultant May Need to Do
- GH
- IGF-1
- IGFBP-3
- OGTT (for serial GH and glucose)
- Glucose
- Glycohemoglobin
- Cortisol, 8 am
- Free T_4
- TSH
- ACTH stimulation test, 1-hour
- Insulin tolerance test
- CRH stimulation test (for ACTH and cortisol)
- GHRH
- Prolactin
- Radiograph, chest
- ECG
- Visual field testing
- Osmolality
  - Serum
  - Urine
- Ultrasound, biliary
- MR, cranial with contrast

Follow-up Visits Generally Required
- Co-management, see *Advice for Referral*

Suggested Readings
Melmed S. Acromegaly. N Engl J Med 1990;322:966–977.
Ezzat S, Wilkins GE, Patel Y, et al. The diagnosis and management of acromegaly: a Canadian consensus report. [Review] [60 refs]. Clin Invest Med 1996;19:259–270.
Chang-DeMoranville BM, Jackson IM. Diagnosis and endocrine testing in acromegaly. Endocrinol Metab Clin North Am 1992;21:649–668.
Molitch ME. Clinical manifestations of acromegaly. [Review]. Endocrinol Metab Clin North Am 1992;21:597–614.
Melmed S. Etiology of pituitary acromegaly. [Review]. Endocrinol Metab Clin North Am 1992;21:539–551.
Sheppard MC, Stewart PM. Treatment options for acromegaly. [Review] [10 refs]. Metabolism 1996;45(Suppl 1):63–64.
Consensus statement: benefits versus risks of medical therapy for acromegaly. Acromegaly Therapy Consensus Development Panel. Am J Med 1994;97:468–473.

See Also
- Multiple endocrine neoplasia I
- Hypopituitarism

Adrenal Insufficiency

Indications and Timing for Referral

- Hypotension
- Severe hyperkalemia
- Clinically significant dehydration
- Fever
- Hyponatremia
- Hypoglycemia
- Abdominal pain, nausea and vomiting

Timing: Urgent (less than 24 hours)

- Diagnostic uncertainty
- Etiology unclear
- Assistance with management

Timing: Expedited (less than 1 week)

Advice for Referral

- ACTH-stimulated or basal cortisol level vital before treatment with glucocorticoids.
- Criteria for adrenal insufficiency are not established for 24-hour urine tests.
- Complete medication history is vital.
- When caused by pituitary disease, see *Hypopituitarism*.
- Consideration should be given to having such patients co-managed with an endocrinologist.

Tests to Prepare for Consult

- Electrolytes (Na, K, Cl, CO_2)
- Glucose
- Calcium
- BUN
- CBC
- ACTH level, plasma
- ACTH stimulation test or 8 am cortisol

Tests Not Useful Before Consult

- 17-hydroxysteroids, 24-hour urine
- 17-ketosteroids, 24-hour urine

Tests Consultant May Need to Do

- CBC
- Calcium
- ALT, AST, alkaline phosphatase
- LH, FSH
- Estradiol, in women
- Testosterone, in men
- TSH
- Very long chain fatty acids
- Aldosterone
- Human immunodeficiency virus (HIV) antibody testing
- Anti-TPO antibody
- PPD
- ACTH stimulation test
  - 1-hour
  - 3-day
- CT scan, abdomen
- Renin, plasma activity or direct assay
- Vitamin B_{12}, serum
- Anti-adrenal antibodies

Follow-up Visits Generally Required

- Co-management, see *Advice for Referral*

ENDOCRINOLOGY AND METABOLISM

Adrenal Insufficiency (continued)

Suggested Readings

Oelkers W, Diederich S, Bahr V. Diagnosis and therapy surveillance in Addison's disease: rapid adrenocorticotropin (ACTH) test and measurement of plasma ACTH, renin activity, and aldosterone. J Clin Endocrinol Metab 1992;75:259–264.

Grinspoon SK, Biller BM. Clinical review 62: Laboratory assessment of adrenal insufficiency. [Review]. J Clin Endocrinol Metab 1994;79:923–931.

Werbel SS, Ober KP. Acute adrenal insufficiency. [Review] [139 refs]. Endocrinol Metab Clin North Am 1993;22:303–328.

Stoffer SS, Krakauer JC. Induction of adrenal suppression by megestrol acetate [letter; comment]. Ann Intern Med 1996;124:613–614.

See Also

- Hypopituitarism
- Glucocorticoid taper

THE CONSULTATION GUIDE

Adrenal Mass, Radiologically Detected

Indications and Timing for Referral

- Etiology unclear
- Diagnostic uncertainty
- To determine clinical significance

Timing: Routine (less than 4 weeks)

Advice for Referral

- False-positive overnight dexamethasone suppression tests may occur in settings of obesity, stress, or use of phenytoin or estrogen.

Tests to Prepare for Consult

- Potassium
- Metanephrines or catecholamines, 24-hour urine
- Overnight dexamethasone suppression test, 1 mg

Tests Not Useful Before Consult

- 17-ketosteroids, 24-hour urine
- Angiography

Tests Consultant May Need to Do

- Aldosterone, 24-hour urine
- Aldosterone, serum
- Renin, plasma activity or direct assay
- Free cortisol or overnight dexamethasone suppression test, 1 mg
- Estradiol, in women
- Testosterone, in men
- DHEA-S
- Androstanediol glucuronide

Follow-up Visits Generally Required

- One

Suggested Readings

Kloos RT, Gross MD, Francis IR, et al. Incidentally discovered adrenal masses. [Review] [253 refs]. Endocr Rev 1995;16:460–484.

Chidiac RM, Aron DC. Incidentalomas. A disease of modern technology. [Review] [155 refs]. Endocrinol Metab Clin North Am 1997;26:233–253.

Cook DM, Loriaux DL. The incidental adrenal mass. [Review] [30 refs]. Am J Med 1996;101:88–94.

Korobkin M, Francis IR, Kloos RT, Dunnick NR. The incidental adrenal mass. [Review] [54 refs]. Radiol Clin North Am 1996;34:1037–1054.

Ross NS, Aron DC. Hormonal evaluation of the patient with and incidentally discovered adrenal mass. N Engl J Med 1990;323:1401–1405.

See Also

- Hyperaldosteronism, primary
- Cushing's syndrome
- Hypertension
- Pheochromocytoma
- Multiple endocrine neoplasia II

ENDOCRINOLOGY AND METABOLISM

Amenorrhea, Secondary

Indications and Timing for Referral

- Diagnostic uncertainty
- Assistance with management

Timing: Routine (less than 4 weeks)

Tests to Prepare for Consult

- Beta HCG, serum (quantitative)
- Prolactin
- LH, FSH
- Testosterone
- Estradiol
- TSH (assay sensitivity <0.1 mU/L)

Tests Not Useful Before Consult

- Radiograph, skull
- Sellar tomograms

Tests Consultant May Need to Do

- Free T_4
- DHEA-S
- Free testosterone
- Free cortisol or overnight dexamethasone suppression test, 1 mg
- Ultrasound, pelvic
- MR, cranial

Follow-up Visits Generally Required

- Two

Suggested Readings

Rebar RW, Cedars MI. Hypergonadotropic forms of amenorrhea in young women. [Review]. Endocrinol Metab Clin North Am 1992;21:173–191.

Speroff L. Premature ovarian failure. [Review] [41 refs]. Adv Endocrinol Metab 1995;6:233–258.

Warren JP. Clinical review 77: evaluation of secondary amenorrhea. J Clin Endocrinol Metab 1996;81:437–442.

Aloi JA. Evaluation of amenorrhea. Compr Ther 1995;21:575–578.

See Also

- Hirsutism
- Anovulatory syndrome, chronic
- Menopause, premature
- Delayed puberty, female
- Hypopituitarism
- Polycystic ovaries

Anovulatory Syndrome, Chronic

Indications and Timing for Referral
- Diagnostic uncertainty
- Assistance with management

Timing: Routine (less than 4 weeks)

Advice for Referral
- Records of all previous endocrine testing are vital.
- If induction of pregnancy is required, co-management with an endocrinologist or gynecologist is appropriate.

Tests to Prepare for Consult
- Testosterone
- LH, FSH
- Estradiol
- Prolactin
- TSH (assay sensitivity <0.1 mU/L)

Tests Not Useful Before Consult
- None

Tests Consultant May Need to Do
- Free testosterone
- DHEA-S
- Free cortisol, 24-hour urine, or overnight dexamethasone suppression test, 1 mg
- ACTH stimulation test (17-hydroxyprogesterone)
- Ultrasound, pelvic
- MR, cranial

Follow-up Visits Generally Required
- Two, see *Advice for Referral*

Suggested Readings
Dunaif A. Insulin resistance and ovarian hyperandrogenism. The Endocrinologist 1992;2:248–260.

Franks S. Medical progress: Polycystic ovary syndrome. N Engl J Med 1995;333:853–861.

Barbieri RL. Polycystic ovarian disease. [Review]. Annu Rev Med 1991;42:199–204.

Hall JE. Polycystic ovarian disease as a neuroendocrine disorder of the female reproductive axis. [Review]. Endocrinol Metab Clin North Am 1993;22:75–92.

See Also
- Amenorrhea, secondary
- Hirsutism
- Polycystic ovaries
- Delayed puberty, female

ENDOCRINOLOGY AND METABOLISM

Carcinoid Syndrome

Indications and Timing for Referral

- Confirm diagnosis
- Assistance with management

Timing: Routine (less than 4 weeks)

Advice for Referral

- Serious consideration should be given to having such patients co-managed with an endocrinologist or oncologist.

Tests to Prepare for Consult

- 5'-HIAA, 24-hour urine
- ALT, AST, alkaline phosphatase
- Creatinine

Tests Not Useful Before Consult

- None

Tests Consultant May Need to Do

- CEA
- Histamine level
- Serotonin, plasma
- Echocardiogram
- CT or MR, abdomen
- CT scan, thorax

Follow-up Visits Generally Required

- Co-management, see *Advice for Referral*

Suggested Readings

Bax ND, Woods HF, Batchelor A, Jennings M. Clinical manifestations of carcinoid disease. [Review] [33 refs]. World J Surg 1996;20:142–146.

Kvols LK. Therapy of the malignant carcinoid syndrome. [Review]. Endocrinol Metab Clin North Am 1989;18:557–568.

Vinik AI, McLeod MK, Fig LM, et al. Clinical features, diagnosis, and localization of carcinoid tumors and their management. [Review]. Gastroenterol Clin North Am 1989;18:865–896.

Roberts LJ 2d. Carcinoid syndrome and disorders of systemic mast-cell activation including systemic mastocytosis. [Review]. Endocrinol Metab Clin North Am 1988;17:415–436.

See Also

- Flushing

Cushing's Syndrome

Indications and Timing for Referral

- Clinical evidence of expanding sellar or adrenal mass lesion
- Severe hypokalemia
- Psychosis
- Signs of infection
- Severe hypercortisolism

Timing: Urgent (less than 24 hours) or Expedited (less than 1 week)

- Diagnostic uncertainty
- Unclear etiology
- Assistance with management

Timing: Routine (less than 4 weeks)

Advice for Referral

- Urine for free cortisol should include creatinine level to assess completeness of collection.
- Imaging of pituitary should be deferred until biochemical diagnosis is established.
- Long-term management should include bone mineral density testing.
- Serious consideration should be given to having such patients co-managed with an endocrinologist.

Tests to Prepare for Consult

- Electrolytes (Na, K, Cl, CO_2)
- Glucose
- Creatinine
- Free cortisol, 24-hour urine
- Creatinine, 24-hour urine

Tests Not Useful Before Consult

- Radiograph, skull
- MR, cranial

Tests Consultant May Need to Do

- Dexamethasone suppression tests
  - Low-dose, 2-day
  - High-dose, 2-day
  - High-dose (8 mg), overnight
- ACTH level, plasma
- Prolactin
- LH, FSH
- Estradiol
- Testosterone, in men
- Free testosterone
- IGF-1
- GH
- Radiograph, chest
- Visual field testing
- CRH stimulation test (ACTH and cortisol)
- DHEA-S
- CT scan
  - Thorax
  - Adrenal
- MR, cranial with contrast
- Inferior petrosal sinus catheterization

Cushing's Syndrome (continued)

Follow-up Visits Generally Required
- Co-management, see *Advice for Referral*

Suggested Readings
Tsigos C, Chrousos GP. Differential diagnosis and management of Cushing's syndrome. [Review] [52 refs]. Annu Rev Med 1996;47:443–461.
Biller BM. Pathogenesis of pituitary Cushing's syndrome. Pituitary versus hypothalamic. [Review]. Endocrinol Metab Clin North Am 1994;23:547–554.
Findling JW, Doppman JL. Biochemical and radiologic diagnosis of Cushing's syndrome. [Review]. Endocrinol Metab Clin North Am 1994;23:511–537.
Dickstein G, DeBold CR, Gaitan D, et al. Plasma corticotropin and cortisol responses to ovine corticotropin-releasing hormone (CRH), arginine vasopressin (AVP), CRH plus AVP, and CRH plus metyrapone in patients with Cushing's disease. J Clin Endocrinol Metab 1996;81:2934–2941.
Oldfield EH, Doppman JL, Nieman LK, et al. Petrosal sinus sampling with and without corticotropin-releasing hormone for the differential diagnosis of Cushing's syndrome. N Engl J Med 1991;325:897–905.
Tyrrell JB, Wilson CB. Cushing's disease. Therapy of pituitary adenomas. [Review]. Endocrinol Metab Clin North Am 1994;23:925–938.

See Also
- Multiple endocrine neoplasia I
- Pituitary tumor
- Adrenal mass, radiologically detected
- Hirsutism
- Hypertension

THE CONSULTATION GUIDE

Delayed Puberty, Female

Indications and Timing for Referral

- Diagnostic uncertainty
- Assistance with management

Timing: Routine (less than 4 weeks)

Advice for Referral

- If organic etiology is discovered or prolonged hormonal therapy is begun, co-management with an endocrinologist is usually appropriate.

Tests to Prepare for Consult

- CBC
- BUN, creatinine
- ALT, AST, alkaline phosphatase
- LH, FSH
- Estradiol
- Prolactin
- Free T_4
- TSH (assay sensitivity <0.1 mU/L)
- Radiograph, hand, for bone age

Tests Not Useful Before Consult

- Radiograph, skull
- Sellar tomograms

Tests Consultant May Need to Do

- Karyotype
- Testosterone
- Ultrasound, pelvic
- GH
- IGF-1
- IGFBP-3
- MR, cranial

Follow-up Visits Generally Required

- Two, see *Advice for Referral*

Suggested Readings

Kulin HE. Delayed puberty. [Review] [17 refs]. J Clin Endocrinol Metab 1996;81:3460–3464.

Styne DM. New aspects in the diagnosis and treatment of pubertal disorders. [Review] [197 refs]. Pediatr Clin North Am 1997;44:505–529.

Albanese A, Stanhope R. Investigation of delayed puberty. Clin Endocrinol (Oxf) 1995;43:105–110.

Rosenfield RL. Clinical review 6: Diagnosis and management of delayed puberty. [Review]. J Clin Endocrinol Metab 1990;70:559–562.

See Also

- Amenorrhea, secondary
- Hirsutism
- Anovulatory syndrome, chronic
- Polycystic ovaries
- Hyperprolactinemia

ENDOCRINOLOGY AND METABOLISM

Delayed Puberty, Male

Indications and Timing for Referral

- Diagnostic uncertainty
- Assistance with management

Timing: Routine (less than 4 weeks)

Advice for Referral

- If organic etiology is discovered or prolonged hormonal therapy is begun, co-management with an endocrinologist is usually appropriate.

Tests to Prepare for Consult

- CBC
- BUN, creatinine
- ALT, AST, alkaline phosphatase
- LH, FSH
- Testosterone
- Prolactin
- Free T_4
- TSH (assay sensitivity <0.1 mU/L)
- Radiograph, hand, for bone age

Tests Not Useful Before Consult

- Radiograph, skull
- Sellar tomograms

Tests Consultant May Need to Do

- Estradiol
- Karyotype
- HCG stimulation test
- GH
- IGF-1
- IGFBP-3
- MR, cranial

Follow-up Visits Generally Required

- Two, see *Advice for Referral*

Suggested Readings

Styne DM. New aspects in the diagnosis and treatment of pubertal disorders. [Review] [197 refs]. Pediatr Clin North Am 1997;44:505–529.

Kulin HE. Delayed puberty. [Review] [17 refs]. J Clin Endocrinol Metab 1996;81:3460–3464.

Albanese A, Stanhope R. Investigation of delayed puberty. Clin Endocrinol (Oxf) 1995;43:105–110.

Rosenfield RL. Clinical review 6: Diagnosis and management of delayed puberty. [Review]. J Clin Endocrinol Metab 1990;70:559–562.

See Also

- Impotence
- Gynecomastial
- Hyperprolactinemia
- Hypogonadism, male

THE CONSULTATION GUIDE

Diabetes Insipidus

Indications and Timing for Referral

- Clinically significant dehydration
- Severe symptoms
- Sudden onset
- Rapidly progressive
- Significant serum electrolyte imbalance

Timing: Urgent (less than 24 hours)

- Diagnostic uncertainty
- Etiology unclear
- Assistance with management

Timing: Routine (less than 4 weeks)

Advice for Referral

- Water deprivation may be dangerous in patients with diabetes insipidus.
- Serious consideration should be given to having such patients co-managed with an endocrinologist.

Tests to Prepare for Consult

- Glucose
- Electrolytes (Na, K, Cl, CO_2)
- Calcium
- BUN, creatinine
- Albumin, total protein
- Urinalysis with microscopic
- Urine specific gravity
- Creatinine, 24-hour urine, for clearance
- Protein, 24-hour urine
- Volume, 24-hour urine
- Serum and urine osmolarity, fasting, simultaneous

Tests Not Useful Before Consult

- None

Tests Consultant May Need to Do

- LH, FSH
- Estradiol, in women
- Testosterone, in men
- Free T_4
- TSH
- ACTH stimulation test, 1 hour
- Insulin tolerance test
- MR, cranial with contrast

Follow-up Visits Generally Required

- Co-management, see *Advice for Referral*

Suggested Readings

Buonocore CM, Robinson AG. The diagnosis and management of diabetes insipidus during medical emergencies. [Review]. Endocrinol Metab Clin North Am 1993;22:411–423.

Robertson GL. Differential diagnosis of polyuria. [Review]. Annu Rev Med 1988;39:425–442.

Adam P. Evaluation and management of diabetes insipidus. [Review] [16 refs]. Am Fam Physician 1997;55:2146–2153.

Singer I, Oster JR, Fishman LM. The management of diabetes insipidus in adults. [Review] [38 refs]. Arch Intern Med 1997;157:1293–1301.

Ciric I, Ragin A, Baumgartner C, Pierce D. Complications of transsphenoidal surgery: results of a national survey, review of the literature, and personal experience. Neurosurgery 1997;40:225–236.

ENDOCRINOLOGY AND METABOLISM

Diabetes Mellitus, Glycemic Control

Indications and Timing for Referral

- Assistance with management, especially:
  - Uncontrolled symptoms
  - Type I diabetes
  - During or before planned pregnancy
  - Recurrent hypoglycemia
  - Glycohemoglobin greater than 20% above upper limit of normal for assay

Timing: Routine (less than 4 weeks)

Advice for Referral

- Follow-up may be none or co-management based on support required to achieve patient's goals for glycemic control.

Tests to Prepare for Consult

- Glycohemoglobin
- Electrolytes (Na, K, Cl, CO$_2$)
- BUN, creatinine
- UA with microalbumin
- Lipid profile, fasting (cholesterol, HDL, TG)

Tests Not Useful Before Consult

- None

Tests Consultant May Need to Do

- Fructosamine or protein-bound glucose
- Creatinine, 24-hour urine, for clearance
- Protein or microalbumin, 24-hour urine
- Free cortisol or overnight dexamethasone suppression test, 1 mg
- IGF-1
- TSH
- ECG with prolonged rhythm strip
- Arterial Doppler study
- Nerve conduction study

Follow-up Visits Generally Required

- See *Advice for Referral*

Suggested Readings

Nathan DM. The pathophysiology of diabetic complications—how much does the glucose hypothesis explain. Ann Intern Med 1996;124:86–89.

Laine C, Caro JF. Preventing complications in diabetes mellitus—the role of the primary care physician. Med Clin North Am 1996;80:457–474.

Nathan DM. Long-term complications of diabetes mellitus. [Review]. N Engl J Med 1993;328:1676–1685.

Clark CM Jr, Lee DA. Prevention and treatment of the complications of diabetes mellitus. [Review]. N Engl J Med 1995;332:1210–1217.

Goldstein DE, Little RR, Lorenz RA, et al. Tests of glycemia in diabetes. Diabetes Care 1995;18:896–908.

Schade DS, Burge MR. Brittle diabetes: etiology and treatment. [Review] [84 refs]. Adv Endocrinol Metab 1995;6:289–319.

Diabetes Mellitus, Glycemic Control (*continued*)

Selected Guidelines

American Diabetes Association. Clinical practice recommendations 1997. Diabetes Care 1997;20(Suppl 1):S1–S70.

Tinker LF, Heins JM, Holler HJ. Commentary and translation: 1994 nutrition recommendations for diabetes. Diabetes Care and Education, a Practice Group of the American Dietetic Association [see comments]. J Am Diet Assoc 1994;94:507–511.

See Also

- Diabetic nephropathy
- Diabetes, with gastrointestinal complications
- Diabetic neuropathy

Diabetes, with Gastrointestinal Complications

Indications and Timing for Referral
- Patient's oral intake is critically or seriously impaired

Timing: Urgent (less than 24 hours) or Expedited (less than 1 week)

- Control of symptoms

Timing: Routine (less than 4 weeks)

Advice for Referral
- Follow-up may be none or co-management based on support required to achieve patient's goals for glycemic control.
- Factors favoring referral to gastroenterologist include:
  - Unclear etiology
  - Primarily gastrointestinal contributing factors are present
- Factors favoring referral to endocrinologist include:
  - Associated poor glycemic control

Tests to Prepare for Consult
- Glycohemoglobin
- Electrolytes (Na, K, Cl, CO_2)
- CBC
- Lipid profile, fasting (cholesterol, HDL, TG)
- Creatinine
- UA with microalbumin
- ECG

Tests Not Useful Before Consult
- None

Tests Consultant May Need to Do
- Qualitative fecal fat and fiber
- Prothrombin time
- Beta-carotene
- Gastric emptying study
- ECG with prolonged rhythm strip

Follow-up Visits Generally Required
- See *Advice for Referral*

Suggested Readings
Camilleri M. Gastrointestinal problems in diabetes. [Review] [54 refs]. Endocrinol Metab Clin North Am 1996;25:361–378.

Kong MFSC, Macdonald IA, Tattersall RB. Gastric emptying in diabetes [Review]. Diabetic Medicine 1996;13:112–119.

Valdovinos MA, Camilleri M, Zimmerman BR. Chronic diarrhea in diabetes mellitus: mechanisms and an approach to diagnosis and treatment. [Review]. Mayo Clin Proc 1993;68:691–702.

Ogbonnaya KI, Arem R. Diabetic diarrhea. Pathophysiology, diagnosis, and management [see comments]. [Review]. Arch Intern Med 1990;150:262–267.

See Also
- Diabetes mellitus, glycemic control
- Diabetic nephropathy
- Diabetic neuropathy

THE CONSULTATION GUIDE

Diabetic Nephropathy

Indications and Timing for Referral

- Renal insufficiency present
- Patient also has uncontrolled hypertension (HTN)
- High-grade proteinuria is present
- Assistance with management

Timing: Routine (less than 1 week)

Advice for Referral

- Follow-up may be none or co-management based on support required to achieve patient's goals for glycemic control.
- Factors favoring referral to nephrologist include:
  - Creatinine clearance under 30 mL/min
  - Rapidly progressive decrease in creatinine clearance
- Factors favoring referral to endocrinologist include:
  - Associated poor glycemic control

Tests to Prepare for Consult

- Glycohemoglobin
- Electrolytes (Na, K, Cl, CO_2)
- Albumin, total protein
- Calcium, phosphorus
- BUN, creatinine
- UA with microalbumin
- CBC
- Lipid profile, fasting (cholesterol, HDL, TG)
- Creatinine, 24-hour urine, for clearance
- Protein, 24-hour urine

Tests Not Useful Before Consult

- IVP

Tests Consultant May Need to Do

- Ultrasound, renal
- TSH
- ECG
- Nerve conduction study

Follow-up Visits Generally Required

- See *Advice for Referral*

Suggested Readings

Lapuz MH. Diabetic nephropathy. [Review] [49 refs]. Med Clin North Am 1997;81:679–688.

Molitch ME. The relationship between glucose control and the development of diabetic nephropathy in type I diabetes. [Review] [72 refs]. Semin Nephrol 1997;17:101–113.

Adler S, Nast C, Artishevsky A. Diabetic nephropathy: pathogenesis and treatment. [Review]. Annu Rev Med 1993;44:303–315.

Rodby RA. Type II diabetic nephropathy: its clinical course and therapeutic implications. [Review] [93 refs]. Semin Nephrol 1997;17:132–147.

Clark CM Jr, Lee DA. Prevention and treatment of the complications of diabetes mellitus. [Review]. N Engl J Med 1995;332:1210–1217.

Deckert T, Kofoed-Enevoldsen A, Norgaard K, et al. Microalbuminuria. Implications for micro- and macrovascular disease. [Review]. Diabetes Care 1992;15:1181–1191.

Maher JF. Diabetic nephropathy: early detection, prevention and management. [Review]. Am Fam Physician 1992;45:1661–1668.

ENDOCRINOLOGY AND METABOLISM

Diabetic Nephropathy (*continued*)

Selected Guidelines

Consensus development conference on the diagnosis and management of nephropathy in patients with diabetes mellitus. American Diabetes Association and the National Kidney Foundation. [Review]. Diabetes Care 1994;17:1357–1361.

Bennett PH, Haffner S, Kasiske BL, et al. Screening and management of microalbuminuria in patients with diabetes mellitus: recommendations to the Scientific Advisory Board of the National Kidney Foundation from an ad hoc committee of the Council on Diabetes Mellitus of the National Kidney Foundation. Am J Kidney Dis 1995;25:107–112.

American Diabetes Association: clinical practice recommendations 1997. Diabetes Care 1997;20(Suppl 1):S1–S70.

See Also

- Diabetes mellitus, glycemic control
- Diabetic neuropathy
- Diabetes, with gastrointestinal complications
- Synonym: Diabetic glomerulonephropathy

Diabetic Neuropathy

Indications and Timing for Referral

- Assistance with management (e.g., control of symptoms)
- Possible other etiology
- Prevention of progression

Timing: Routine (less than 4 weeks)

Advice for Referral

- Follow-up may be none or co-management based on support required to achieve patient's goals for glycemic control.
- Factors favoring referral to neurologist include:
  - Etiology of neurologic problem(s) is uncertain
- Factors favoring referral to endocrinologist include:
  - Associated poor glycemic control

Tests to Prepare for Consult

- Glycohemoglobin
- Electrolytes (Na, K, Cl, CO_2)
- Creatinine
- UA with microalbumin
- Lipid profile, fasting (cholesterol, HDL, TG)
- TSH
- ECG

Tests Not Useful Before Consult

- None

Tests Consultant May Need to Do

- Vitamin B_{12}, serum
- RPR or VDRL
- Serum folate level
- Protein, 24-hour urine
- Creatinine, 24-hour urine, for clearance
- IEP
  - Serum
  - Urine
- Testosterone, in men
- Nerve conduction study
- ECG with prolonged rhythm strip

Follow-up Visits Generally Required

- See *Advice for Referral*

Suggested Readings

Valensi P, Giroux C, Seeboth-Ghalayini B, Attali JR. Diabetic peripheral neuropathy: effects of age, duration of diabetes, glycemic control, and vascular factors. J Diabetes Complications 1997;11:27–34.

Clark CM Jr, Lee DA. Prevention and treatment of the complications of diabetes mellitus. [Review]. N Engl J Med 1995;332:1210–1217.

Greene DA, Sima AF, Pfeifer MA, Albers JW. Diabetic neuropathy. [Review]. Annu Rev Med 1990;41:303–317.

Proceedings of a consensus development conference on standardized measures in diabetic neuropathy. Neurology 1992;42:1825–1839.

Nathan DM. Long-term complications of diabetes mellitus. [Review]. N Engl J Med 1993;328:1676–1685.

See Also

- Diabetes mellitus, glycemic control
- Diabetic nephropathy
- Diabetes, with gastrointestinal complications

ENDOCRINOLOGY AND METABOLISM

Empty Sella Syndrome

Indications and Timing for Referral

- MR or CT showing pituitary mass or other regional abnormality
- Clinical or laboratory evidence of pituitary hormone excess or deficiency

Timing: Routine (less than 4 weeks)

Tests to Prepare for Consult

- MR, cranial with pituitary cuts
- Prolactin
- Free T_4
- TSH (assay sensitivity <0.1 mU/L)
- Testosterone, in men
- CBC
- Glucose
- Sodium

Tests Not Useful Before Consult

- ACTH level, plasma
- Sellar tomograms
- Arteriogram

Tests Consultant May Need to Do

- Cortisol, 8 am
- GH
- IGF-1
- Estradiol, in women
- Testosterone, in men
- LH, FSH
- CRH stimulation test (serial for cortisol and ACTH)
- ACTH stimulation test, 1-hour (for cortisol)
- Insulin tolerance test (for cortisol and GH)

Follow-up Visits Generally Required

- Two

Suggested Readings

Bjerre P. The empty sella. A reappraisal of etiology and pathogenesis [see comments]. [Review]. Acta Neurologica Scandinavica 1994;Supplementum 1990;13–25.

Felsberg GJ, Tien RD. Sellar and parasellar lesions involving the skull base. [Review]. Neuroimaging Clin North Am 1994;4:543–560.

Chakeres DW, Curtin A, Ford G. Magnetic resonance imaging of pituitary and parasellar abnormalities. [Review]. Radiol Clin North Am 1989;27:265–281.

Selected Guidelines

Magnetic resonance imaging of the brain and spine: a revised statement. American College of Physicians [comment] [see comments]. Ann Intern Med 1994;120:872–875.

See Also

- Sella turcica, enlarged
- Pituitary tumor

Flushing

Indications and Timing for Referral

- Diagnostic uncertainty
- Assistance with management

Timing: Routine (less than 4 weeks)

Advice for Referral

- Complete medication history is vital (e.g., nicotinic acid).
- Factors favoring referral to allergy and immunology include:
  - Other clinical evidence of allergic diathesis
- Factors favoring referral to endocrinology and metabolism include:
  - Clinical or laboratory evidence of hypogonadism
  - Thyroid nodule
- Factors favoring referral to oncology include:
  - Clinical or laboratory evidence of carcinoid or systemic mastocytosis

Tests to Prepare for Consult

- TSH (assay sensitivity <0.1 mU/L)
- Testosterone, in men
- FSH, in women

Tests Not Useful Before Consult

- None

Tests Consultant May Need to Do

- LH, FSH
- 5'-HIAA, 24-hour urine
- Histamine level
- Serotonin, plasma
- Creatinine, 24-hour urine
- Metanephrines, 24-hour urine
- Histamine, 24-hour urine
- Calcitonin
- Skin biopsy
- Bone marrow biopsy

Follow-up Visits Generally Required

- One

Suggested Readings

Ray D, Williams G. Pathophysiological causes and clinical significance of flushing. [Review] [18 refs]. Br J Hosp Med 1993;50:594–598.

Wilkin JK. The red face: flushing disorders. [Review] [103 refs]. Clin Dermatol 1993;11:211–213.

Fellner MJ, Ledesma GN. The red face: drugs, chemicals and other causes. [Review]. Clin Dermatol 1993;11:315–318.

Friedman BS, Germano P, Miletti J, Metcalfe DD. A clinicopathologic study of ten patients with recurrent unexplained flushing. J Allergy Clin Immunol 1994;93:53–60.

Shakir KM, Jasser MZ, Yoshihashi AK, et al. Pseudocarcinoid syndrome associated with hypogonadism and response to testosterone therapy. Mayo Clin Proc 1996;71:1145–1149.

Roberts LJ 2d. Carcinoid syndrome and disorders of systemic mast-cell activation including systemic mastocytosis. [Review]. Endocrinol Metab Clin North Am 1988;17:415–436.

See Also

- Carcinoid syndrome
- Amenorrhea, secondary
- Vasculitis with cutaneous lesions
- Menopausal hormone replacement
- Menopause, premature

ENDOCRINOLOGY AND METABOLISM

Galactorrhea

Indications and Timing for Referral

- Associated hyperprolactinemia
- Assistance with management

Timing: Routine (less than 4 weeks)

Advice for Referral

- Galactorrhea with a normal serum prolactin level is a common and benign finding in women with a previous pregnancy.
- If hyperprolactinemia is found, see *Hyperprolactinemia*.

Tests to Prepare for Consult

- Prolactin

Tests Not Useful Before Consult

- Radiograph, skull
- Sellar tomograms
- MR, cranial

Tests Consultant May Need to Do

- None

Follow-up Visits Generally Required

- One

Suggested Readings

Fiorica JV. Nipple discharge. [Review] [13 refs]. Obstet Gynecol Clin North Am 1994;21:453–460.

Yazigi RA, Quintero CH, Salameh WA. Prolactin disorders. [Review] [100 refs]. Fertil Steril 1997;67:215–225.

Blackwell RE. Hyperprolactinemia. Evaluation and management. [Review]. Endocrinol Metab Clin North Am 1992;21:105–124.

See Also

- Hyperprolactinemia

THE CONSULTATION GUIDE

Glucocorticoid Taper

Indications and Timing for Referral

- Signs of adrenal insufficiency are present

Timing: Urgent (less than 24 hours) or Expedited (less than 1 week)

- Assistance in determining whether underlying adrenal insufficiency is present
- Assistance with accomplishment of taper

Timing: Routine (less than 4 weeks)

Advice for Referral

- Complete history of glucocorticoid treatment is vital, including indications for use, and preparations and doses used.

Tests to Prepare for Consult

- Sodium
- ACTH stimulation test or 8 am cortisol

Tests Not Useful Before Consult

- ACTH level, plasma
- Free cortisol, 24-hour urine
- 17-hydroxysteroids, 24-hour urine
- 17-ketosteroids, 24-hour urine

Tests Consultant May Need to Do

- ACTH stimulation test, 1-hour
- CRH stimulation test (for ACTH and cortisol)

Follow-up Visits Generally Required

- Two

Suggested Readings

Baxter JD, Tyrrell JB. Evaluation of the hypothalamic-pituitary-adrenal axis: importance in steroid therapy, AIDS, and other stress syndromes. [Review] [91 refs]. Adv Intern Med 1994;39:667–696.

Grinspoon SK, Biller BM. Clinical review 62: Laboratory assessment of adrenal insufficiency. [Review] [35 refs]. J Clin Endocrinol Metab 1994;79:923–931.

Holland EG, Taylor AT. Glucocorticoids in clinical practice. [Review]. J Fam Pract 1991;32:512–519.

See Also

- Adrenal insufficiency

Goiter, Simple/Diffuse

Indications and Timing for Referral
- Diagnostic uncertainty
- Assistance with management of local compressive symptoms or cosmetic concerns

Timing: Routine (less than 4 weeks)

Tests to Prepare for Consult
- TSH (assay sensitivity <0.1 mU/L)
- Anti-TPO antibody

Tests Not Useful Before Consult
- None

Tests Consultant May Need to Do
- Free T_4
- Triiodothyronine (T_3)
- ESR
- Calcitonin
- Radiograph, chest
- Radionuclide uptake and scan
- Sonogram, thyroid
- CT or MR, neck and/or chest
- Fine needle aspiration biopsy

Follow-up Visits Generally Required
- One

Suggested Readings
Greenspan FS. The problem of the nodular goiter. [Review]. Med Clin North Am 1991;75:195–209.

Ladenson PW. Optimal laboratory testing for diagnosis and monitoring of thyroid nodules, goiter, and thyroid cancer. [Review] [27 refs]. Clin Chem 1996;42:183–187.

Hurley DL, Gharib H. Evaluation and management of multinodular goiter. Otolaryngol Clin North Am 1996;29:527–540.

Gharib H. Diffuse nontoxic and multinodular goiter. Curr Ther Endocrinol Metab 1994;5:99–101.

Huysmans D, Hermus A, Edelbroek M, et al. Radioiodine for nontoxic multinodular goiter. Thyroid 1997;7:235–239.

See Also
- Hypothyroidism
- Thyrotoxicosis
- Thyroid nodule

Gynecomastia

Indications and Timing for Referral

- Unclear etiology
- Assistance with management

Timing: Routine (less than 4 weeks)

Advice for Referral

A complete medication history is vital.

Tests to Prepare for Consult

- Testosterone
- Creatinine
- ALT, AST, alkaline phosphatase
- TSH (assay sensitivity <0.1 mU/L)
- Prolactin

Tests Not Useful Before Consult

- None

Tests Consultant May Need to Do

- Estradiol
- Beta HCG, serum
- LH, FSH
- Karyotype
- Toxicology screen
- Mammogram
- Ultrasound, testicular
- CT scan, adrenal
- MR, cranial

Follow-up Visits Generally Required

- One

Suggested Readings

Glass AR. Gynecomastia. [Review]. Endocrinol Metab Clin North Am 1994;23:825–837.

Braunstein GD. Gynecomastia [see comments]. [Review]. N Engl J Med 1993;328:490–495.

Neuman JF. Evaluation and treatment of gynecomastia. [Review] [28 refs]. Am Fam Physician 1997;55:1835–1844.

Thompson DF, Carter JR. Drug-induced gynecomastia. [Review] [86 refs]. Pharmacotherapy 1993;13:37–45.

See Also

- Impotence
- Hypogonadism, male

High Density Lipoprotein (HDL) Cholesterol, Low

Indications and Timing for Referral

- Interpretation of clinical significance and/or management
- Assistance with management

Timing: Routine (less than 4 weeks)

Tests to Prepare for Consult

- Lipid profile, fasting (cholesterol, HDL, TG)
- Glucose
- TSH (assay sensitivity <0.1 mU/L)

Tests Not Useful Before Consult

- None

Tests Consultant May Need to Do

- Lipid profile, fasting (cholesterol, HDL, TG)
- Glycohemoglobin
- LDL, direct measurement
- Apolipoprotein B
- Lp_a

Follow-up Visits Generally Required

- One

Suggested Readings

Rosenson RS. Low levels of high-density lipoprotein cholesterol (hypoalphalipoproteinemia). An approach to management. [Review]. Arch Intern Med 1993;153:1528–1538.

Grundy SM, Goodman DW, Rifkind BM, Cleeman JI. The place of HDL in cholesterol management. A perspective from the National Cholesterol Educational Program [published erratum appears in Arch Intern Med 1989;149:940] [comment] [see comments]. [Review]. Arch Intern Med 1989;149:505–510.

Pasternak RC, Brown LE, Stone PH, et al. Effect of combination therapy with lipid-reducing drugs in patients with coronary heart disease and "normal" cholesterol levels. A randomized, placebo-controlled trial. Harvard Atherosclerosis Reversibility Project (HARP) Study Group. Ann Intern Med 1996;125:529–540.

Selected Guidelines

U.S. Preventive Services Task Force. Screening for high blood cholesterol and other lipid abnormalities. In: DiGuiseppi C, Atkins D, Woolf S, eds. Guide to clinical preventive services. 2nd ed. Baltimore: Williams & Wilkins, 1996;15–38.

Guidelines for using serum cholesterol, high-density lipoprotein cholesterol, and triglyceride levels as screening tests for preventing coronary heart disease in adults. American College of Physicians. Part 1 [see comments]. Ann Intern Med 1996;124:515–517.

Triglyceride, high density lipoprotein, and coronary heart disease. NIH Consens Statement 1992;10:1–28.

See Also

- Hypercholesterolemia
- Hypertriglyceridemia

THE CONSULTATION GUIDE

Hirsutism

Indications and Timing for Referral

- Diagnostic uncertainty
- Assistance with management

Timing: Routine (less than 4 weeks)

Tests to Prepare for Consult

- Testosterone
- Free testosterone
- DHEA-S

Tests Not Useful Before Consult

- 17-hydroxysteroids, 24-hour urine
- 17-ketosteroids, 24-hour urine

Tests Consultant May Need to Do

- LH, FSH
- Free testosterone
- Prolactin
- Glucose
- Lipid profile, fasting (cholesterol, HDL, TG)
- Insulin
- Free cortisol, 24-hour urine, or overnight dexamethasone suppression test, 1 mg
- ACTH stimulation test (17-hydroxyprogesterone)
- Androstanediol glucuronide
- Ultrasound, ovarian
- CT scan, adrenal

Follow-up Visits Generally Required

- Two

Suggested Readings

Rittmaster RS. Hirsutism [see comments]. [Review] [30 refs]. Lancet 1997;349:191–195.

O'Driscoll JB, Mamtora H, Higginson J, et al. A prospective study of the prevalence of clear-cut endocrine disorders and polycystic ovaries in 350 patients presenting with hirsutism or androgenic alopecia. Clin Endocrinol (Oxf) 1994;41:231–236.

Lucky AW. Hormonal correlates of acne and hirsutism. [Review]. Am J Med 1995;98(Suppl 1A):89S–94S.

Ehrmann DA, Rosenfield RL. Clinical review 10: An endocrinologic approach to the patient with hirsutism. [Review]. J Clin Endocrinol Metab 1990;71:1–4.

Conn JJ, Jacobs HS. The clinical management of hirsutism. [Review] [94 refs]. Eur J Endocrinol 1997;136:339–348.

See Also

- Delayed puberty, female
- Amenorrhea, secondary
- Anovulatory syndrome, chronic
- Polycystic ovaries

ENDOCRINOLOGY AND METABOLISM

Hyperaldosteronism, Primary

Indications and Timing for Referral
- Signigicant hypokalemia or uncontrolled hypertension are present

Timing: Urgent (less than 24 hours) or Expedited (less than 1 week)

- Diagnostic uncertainty
- Unclear etiology
- Assistance with management

Timing: Routine (less than 4 weeks)

Advice for Referral
- Renin and aldosterone should be measured simultaneously under defined conditions of posture and sodium intake.
- Testing should be performed with patient off diuretics for 2 weeks if possible.
- Careful history of medications and possible licorice intake is important.

Tests to Prepare for Consult
- Electrolytes (Na, K, Cl, CO_2)
- BUN, creatinine
- Aldosterone
- Renin, plasma activity or direct assay

Tests Not Useful Before Consult
- None

Tests Consultant May Need to Do
- Magnesium
- Urine sodium
- Urine potassium
- ECG
- Aldosterone, 24-hour urine
- Furosemide stimulation test
- Saline suppression test
- Captopril suppression test

- Free cortisol, 24-hour urine, or overnight dexamethasone suppression test, 1 mg
- CT scan, abdomen
- 18-hydroxycorticosterone
- Creatinine, 24-hour urine

Follow-up Visits Generally Required
- Two

Suggested Readings
Vallotton MB. Primary aldosteronism. Part I. Diagnosis of primary hyperaldosteronism. [Review] [31 refs]. Clin Endocrinol (Oxf) 1996;45:47–52.

Vallotton MB. Primary aldosteronism. Part II. Differential diagnosis of primary hyperaldosteronism and pseudoaldosteronism. [Review] [73 refs]. Clin Endocrinol (Oxf) 1996;45:53–60.

Blumenfeld JD, Sealey JE, Schlussel Y, et al. Diagnosis and treatment of primary hyperaldosteronism [see comments]. Ann Intern Med 1994;121:877–885.

Bravo EL. Primary aldosteronism. Issues in diagnosis and management. [Review] [27 refs]. Endocrinol Metab Clin North Am 1994;23:271–283.

Melby JC. Diagnosis of hyperaldosteronism. [Review]. Endocrinol Metab Clin North Am 1991;20:247–255.

Young WF Jr, Hogan MJ, Klee GG, et al. Primary aldosteronism: diagnosis and treatment. [Review]. Mayo Clin Proc 1990;65:96–110.

Doppman JL, Gill JR, Miller DL, et al. Distinction between hyperaldosteronism due to bilateral hyperplasia and unilateral aldosteronoma: reliability of CT. Radiology 1992;184:677–682.

See Also
- Hypertension
- Adrenal mass, radiologically detected

THE CONSULTATION GUIDE

Hypercalcemia

Indications and Timing for Referral

- Calcium level is greater than 14 mg/dL
- Significant mental status changes, potentially attributable to hypercalcemia

Timing: Immediate or Urgent (less than 24 hours)

- Etiology unclear
- Diagnostic uncertainty
- Assistance with management

Timing: Routine (less than 4 weeks)

Advice for Referral

- If parathyroid hormone (PTH) elevated, or in upper half of normal range, see *Hyperparathyroidism*.
- If PTH low, see *Hypercalcemia with Low PTH*.
- If patient has previous history of malignancy, consider possibility of recurrent neoplasm.

Tests to Prepare for Consult

- Calcium, phosphorus
- Albumin, total protein
- Alkaline phosphatase
- PTH, intact

Tests Not Useful Before Consult

- None

Tests Consultant May Need to Do

- Calcium, ionized
- Calcium, 24-hour urine
- Creatinine, 24-hour urine

Follow-up Visits Generally Required

- Two

Suggested Readings

Potts JT Jr. Hyperparathyroidism and other hypercalcemic disorders. [Review] [252 refs]. Adv Intern Med 1996;41:165–212.

Deftos LJ. Hypercalcemia: mechanisms, differential diagnosis, and remedies. [Review] [9 refs]. Postgrad Med 1996;100:119–121.

Bilezikian JP. Clinical review 51: Management of hypercalcemia. [Review]. J Clin Endocrinol Metab 1993;77:1445–1449.

Edelson GW, Kleerekoper M. Hypercalcemic crisis. [Review]. Med Clin North Am 1995;79:79–92.

Wysolmerski JJ, Broadus AE. Hypercalcemia of malignancy: the central role of parathyroid hormone-related protein. [Review]. Annu Rev Med 1994;45:189–200.

Pont A. Unusual causes of hypercalcemia. [Review]. Endocrinol Metab Clin North Am 1989;18:753–764.

Selected Guidelines

NIH conference. Diagnosis and management of asymptomatic primary hyperparathyroidism: consensus development conference statement. [Review]. Ann Intern Med 1991;114:593–597.

See Also

- Hypercalcemia, low PTH
- Hyperparathyroidism
- Multiple endocrine neoplasia I
- Multiple endocrine neoplasia II

Hypercalcemia, Low PTH

Indications and Timing for Referral

- Calcium level is greater than 14 mg/dL
- Significant mental status changes, potentially attributable to hypercalcemia

Timing: Immediate or Urgent (less than 24 hours)

- Etiology unclear
- Assistance with management

Timing: Routine (less than 4 weeks)

Advice for Referral

- Complete medication history is vital (e.g., vitamins).

Tests to Prepare for Consult

- CBC
- PTH, intact
- Albumin, total protein
- Calcium, phosphorus
- ALT, AST, alkaline phosphatase
- Creatinine
- TSH (assay sensitivity <0.1 mU/L)
- Urinalysis with microscopic
- Radiograph, chest

Tests Consultant May Need to Do

- PTH-RP
- 1,25-dihydroxyvitamin D_3
- 25-hydroxyvitamin D_3
- Beta-carotene
- Vitamin A level
- PPD
- IEP
  - Serum
  - Urine
- ACTH stimulation test, 1-hour
- Angiotensin-converting enzyme
- Free T_4
- T_3
- Calcium, 24-hour urine
- Bone scan
- Skeletal survey
- Mammogram
- Ultrasound, renal
- CT scan, abdomen
- Creatinine, 24-hour urine

Follow-up Visits Generally Required

- Two

Suggested Readings

Wysolmerski JJ, Broadus AE. Hypercalcemia of malignancy: the central role of parathyroid hormone-related protein. [Review]. Annu Rev Med 1994;45:189–200.

Pont A. Unusual causes of hypercalcemia. [Review]. Endocrinol Metab Clin North Am 1989;18:753–764.

Deftos LJ. Hypercalcemia: mechanisms, differential diagnosis, and remedies. [Review] [9 refs]. Postgrad Med 1996;100:119–121.

Bilezikian JP. Clinical review 51: Management of hypercalcemia. [Review]. J Clin Endocrinol Metab 1993;77:1445–1449.

See Also

- Hyperparathyroidism
- Hypercalcemia

THE CONSULTATION GUIDE

Hypercholesterolemia

Indications and Timing for Referral

- Failure of conventional dietary and pharmacologic therapies
- Assistance with management

Timing: Routine (less than 4 weeks)

Tests to Prepare for Consult

- Lipid profile, fasting (cholesterol, HDL, TG)
- Glucose
- Creatinine
- ALT, AST, alkaline phosphatase
- TSH
- ECG

Tests Not Useful Before Consult

- None

Tests Consultant May Need to Do

- Lipid profile, fasting (cholesterol, HDL, TG)
- Apolipoprotein B
- Lipoproteins, ultracentrifugation
- Lp_a
- Glucose, fasting

Follow-up Visits Generally Required

- Two

Suggested Readings

Levine GN, Keaney JF Jr, Vita JA. Cholesterol reduction in cardiovascular disease. Clinical benefits and possible mechanisms [comment]. [Review]. N Engl J Med 1995;332:512–521.

Denke MA. Cholesterol-lowering diets. A review of the evidence. [Review]. Arch Intern Med 1995;155:17–26.

Stone NJ, Nicolosi RJ, Kris-Etherton P, et al. AHA conference proceedings. Summary of the scientific conference on the efficacy of hypocholesterolemic dietary interventions. American Heart Association. Circulation 1996;94:3388–3391.

Schectman G, Hiatt J. Drug therapy for hypercholesterolemia in patients with cardiovascular disease—factors limiting achievement of lipid goals. Am J Med 1996;100:197–204.

Johannesson M, Jonsson B, Kjekshus J, et al. Cost effectiveness of simvastatin treatment to lower cholesterol levels in patients with coronary heart disease. Scandinavian Simvastatin Survival Study Group. N Engl J Med 1997;336:332–336.

Selected Guidelines

U.S. Preventive Services Task Force. Screening for high blood cholesterol and other lipid abnormalities. In: DiGuiseppi C, Atkins D, Woolf S, eds. Guide to Clinical Preventive Services. 2nd ed. Baltimore: Williams & Wilkins, 1996:15–38.

Summary of the second report of the National Cholesterol Education Program (NCEP) Expert Panel on Detection, Evaluation, and Treatment of High Blood Cholesterol in Adults (Adult Treatment Panel II). JAMA 1993;269:3015–3023.

Guidelines for using serum cholesterol, high-density lipoprotein cholesterol, and triglyceride levels as screening tests for preventing coronary heart disease in adults. American College of Physicians. Part 1 [see comments]. Ann Intern Med 1996;124:515–517.

See Also

- Obesity
- Hypertriglyceridemia
- HDL cholesterol, low

ENDOCRINOLOGY AND METABOLISM

Hyperparathyroidism

Indications and Timing for Referral

- Calcium level is greater than 14 mg/dL
- Significant mental status changes, potentially attributable to hypercalcemia

Timing: Immediate or Urgent (less than 24 hours)

- Confirm diagnosis
- Assistance with management

Timing: Routine (less than 4 weeks)

Advice for Referral

- Preoperative localization procedures are generally not indicated before first neck exploration.
- Preoperative localization procedures are generally indicated if neck surgery is to be performed in patient with previous neck surgery.
- Optimal bone mineral density assessment requires dual energy x-ray densitometry.
- If familial hyperparathyroidism or other clinical findings suggest it, see Multiple Endocrine Neoplasia I or II.

Tests to Prepare for Consult

- Calcium, phosphorus
- Albumin, total protein
- Alkaline phosphatase
- PTH, intact

Tests Not Useful Before Consult

- Skeletal survey

Tests Consultant May Need to Do

- Bone mineral density
- Calcium, 24-hour urine
- Creatinine, 24-hour urine, for clearance
- Plain film, abdomen
- Ultrasound, abdomen
- Magnesium
- Osteocalcin
- Bone specific alkaline phosphatase
- Pyridinium and deoxypyridinium cross-links
- N-terminal telopeptide

Follow-up Visits Generally Required

- Two

Hyperparathyroidism (*continued*)

Suggested Readings

Silverberg SJ, Bilezikian JP. Evaluation and management of primary hyperparathyroidism [see comments]. [Review] [7 refs]. J Clin Endocrinol Metab 1996;81:2036–2040.

Potts JT Jr. Hyperparathyroidism and other hypercalcemic disorders. [Review] [252 refs]. Adv Intern Med 1996;41:165–212.

Wermers RA, Khosla S, Atkinson EJ, et al. The rise and fall of primary hyperparathyroidism: a population-based study in Rochester, Minnesota, 1965–1992. Ann Intern Med 1997;126:433–440.

Grey AB, Stapleton JP, Evans MC, et al. Effect of hormone replacement therapy on bone mineral density in postmenopausal women with mild primary hyperparathyroidism. A randomized, controlled trial [see comments]. Ann Intern Med 1996;125:360–368.

Strewler GJ. Indications for surgery in patients with minimally symptomatic primary hyperparathyroidism. [Review]. Surg Clin North Am 1995;75:439–447.

Selected Guidelines

NIH conference. Diagnosis and management of asymptomatic primary hyperparathyroidism: consensus development conference statement. [Review]. Ann Intern Med 1991;114:593–597.

See Also

- Multiple endocrine neoplasia II
- Hypercalcemia, low PTH
- Multiple endocrine neoplasia I
- Hypercalcemia

ENDOCRINOLOGY AND METABOLISM

Hyperprolactinemia

Indications and Timing for Referral
- Associated pituitary mass (see *Pituitary Tumor*)
- Diagnostic uncertainty
- Assistance with management

Timing: Routine (less than 4 weeks)

Advice for Referral
- Repeat prolactin level if less than 50 ng/dL.
- MR needed unless patient on medications associated with hyperprolactinemia.
- MR may be appropriate before referral if hCG negative and TSH normal.
- Complete medication history is vital (e.g., metoclopramide, antihypertensives, psychotropic medications).
- Optimal bone mineral density assessment requires dual energy densitometry.

Tests to Prepare for Consult
- Prolactin
- Beta HCG, serum
- TSH (assay sensitivity <0.1 mU/L)
- Creatinine

Tests Not Useful Before Consult
- ACTH, plasma
- Radiograph, skull
- Sellar tomograms

Tests Consultant May Need to Do
- Prolactin
- Progesterone
- LH, FSH
- Estradiol
- Testosterone, in men
- Growth hormone
- IGF-1
- ACTH stimulation test, 1-hour
- Insulin tolerance test
- OGTT (for serial GH and glucose)
- CRH stimulation test (for ACTH and cortisol)
- Bone mineral density
- MR, cranial with contrast

Follow-up Visits Generally Required
- Two

Suggested Readings
Yazigi RA, Quintero CH, Salameh WA. Prolactin disorders. [Review] [100 refs]. Fertil Steril 1997;67:215–225.

Molitch ME. Pathologic hyperprolactinemia. [Review]. Endocrinol Metab Clin North Am 1992;21:877–901.

Blackwell RE. Hyperprolactinemia. Evaluation and management. [Review]. Endocrinol Metab Clin North Am 1992;21:105–124.

Jeffcoate WJ, Pound N, Sturrock ND, Lambourne J. Long-term follow-up of patients with hyperprolactinaemia. Clin Endocrinol (Oxf) 1996;45:299–303.

Dalkin AC, Marshall JC. Medical therapy of hyperprolactinemia. [Review]. Endocrinol Metab Clin North Am 1989;18:259–276.

Feigenbaum SL, Downey DE, Wilson CB, Jaffe RB. Transsphenoidal pituitary resection for preoperative diagnosis of prolactin-secreting pituitary adenoma in women—long term follow-up. J Clin Endocrinol Metab 1996;81:1711–1719.

See Also
- Multiple endocrine neoplasia I
- Pituitary tumor
- Amenorrhea, secondary
- Acromegaly
- Galactorrhea

Hypertension

Indications and Timing for Referral

- Severe hypertension
- Associated neurologic changes
- Related subacute cardiovascular complications, e.g., exacerbation of heart failure
- Imminently planned radiologic or surgical procedure in patient with poor blood pressure control

Timing: Immediate, Urgent (less than 24 hours) or Expedited (less than 1 week)

- Need assistance in excluding underlying endocrinopathy or other cause of secondary hypertension

Timing: Routine (less than 4 weeks)

Advice for Referral

- See *Pheochromocytoma*, if suspected.

Tests to Prepare for Consult

- BUN, creatinine
- Electrolytes (Na, K, Cl, CO_2)
- Metanephrines, 24-hour urine
- Creatinine, 24-hour urine, for clearance

Tests Not Useful Before Consult

- None

Tests Consultant May Need to Do

- Aldosterone
- Renin, plasma activity or direct assay
- Catecholamines, 24-hour urine
- Catecholamines, plasma
- MR or CT, adrenal
- Creatinine, 24-hour urine

Follow-up Visits Generally Required

- One

Suggested Readings

Chalmers J. Treatment guidelines in hypertension: current limitations and future solutions. [Review] [38 refs]. J Hypertens Suppl 1996;14:S3–S8.

Davidson RA, Wilcox CS. Newer tests for the diagnosis of renovascular disease [published erratum appears in JAMA 1993;269:1508]. [Review]. JAMA 1992;268:3353–3358.

Akpunonu BE, Mulrow PJ, Hoffman EA. Secondary hypertension: evaluation and treatment. Dis Mon 1996;42:609–722.

Selected Guidelines

Automated ambulatory blood pressure devices and self-measured blood pressure monitoring devices: their role in the diagnosis and management of hypertension. American College of Physicians [comment]. Ann Intern Med 1993;118:889–892.

See Also

- Adrenal mass, radiologically detected
- Pheochromocytoma
- Hyperaldosteronism, primary
- Thyrotoxicosis

Hypertriglyceridemia

Indications and Timing for Referral

- Associated with pancreatitis

Timing: Immediate or Urgent (less than 24 hours)

- Failure of conventional dietary and pharmacologic therapies
- Assistance with management

Timing: Routine (less than 4 weeks)

Advice for Referral

- Complete medication history is vital.

Tests to Prepare for Consult

- Lipid profile, fasting (cholesterol, HDL, TG)
- Glucose
- Creatinine
- ALT, AST, alkaline phosphatase
- TSH
- Urinalysis with microscopic
- ECG

Tests Not Useful Before Consult

- None

Tests Consultant May Need to Do

- Lipid profile, fasting (cholesterol, HDL, TG)
- Amylase
- Glycohemoglobin
- LDL, direct measurement
- Lipoproteins, ultracentrifugation
- Lp_a
- GGT

Follow-up Visits Generally Required

- Two

Suggested Readings

Ginsberg HN. Is hypertriglyceridemia a risk factor for atherosclerotic cardiovascular disease? A simple question with a complicated answer [editorial]. Ann Intern Med 1997;126:912–914.

Grundy SM, Vega GL. Two different views of the relationship of hypertriglyceridemia to coronary heart disease. Implications for treatment. [Review]. Arch Intern Med 1992;152:28–34.

Bakker-Arkema RG, Davidson MH, Goldstein RJ, et al. Efficacy and safety of a new HMG-CoA reductase inhibitor, atorvastatin, in patients with hypertriglyceridemia. JAMA 1996;275:128–133.

Selected Guidelines

U.S. Preventive Services Task Force. Screening for high blood cholesterol and other lipid abnormalities. In: DiGuiseppi C, Atkins D, Woolf S, eds. Guide to Clinical Preventive Services. 2nd ed. Baltimore: Williams & Wilkins, 1996:15–38.

Guidelines for using serum cholesterol, high-density lipoprotein cholesterol, and triglyceride levels as screening tests for preventing coronary heart disease in adults. American College of Physicians. Part 1 [see comments]. Ann Intern Med 1996;124:515–517.

Triglyceride, high density lipoprotein, and coronary heart disease. NIH Consens Statement 1992;10:1–28.

See Also

- Hypercholesterolemia
- HDL cholesterol, low

Hypoaldosteronism

Indications and Timing for Referral

- Hypotension or significant hyperkalemia are presented

Timing: Immediate or Urgent (less than 24 hours)

- Diagnostic uncertainty
- Assistance with management

Timing: Routine (less than 4 weeks)

Advice for Referral

- Renin and aldosterone should be measured simultaneously under defined conditions of posture and sodium intake.
- A complete medication history is vital.

Tests to Prepare for Consult

- Electrolytes (Na, K, Cl, CO_2)
- Glucose
- BUN, creatinine
- Renin, plasma activity or direct assay
- Aldosterone
- Urinalysis with microscopic

Tests Not Useful Before Consult

- ACTH level, plasma
- CT scan, adrenal

Tests Consultant May Need to Do

- ACTH stimulation test (for cortisol and aldosterone)
- Glycohemoglobin
- Uric acid
- Arterial blood gas
- ECG
- HIV antibody testing

Follow-up Visits Generally Required

- Two

Suggested Readings

White PC. Disorders of aldosterone biosynthesis and action. [Review] [63 refs]. N Engl J Med 1994;331:250–258.

Gittler RD, Fajans SS. Primary aldosteronism (Conn's syndrome). J Clin Endocrinol Metab 1995;80:3438–3441.

McKenna TJ, Sequeira SJ, Heffernan A, et al. Diagnosis under random conditions of all disorders of the renin-angiotensin-aldosterone axis, including primary hyperaldosteronism. J Clin Endocrinol Metab 1991;73:952–957.

See Also

- Hyperkalemia

ENDOCRINOLOGY AND METABOLISM

Hypocalcemia

Indications and Timing for Referral

- Tetany or seizures are present

Timing: Immediate or Urgent (less than 24 hours)

- Diagnostic uncertainty
- Etiology unclear

Timing: Routine (less than 4 weeks)

Advice for Referral

- If PTH is low, or in the lower half of the normal range, see *Hypoparathyroidism*.
- If PTH is elevated, see *Hypocalcemia with Elevated PTH*.

Tests to Prepare for Consult

- Calcium, phosphorus
- Alkaline phosphatase
- Albumin, total protein
- Creatinine
- PTH, intact

Tests Not Useful Before Consult

- None

Tests Consultant May Need to Do

- None

Follow-up Visits Generally Required

- None

Suggested Readings

Reber PM, Heath H 3rd. Hypocalcemic emergencies. [Review] [76 refs]. Med Clin North Am 1995;79:93–106.

Guise TA, Mundy GR. Clinical review 69: Evaluation of hypocalcemia in children and adults. [Review] [25 refs]. J Clin Endocrinol Metab 1995;80:1473–1478.

Bourke E, Delaney V. Assessment of hypocalcemia and hypercalcemia. [Review] [115 refs]. Clin Lab Med 1993;13:157–181.

Shaker JL, Brickner RC, Findling JW, et al. Hypocalcemia and skeletal disease as presenting features of celiac disease. Arch Intern Med 1997;157:1013–1016.

Pearce SH, Williamson C, Kifor O, et al. A familial syndrome of hypocalcemia with hypercalciuria due to mutations in the calcium-sensing receptor [see comments]. N Engl J Med 1996;335:1115–1122.

Singer FR. Medical management of nonparathyroid hypercalcemia and hypocalcemia. [Review] [37 refs]. Otolaryngol Clin North Am 1996;29:701–710.

See Also

- Hypoparathyroidism
- Hypocalcemia with elevated PTH

Hypocalcemia with Elevated PTH

Indications and Timing for Referral

- Tetany or seizures are present

Timing: Immediate or Urgent (less than 24 hours)

- Diagnostic uncertainty
- Assistance with management

Timing: Routine (less than 4 weeks)

Advice for Referral

- Complete medication history is vital (e.g., anti-seizure medications).
- See also *Steatorrhea* and *Malabsorption*.

Tests to Prepare for Consult

- Calcium, phosphorus
- PTH, intact
- Creatinine
- ALT, AST, alkaline phosphatase
- Albumin, total protein
- Magnesium

Tests Not Useful Before Consult

- None

Tests Consultant May Need to Do

- Urinalysis with microscopic
- 1,25-dihydroxyvitamin D_3
- 25-hydroxyvitamin D_3
- Qualitative fecal fat and fiber, stool
- Prothrombin time
- Radiographs, skeletal
- PTH stimulation test
- Amylase
- Lipase
- Calcium, 24-hour urine
- Creatinine, 24-hour urine

Follow-up Visits Generally Required

- Two

Suggested Readings

Bourke E, Delaney V. Assessment of hypocalcemia and hypercalcemia. [Review] [115 refs]. Clin Lab Med 1993;13:157–181.

Guise TA, Mundy GR. Clinical review 69: Evaluation of hypocalcemia in children and adults. [Review] [25 refs]. J Clin Endocrinol Metab 1995;80:1473–1478.

Reber PM, Heath H 3rd. Hypocalcemic emergencies. [Review] [76 refs]. Med Clin North Am 1995;79:93–106.

Singer FR. Medical management of nonparathyroid hypercalcemia and hypocalcemia. [Review] [37 refs]. Otolaryngol Clin North Am 1996;29:701–710.

See Also

- Hypoparathyroidism
- Hypocalcemia
- Steatorrhea
- Malabsorption

ENDOCRINOLOGY AND METABOLISM

Hypogonadism, Male

Indications and Timing for Referral
- Unclear etiology
- Assistance with management

Timing: Routine (less than 4 weeks)

Advice for Referral
- Testosterone level should be compared to age-adjusted reference range as normal levels decrease with age in men.

Tests to Prepare for Consult
- CBC
- BUN, creatinine
- Glucose
- ALT, AST, alkaline phosphatase
- Testosterone × 2
- LH, FSH
- TSH (assay sensitivity <0.1 mU/L)
- Prolactin

Tests Not Useful Before Consult
- None

Tests Consultant May Need to Do
- Free testosterone
- Free T_4
- Karyotype
- ACTH stimulation test, 1-hour
- Free cortisol, 24-hour urine, or overnight dexamethasone suppression test, 1 mg
- Creatinine, 24-hour urine
- Bone mineral density
- MR, cranial
- Insulin tolerance test

Follow-up Visits Generally Required
- One

Suggested Readings
Whitcomb RW, Crowley WF Jr. Male hypogonadotropic hypogonadism. [Review]. Endocrinol Metab Clin North Am 1993;22:125–143.

Plymate S. Hypogonadism. [Review]. Endocrinol Metab Clin North Am 1994;23:749–772.

Winters SJ. Endocrine evaluation of testicular function. [Review] [83 refs]. Endocrinol Metab Clin North Am 1994;23:709–723.

Rugarli EI, Ballabio A. Kallmann syndrome. From genetics to neurobiology. [Review]. JAMA 1993;270:2713–2716.

Schwartz ID, Root AW. The Klinefelter syndrome of testicular dysgenesis. [Review]. Endocrinol Metab Clin North Am 1991;20:153–163.

Shakir KM, Jasser MZ, Yoshihashi AK, et al. Pseudocarcinoid syndrome associated with hypogonadism and response to testosterone therapy. Mayo Clin Proc 1996;71:1145–1149.

Meikle AW, Arver S, Dobs AS, et al. Pharmacokinetics and metabolism of a permeation-enhanced testosterone transdermal system in hypogonadal men: influence of application site—a clinical research center study. J Clin Endocrinol Metab 1996;81:1832–1840.

Matsumoto AM. Hormonal therapy of male hypogonadism. [Review]. Endocrinol Metab Clin North Am 1994;23:857–875.

See Also
- Gynecomastia
- Impotence

Hypoglycemia, Fasting

Indications and Timing for Referral

- Recurrent hypoglycemia cannot be controlled

Timing: Urgent (less than 24 hours) or Expedited (less than 1 week)

- Uncertainty whether symptoms are caused by true hypoglycemia
- Glucose less than 50 mg/dL with symptoms relieved by consumption of carbohydrates
- Etiology of hypoglycemia unclear

Timing: Routine (less than 4 weeks)

Advice for Referral

- Complete medication history is vital.

Tests to Prepare for Consult

- Blood glucose during symptoms
- Creatinine
- ALT, AST, alkaline phosphatase

Tests Not Useful Before Consult

- OGTT

Tests Consultant May Need to Do

- Glucose
- Insulin
- C-peptide
- Anti-insulin antibody
- ACTH stimulation test, 1-hour
- Free T_4
- TSH (assay sensitivity <0.1 mU/L)
- MR, abdomen
- Octreotide scan

Follow-up Visits Generally Required

- Two

Suggested Readings

Service FJ. Hypoglycemic disorders [see comments]. N Engl J Med 1995;332:1144–1152.

Marks V, Teale JD. Tumours producing hypoglycaemia. [Review]. Diabetes Metab Rev 1991;7:79–91.

Comi RJ. Approach to acute hypoglycemia. [Review]. Endocrinol Metab Clin North Am 1993;22:247–262.

Hypoglycemia in the diabetes control and complications trial. The Diabetes Control and Complications Trial Research Group. Diabetes 1997;46:271–286.

Cryer PE, Fisher JN, Shamoon H. Hypoglycemia. [Review] [233 refs]. Diabetes Care 1994;17:734–755.

See Also

- Multiple endocrine neoplasia I
- Hypoglycemia, reactive

Hypoglycemia, Reactive

Indications and Timing for Referral

- Etiology of symptoms unclear

Timing: Routine (less than 4 weeks)

Tests to Prepare for Consult

- Blood glucose during symptoms

Tests Not Useful Before Consult

- OGTT

Tests Consultant May Need to Do

- Gastric emptying study

Follow-up Visits Generally Required

- One

Suggested Readings

Service FJ. Hypoglycemia. [Review]. Med Clin North Am 1995;79:1–8.

Hofeldt FD. Reactive hypoglycemia. [Review]. Endocrinol Metab Clin North Am 1989;18:185–201.

Comi RJ. Approach to acute hypoglycemia. [Review]. Endocrinol Metab Clin North Am 1993;22:247–262.

Cryer PE, Fisher JN, Shamoon H. Hypoglycemia. [Review] [233 refs]. Diabetes Care 1994;17:734–755.

See Also

- Hypoglycemia, fasting

Hypoparathyroidism

Indications and Timing for Referral

- Confirm diagnosis
- Assistance with management

Timing: Routine (less than 4 weeks)

Advice for Referral

- Consideration should be given to having such patients co-managed with an endocrinologist.

Tests to Prepare for Consult

- Calcium, phosphorus
- Albumin, total protein
- Alkaline phosphatase
- Magnesium
- PTH, intact

Tests Not Useful Before Consult

- Skeletal survey

Tests Consultant May Need to Do

- CBC
- ALT, AST, alkaline phosphatase
- Glucose
- 1,25-dihydroxyvitamin D_3
- 25-hydroxyvitamin D_3
- Calcium, 24-hour urine
- Creatinine, 24-hour urine
- TSH
- LH, FSH
- Estradiol, in women
- Testosterone, in men
- ACTH stimulation test, 1-hour
- Vitamin B_{12}, serum
- PTH, intact
- Ferritin
- Magnesium
- Radiograph, skull
- CT scan, cranial

Follow-up Visits Generally Required

- Co-management, see *Advice for Referral*

Suggested Readings

Rude RK. Hypocalcemia and hypoparathyroidism. [Review] [4 refs]. Curr Ther Endocrinol Metab 1997;6:546–551.

Bourke E, Delaney V. Assessment of hypocalcemia and hypercalcemia. [Review] [115 refs]. Clin Lab Med 1993;13:157–181.

Guise TA, Mundy GR. Clinical review 69: Evaluation of hypocalcemia in children and adults. [Review] [25 refs]. J Clin Endocrinol Metab 1995;80:1473–1478.

Reber PM, Heath H 3rd. Hypocalcemic emergencies. [Review] [76 refs]. Med Clin North Am 1995;79:93–106.

Lehmann R, Leuzinger B, Salomon F. Symptomatic hypoparathyroidism in acquired immunodeficiency syndrome. Horm Res 1994;42:295–299.

See Also

- Hypocalcemia
- Hypocalcemia with elevated PTH

ENDOCRINOLOGY AND METABOLISM

Hypopituitarism

Indications and Timing for Referral

- Change in vision
- Severe headaches
- Clinical or laboratory evidence of adrenal insufficiency or severe hypothyroidism

Timing: Urgent (less than 24 hours) or Expedited (less than 1 week)

- Assistance with management

Timing: Routine (less than 4 weeks)

Advice for Referral

- Serious consideration should be given to having such patients co-managed with an endocrinologist.

Tests to Prepare for Consult

- BUN
- Potassium, sodium
- CBC

Tests Not Useful Before Consult

- ACTH stimulation test
- Radiograph, skull
- Sellar tomograms

Tests Consultant May Need to Do

- ACTH stimulation test, 1-hour
- Free T_4
- TSH
- Prolactin
- GH
- IGF-1
- Cortisol, 8 am
- LH, FSH
- Estradiol, in women
- Testosterone, in men
- Bone mineral density
- CRH stimulation test (for ACTH and cortisol)
- Insulin tolerance test
- MR, cranial with contrast
- Arginine stimulation test (for GH)
- L-dopa stimulation test (for GH)

Follow-up Visits Generally Required

- Co-management, see *Advice for Referral*

Suggested Readings

Vance ML. Hypopituitarism [published erratum appears in N Engl J Med 1994;331:487]. [Review] [59 refs]. N Engl J Med 1994;330:1651–1662.

Bates AS, Vanthoff W, Jones PJ, Clayton RN. The effect of hypopituitarism on life expectancy. J Clin Endocrinol Metab 1996;81:1169–1172.

Meling TR, Nylen ES. Growth hormone deficiency in adults: a review. [Review] [124 refs]. Am J Med Sci 1996;311:153–166.

Streeten DHP, Anderson GH, Bonaventura MM. The potential for serious consequences from misinterpreting normal responses to the rapid adrenocorticotropin test. J Clin Endocrinol Metab 1996;81:285–290.

Johannsson G, Rosen T, Bosaeus I, et al. Two years of growth hormone (GH) treatment increases bone mineral content and density in hypopituitary patients with adult-onset GH deficiency. J Clin Endocrinol Metab 1996;81:2865–2873.

See Also

- Empty sella syndrome
- Pituitary tumor
- Hypothyroidism
- Menopause, premature
- Amenorrhea, secondary
- Hypogonadism, male
- Adrenal insufficiency

Hypothyroidism

Indications and Timing for Referral

- Confusing laboratory tests
- Unsatisfactory response to initial T_4 therapy
- Associated cardiovascular disease
- Suspicion of central hypothyroidism

Timing: Routine (less than 4 weeks)

Tests to Prepare for Consult

- TSH (assay sensitivity <0.1 mU/L)
- Free T_4

Tests Not Useful Before Consult

- Sonogram, thyroid
- Radionuclide uptake and scan, thyroid

Tests Consultant May Need to Do

- TSH (assay sensitivity <0.1 mU/L)
- Free T_4
- Free T_4, by dialysis
- Anti-TPO antibody
- TRH test (for TSH)
- Vitamin B_{12}, serum
- Cortisol
- ACTH stimulation test, 1-hour
- MR or CT, cranial with pituitary cuts
- ECG

Follow-up Visits Generally Required

- Two

Suggested Readings

Lazarus JH. Investigation and treatment of hypothyroidism [see comments]. Clin Endocrinol (Oxf) 1996;44:129–131.

Arem R, Escalante D. Subclinical hypothyroidism: epidemiology, diagnosis, and significance. [Review] [206 refs]. Adv Intern Med 1996;41:213–250.

Surks MI, Ocampo E. Subclinical thyroid disease. Am J Med 1996;100:217–223.

Toft AD. Thyroxine therapy [published erratum appears in N Engl J Med 1994;331:1035]. [Review]. N Engl J Med 1994;331:174–180.

Ladenson PW. Diagnosis of hypothyroidism. In: Braverman LE, Utiger RD, eds. The thyroid: a fundamental and clinical text. 7th ed. Philadelphia: JB Lippincott Co., 1996;878–882.

Selected Guidelines

Singer PA, Cooper DS, Levy EG, et al. Treatment guidelines for patients with hyperthyroidism and hypothyroidism. Standards of Care Committee, American Thyroid Association. JAMA 1995;273:808–812.

See Also

- Hypopituitarism
- Thyroid function tests, abnormal
- Goiter, simple/diffuse

ENDOCRINOLOGY AND METABOLISM

Impotence

Indications and Timing for Referral
- Etiology unclear
- Assistance with treatment of underlying disorder

Timing: Routine (less than 4 weeks)

Advice for Referral
- A complete medication history is vital.
- Factors favoring referral to endocrinologist include:
    - Abnormalities in initial endocrine tests
- Factors favoring referral to urologist include:
    - Assistance with management of neurologic or vascular etiologies

Tests to Prepare for Consult
- CBC
- BUN
- Glucose
- ALT, AST, alkaline phosphatase
- Testosterone
- TSH (assay sensitivity <0.1 mU/L)
- Prolactin

Tests Not Useful Before Consult
- None

Tests Consultant May Need to Do
- LH, FSH
- Free testosterone
- Testosterone
- Glycohemoglobin
- Nocturnal penile tumescence study

Follow-up Visits Generally Required
- Two

Suggested Readings
O'Keefe M, Hunt DK. Assessment and treatment of impotence. [Review]. Med Clin North Am 1995;79:415–434.

Carrier S, Zvara P, Lue TF. Erectile dysfunction. [Review]. Endocrinol Metab Clin North Am 1994;23:773–782.

Hakim LS, Goldstein I. Diabetic sexual dysfunction. [Review] [133 refs]. Endocrinol Metab Clin North Am 1996;25:379–400.

Kirby RS. Impotence: diagnosis and management of male erectile dysfunction [published erratum appears in Br Med J 1994;308:1091]. [Review]. Br Med J 1994;308:957–961.

Selected Guidelines
NIH Consensus Conference. Impotence. NIH Consensus Development Panel on Impotence. [Review]. JAMA 1993;270:83–90.

Montague DK, Barada JH, Belker AM, et al. Clinical guidelines panel on erectile dysfunction: summary report on the treatment of organic erectile dysfunction. The American Urological Association. J Urol 1996;156:2007–2011.

See Also
- Hypogonadism, male
- Gynecomastia

THE CONSULTATION GUIDE

Menopausal Hormone Replacement

Indications and Timing for Referral

- Assistance needed by primary care physician or desired by patient with decision-making regarding relative benefits and risks, and specific regimens for hormonal replacement therapy

Timing: Routine (less than 4 weeks)

Tests to Prepare for Consult

- Lipid profile, fasting (cholesterol, HDL, TG)
- Bone mineral density
- Mammogram
- Pap smear

Tests Not Useful Before Consult

- None

Tests Consultant May Need to Do

- None

Follow-up Visits Generally Required

- One

Suggested Readings

Grodstein F, Stampfer MJ, Colditz GA, et al. Postmenopausal hormone therapy and mortality [see comments]. N Engl J Med 1997;336:1769–1775.

Grodstein F, Stampfer MJ, Manson JE, et al. Postmenopausal estrogen and progestin use and the risk of cardiovascular disease [see comments] [published erratum appears in N Engl J Med 1996;335:1406]. N Engl J Med 1996;335:453–461.

Belchetz PE. Hormonal treatment of postmenopausal women [see comments]. [Review]. N Engl J Med 1994;330:1062–1071.

Grady D, Rubin SM, Petitti DB, et al. Hormone therapy to prevent disease and prolong life in postmenopausal women [see comments]. [Review]. Ann Intern Med 1992;117:1016–1037.

Schneider DL, Barrett-Connor EL, Morton DJ. Timing of postmenopausal estrogen for optimal bone mineral density. The Rancho Bernardo Study. JAMA 1997;277:543–547.

Selected Guidelines

U.S. Preventive Services Task Force. Postmenopausal hormone prophylaxis. In: DiGuiseppi C, Atkins D, Woolf S, eds. Guide to Clinical Preventive Services. 2nd ed. Baltimore: Williams & Wilkins, 1996;829–844.

Moy JG, Realini JP. Guidelines for postmenopausal preventive hormone therapy: a policy review. American College of Physicians [see comments]. J Am Board Fam Pract 1993;6:153–162.

International Consensus Conference on Hormone Replacement Therapy and The Cardiovascular System. Bethesda, Maryland, December 2–4, 1993. [Review]. Fertil Steril 1994;62(Suppl 2):iii–vi.

See Also

- Menopause, premature

ENDOCRINOLOGY AND METABOLISM

Menopause, Premature

Indications and Timing for Referral

- Etiology unclear
- Assistance with management

Timing: Routine (less than 4 weeks)

Tests to Prepare for Consult

- LH, FSH
- Estradiol
- Prolactin
- TSH (assay sensitivity <0.1 mU/L)

Tests Not Useful Before Consult

- None

Tests Consultant May Need to Do

- Electrolytes (Na, K, Cl, CO_2)
- Albumin, total protein
- Calcium
- PTH
- Lipid profile, fasting (cholesterol, HDL, TG)
- Karyotype
- ACTH stimulation test, 1-hour
- Bone mineral density
- Ultrasound, ovarian

Follow-up Visits Generally Required

- Two

Suggested Readings

Speroff L. Premature ovarian failure. [Review] [41 refs]. Adv Endocrinol Metab 1995;6:233–258.

Rebar RW, Cedars MI. Hypergonadotropic forms of amenorrhea in young women. [Review]. Endocrinol Metab Clin North Am 1992;21:173–191.

Belchetz PE. Hormonal treatment of postmenopausal women [see comments]. [Review]. N Engl J Med 1994;330:1062–1071.

Steingold KA, Matt DW, DeZiegler D, et al. Comparison of transdermal to oral estradiol administration on hormonal and hepatic parameters in women with premature ovarian failure. J Clin Endocrinol Metab 1991;73:275–280.

See Also

- Amenorrhea, secondary
- Menopausal hormone replacement

THE CONSULTATION GUIDE

Multiple Endocrine Neoplasia I

Indications and Timing for Referral

- Suspicion on basis of established diagnosis of one or more components in patient or family member

Timing: Routine (less than 4 weeks)

Advice for Referral

- Serious consideration should be given to having such patients co-managed with an endocrinologist.

Tests to Prepare for Consult

- Albumin, total protein
- Calcium, phosphorus
- Alkaline phosphatase
- Prolactin

Tests Not Useful Before Consult

- None

Tests Consultant May Need to Do

- PTH
- Glucose
- Insulin
- Gastrin
- C-peptide
- Glucagon
- Pancreatic polypeptide
- Somatostatin
- VIP
- CT or MR, abdomen
- IGF-1
- Free cortisol, 24-hour urine, or overnight dexamethasone suppression test, 1 mg
- Creatinine, 24-hour urine
- MR or CT, cranial with pituitary cuts

Follow-up Visits Generally Required

- Co-management, see *Advice for Referral*

Suggested Readings

Gardner DG. Recent advances in multiple endocrine neoplasia syndromes. [Review] [127 refs]. Adv Intern Med 1997;42:597–627.

Mallette LE. Management of hyperparathyroidism in the multiple endocrine neoplasia syndromes and other familial endocrinopathies. [Review]. Endocrinol Metab Clin North Am 1994;23:19–36.

Larsson C, Friedman E. Localization and identification of the multiple endocrine neoplasia type 1 disease gene. [Review]. Endocrinol Metab Clin North Am 1994;23:67–79.

See Also

- Hypercalcemia
- Hyperprolactinemia
- Pituitary tumor
- Hyperparathyroidism
- Acromegaly
- Cushing's syndrome
- Hypoglycemia, fasting

Multiple Endocrine Neoplasia II

Indications and Timing for Referral

- Suspicion on basis of established diagnosis of one or more components in patient or family member

Timing: Routine (less than 4 weeks)

Advice for Referral

- Serious consideration should be given to having such patients co-managed with an endocrinologist.

Tests to Prepare for Consult

- Calcium, phosphorus
- Alkaline phosphatase
- Calcitonin
- Metanephrines, 24-hour urine
- Creatinine, 24-hour urine

Tests Not Useful Before Consult

- None

Tests Consultant May Need to Do

- PTH
- Calcium/pentagastrin stimulation test
- RET proto-oncogene analysis
- Sonogram, thyroid
- CT or MR, abdomen

Follow-up Visits Generally Required

- Co-management, see *Advice for Referral*

Suggested Readings

Gardner DG. Recent advances in multiple endocrine neoplasia syndromes. [Review] [127 refs]. Adv Intern Med 1997;42:597–627.

Heshmati HM, Gharib H, van Heerden JA, Sizmore GW. Advances and controversies in the diagnosis and management of medullary thyroid carcinoma. [Review] [75 refs]. Am J Med 1997;103:60–69.

Ledger GA, Khosla S, Lindor NM, et al. Genetic testing in the diagnosis and management of multiple endocrine neoplasia type II. [Review]. Ann Intern Med 1995;122:118–124.

Wells SA Jr, Donis-Keller H. Current perspectives on the diagnosis and management of patients with multiple endocrine neoplasia type 2 syndromes. [Review]. Endocrinol Metab Clin North Am 1994;23:215–228.

Mallette LE. Management of hyperparathyroidism in the multiple endocrine neoplasia syndromes and other familial endocrinopathies. [Review]. Endocrinol Metab Clin North Am 1994;23:19–36.

See Also

- Hypercalcemia
- Thyroid nodule
- Adrenal mass, radiologically detected
- Pheochromocytoma
- Hypertension, labile/paroxysmal
- Hyperparathyroidism

THE CONSULTATION GUIDE

Obesity

Indications and Timing for Referral

- Suspicion of underlying endocrinopathy

Timing: Routine (less than 4 weeks)

Tests to Prepare for Consult

- TSH (assay sensitivity <0.1 mU/L)
- Glucose, fasting
- Lipid profile, fasting (cholesterol, HDL, TG)

Tests Not Useful Before Consult

- None

Tests Consultant May Need to Do

- Free cortisol, 24-hour urine, or overnight dexamethasone suppression test, 1 mg
- Creatinine, 24-hour urine

Follow-up Visits Generally Required

- None

Suggested Readings

Rosenbaum M, Leibel RL, Hirsch J. Obesity. [Review] [139 refs]. N Engl J Med 1997;337:396–407.

Pi-Sunyer FX. Medical hazards of obesity. [Review]. Ann Intern Med 1993;119:655–660.

Blackburn GL. Comparison of medically supervised and unsupervised approaches to weight loss and control. [Review]. Ann Intern Med 1993;119:714–718.

Long-term pharmacotherapy in the management of obesity. National Task Force on the Prevention and Treatment of Obesity [see comments]. [Review] [117 refs]. JAMA 1996;276:1907–1915.

Wadden TA. Treatment of obesity by moderate and severe caloric restriction. Results of clinical research trials. [Review]. Ann Intern Med 1993;119:688–693.

Very low-calorie diets. National Task Force on the Prevention and Treatment of Obesity, National Institutes of Health [see comments]. [Review]. JAMA 1993;270:967–974.

Blair SN. Evidence for success of exercise in weight loss and control. [Review]. Ann Intern Med 1993;119:702–706.

Selected Guidelines

U.S. Preventive Services Task Force. Screening for obesity. In: DiGuiseppi C, Atkins D, Woolf S, eds. Guide to Clinical Preventive Services. 2nd ed. Baltimore: Williams & Wilkins, 1996:219–230.

NIH conference. Gastrointestinal surgery for severe obesity. Consensus Development Conference Panel. [Review]. Ann Intern Med 1991;115:956–961.

See Also

- Hypercholesterolemia

ENDOCRINOLOGY AND METABOLISM

Osteodystrophy, Renal

Indications and Timing for Referral

- Assistance with management

Timing: Routine (less than 4 weeks)

Advice for Referral

- Follow-up may range from none to co-management depending on the severity of the renal osteodystrophy.

Tests to Prepare for Consult

- Calcium, phosphorus
- Electrolytes (Na, K, Cl, CO_2)
- Alkaline phosphatase
- Albumin, total protein
- Creatinine
- 1,25-dihydroxyvitamin D_3
- 25-hydroxyvitamin D_3
- PTH, intact
- Aluminum, serum

Tests Not Useful Before Consult

- None

Tests Consultant May Need to Do

- Magnesium
- Osteocalcin
- Bone mineral density
- Radiographs, skeletal
- Bone biopsy

Follow-up Visits Generally Required

- See *Advice for Referral*

Suggested Readings

Hruska KA, Teitelbaum SL. Renal osteodystrophy [see comments]. [Review] [75 refs]. N Engl J Med 1995;333:166–174.

Andress DL, Sherrard DJ. The osteodystrophy of chronic renal failure. In: Schrier RW, Gottschalk CW, eds. Diseases of the kidney. 5th ed. Boston: Little Brown, 1993;2759–2788.

McCarthy JT, Kumar R. Renal osteodystrophy. [Review]. Endocrinol Metab Clin North Am 1990;19:65–93.

See Also

- Osteopenia
- Osteomalacia
- Osteoporosis

Osteomalacia

Indications and Timing for Referral

- Confirm diagnosis
- Assistance with management

Timing: Routine (less than 4 weeks)

Advice for Referral

- Optimal bone mineral density assessment requires dual energy x-ray densitometry.
- See also *Steatorrhea* and *Malabsorption*.

Tests to Prepare for Consult

- Electrolytes (Na, K, Cl, CO_2)
- CBC
- Calcium, phosphorus
- Albumin, total protein
- ALT, AST, alkaline phosphatase
- Creatinine
- Urinalysis with microscopic
- PTH, intact

Tests Not Useful Before Consult

- None

Tests Consultant May Need to Do

- 1,25-dihydroxyvitamin D_3
- 25-hydroxyvitamin D_3
- Calcium, 24-hour urine
- Creatinine, 24-hour urine
- Bone mineral density
- Bone specific alkaline phosphatase
- Osteocalcin
- N-terminal telopeptide
- Pyridinium and deoxypyridinium cross-links
- Prothrombin time
- Radiographs, skeletal
- Bone biopsy

Follow-up Visits Generally Required

- Two

Suggested Readings

Bingham CT, Fitzpatrick LA. Noninvasive testing in the diagnosis of osteomalacia. Am J Med 1993;95:519–523.

Econs MJ, Drezner MK. Tumor-induced osteomalacia—unveiling a new hormone [editorial; comment]. N Engl J Med 1994;330:1679–1681.

Bell NH, Key LLJ. Acquired osteomalacia. Curr Ther Endocrinol Metab 1997;6:530–533.

Wolinsky-Friedland M. Drug-induced metabolic bone disease. Endocrinol Metab Clin North Am 1995;24:395–420.

See Also

- Osteopenia
- Osteoporosis
- Osteodystrophy, renal
- Steatorrhea
- Malabsorption

ENDOCRINOLOGY AND METABOLISM

Osteopenia

Indications and Timing for Referral
- Unclear etiology
- Assistance with management

Timing: Routine (less than 4 weeks)

Advice for Referral
- Optimal bone mineral density assessment requires dual energy x-ray densitometry.
- Decreased bone mineral density is defined as greater than 1 standard deviation below young sex-matched controls.

Tests to Prepare for Consult
- Calcium, phosphorus
- Alkaline phosphatase
- CBC
- Creatinine
- TSH (assay sensitivity <0.1 mU/L)
- Testosterone, in men

Tests Not Useful Before Consult
- None

Tests Consultant May Need to Do
- PTH, intact
- 1,25-dihydroxyvitamin D_3
- 25-hydroxyvitamin D_3
- Calcium, 24-hour urine
- Creatinine, 24-hour urine
- IEP
  - Urine
  - Serum
- LH, FSH
- Free cortisol, 24-hour urine, or overnight dexamethasone suppression test, 1 mg
- Bone specific alkaline phosphatase
- Osteocalcin
- N-terminal telopeptide
- Pyridinium and deoxypyridinium cross-links
- Radiograph
  - L-spine
  - T-spine
- Bone biopsy

Follow-up Visits Generally Required
- Two

Suggested Readings
Compston JE, Cooper C, Kanis JA. Bone densitometry in clinical practice. [Review]. Br Med J 1995;310:1507–1510.

Johnston CC Jr, Slemenda CW, Melton LJ 3d. Clinical use of bone densitometry. [Review]. N Engl J Med 1991;324:1105–1109.

Ribot C, Tremollieres F, Pouilles JM. Can we detect women with low bone mass using clinical risk factors?. [Review]. Am J Med 1995;98(Suppl 2A):52S–55S.

Cummings SR, Black D. Bone mass measurements and risk of fracture in Caucasian women: a review of findings from prospective studies. [Review]. Am J Med 1995;98(Suppl 2A):24S–28S.

Michelson D, Stratakis C, Hill L, et al. Bone mineral density in women with depression. N Engl J Med 1996;335:1176–1181.

Selected Guidelines
Screening for postmenopausal osteoporosis. In: U.S. Preventive Services Task Force Guide to Clinical Preventive Services: an Assessment of the Effectiveness of 169 Interventions: Report of the U.S. Preventive Services Task Force Baltimore: Williams & Wilkins, 1989:239–243. 1995; U.S. Preventive Serv-43.

See Also
- Osteodystrophy, renal
- Osteomalacia
- Osteoporosis

Osteoporosis

Indications and Timing for Referral

- Unclear etiology
- Assistance with management

Timing: Routine (less than 4 weeks)

Advice for Referral

- Optimal bone mineral density assessment requires dual energy x-ray densitometry.
- Decreased bone mineral density is defined as greater than 1 standard deviation below young sex-matched controls.
- Osteoporosis is generally defined as greater than 2.0 standard deviations below young sex-matched controls.
- Consideration should be given to having patients with severely diminished or progressively declining bone density co-managed with an endocrinologist, particularly if they are unresponsive to first-line bone-preserving therapies.

Tests to Prepare for Consult

- Calcium, phosphorus
- Alkaline phosphatase
- CBC
- Creatinine
- TSH (assay sensitivity <0.1 mU/L)
- Testosterone, in men

Tests Not Useful Before Consult

- None

Tests Consultant May Need to Do

- PTH, intact
- 1,25-dihydroxyvitamin D_3
- 25-hydroxyvitamin D_3
- LH, FSH
- Prolactin
- IEP
    - Serum
    - Urine
- Calcium, 24-hour urine
- Creatinine, 24-hour urine
- Free cortisol, 24-hour urine, or overnight dexamethasone suppression test, 1 mg
- Bone-specific alkaline phosphatase
- Osteocalcin
- N-terminal telopeptide
- Pyridinium and deoxypyridinium cross-links
- Radiograph
    - L-spine
    - T-spine
- Bone biopsy

Follow-up Visits Generally Required

- See *Advice for Referral*

ENDOCRINOLOGY AND METABOLISM

Osteoporosis (continued)

Suggested Readings

Raisz LG. The osteoporosis revolution. [Review] [56 refs]. Ann Intern Med 1997;126:458–462.

Khosla S, Riggs BL. Treatment options for osteoporosis. Mayo Clin Proc 1995;70:978–982.

Diagnosis, prophylaxis, and treatment of osteoporosis: Consensus Development Conference. Am J Med 1993;94:646–650.

Mitlak BH, Nussbaum SR. Diagnosis and treatment of osteoporosis. [Review]. Annu Rev Med 1993;44:265–277.

Delmas PD, Bjarnason NH, Mitlak BH, et al. Effects of raloxifene on bone mineral density, serum cholesterol concentrations, and uterine endometrium in postmenopausal women. N Engl J Med 1997;337:1641–1647.

Selected Guidelines

U.S. Preventive Services Task Force. Screening for postmenopausal osteoporosis. In: DiGuiseppi C, Atkins D, Woolf S, eds. Guide to clinical preventive services. 2nd ed. Baltimore: Williams & Wilkins, 1996;509–516.

See Also

- Osteopenia
- Osteomalacia
- Renal osteodystrophy

Paget's Disease

Indications and Timing for Referral

- Neurologic complications are present
- Impending fracture is suspected

Timing: Immediate or Urgent (less than 24 hours)

- Confirm diagnosis
- Assistance with management

Timing: Routine (less than 4 weeks)

Advice for Referral

- Follow-up may range from none to co-management depending on the severity of disease and responsiveness to therapy.

Tests to Prepare for Consult

- Alkaline phosphatase
- Calcium, phosphorus
- Albumin, total protein
- Radiographs, affected regions

Tests Not Useful Before Consult

- None

Tests Consultant May Need to Do

- PTH, intact
- Bone-specific alkaline phosphatase
- Osteocalcin
- N-terminal telopeptide
- Pyridinium and deoxypyridinium cross-links
- Bone scan
- Audiogram
- ECG
- PSA

Follow-up Visits Generally Required

- See *Advice for Referral*

Suggested Readings

Delmas PD, Meunier PJ. The management of Paget's disease of bone. [Review] [71 refs]. N Engl J Med 1997;336:558–566.

Merkow RL, Lane JM. Paget's disease of bone. [Review]. Endocrinol Metab Clin North Am 1990;19:177–204.

Bone HG, Kleerekoper M. Clinical review 39: Paget's disease of bone. [Review]. J Clin Endocrinol Metab 1992;75:1179–1182.

ENDOCRINOLOGY AND METABOLISM

Pheochromocytoma

Indications and Timing for Referral

- Hypertensive crisis

Timing: Immediate

- Uncontrolled hypertension
- Imminent surgical or radiologic procedure
- Patient is pregnant

Timing: Urgent (less than 24 hours)

- Diagnostic uncertainty
- Assistance with management

Timing: Expedited (less than 1 week)

Advice for Referral

- Radiocontrast studies may provoke severe hypertensive crisis.
- Urine and plasma sampling may be most informative when obtained during or immediately after symptoms or hypertensive episode.
- Serious consideration should be given to having such patients co-managed with an endocrinologist, particularly during the perioperative period.

Tests to Prepare for Consult

- ECG
- Metanephrines or catecholamines, 24-hour urine
- Creatinine, 24-hour urine

Tests Not Useful Before Consult

- None

Tests Consultant May Need to Do

- Radiograph, chest
- Metanephrines, 24-hour urine
- Catecholamines, 24-hour urine
- Creatinine, 24-hour urine
- Catecholamines, plasma
- Clonidine suppression test (for catechols)
- 5'-HIAA, 24-hour urine
- MIBG scan
- Octreotide scan
- MR or CT, adrenal
- Calcium
- Calcitonin
- PTH
- TSH
- RET proto-oncogene analysis

Follow-up Visits Generally Required

- Co-management, see *Advice for Referral*

Pheochromocytoma (continued)

Suggested Readings

Gifford RW Jr, Manger WM, Bravo EL. Pheochromocytoma. [Review] [46 refs]. Endocrinol Metab Clin North Am 1994;23:387–404.

Francis IR, Korobkin M. Pheochromocytoma. [Review] [48 refs]. Radiol Clin North Am 1996;34:1101–1112.

Young WF Jr, Maddox DE. Spells: in search of a cause. [Review] [26 refs]. Mayo Clin Proc 1995;70:757–765.

Elijovich F. Plasma metanephrines in the diagnosis of pheochromocytoma. Ann Intern Med 1996;124:694–695.

Heron E, Chatellier G, Billaud E, et al. The urinary metanephrine-to-creatinine ratio for the diagnosis of pheochromocytoma [see comments]. Ann Intern Med 1996;125:300–303.

Sheps SG, Jiang NS, Klee GG, van Heerden JA. Recent developments in the diagnosis and treatment of pheochromocytoma. [Review]. Mayo Clin Proc 1990;65:88–95.

See Also

- Hypertension, labile/paroxysmal
- Multiple endocrine neoplasia II
- Adrenal mass, radiologically detected

ENDOCRINOLOGY AND METABOLISM

Pituitary Tumor

Indications and Timing for Referral

- Change in vision
- Severe headaches
- MR or CT evidence of chiasmal involvement
- Clinical or laboratory evidence of adrenal insufficiency or severe hypothyroidism

Timing: Urgent (less than 24 hours) or Expedited (less than 1 week)

- Assistance with management

Timing: Routine (less than 4 weeks)

Advice for Referral

- Visual field testing is appropriate if chiasmal region is involved or a change in vision is noted.
- Presence of macroadenoma generally requires concurrent consultation with Endocrinology and Neurosurgery.
- Co-management by the endocrinologist is usually appropriate through the postoperative period when the patient's hormonal status must be reassessed and residual hormonal imbalances addressed.

Tests to Prepare for Consult

- MR, cranial with pituitary cuts
- Prolactin
- Free T_4
- TSH (assay sensitivity <0.1 mU/L)
- Testosterone, in men
- CBC
- Glucose
- Potassium, sodium

Tests Not Useful Before Consult

- Radiograph, skull
- Sellar tomograms

Tests Consultant May Need to Do

- GH
- IGF-1
- LH, FSH
- Estradiol, in women
- ACTH stimulation test, 1-hour
- CRH stimulation test (serial for cortisol and ACTH)
- Insulin tolerance test (for cortisol and GH)
- Alpha subunit
- TRH test
- Free cortisol, 24-hour urine
- Creatinine, 24-hour urine
- Overnight dexamethasone suppression test
  - 1 mg
  - 8 mg
- OGTT (1-hour, for GH)

Follow-up Visits Generally Required

- Co-management, see *Advice for Referral*

Pituitary Tumor (*continued*)

Suggested Readings

Aron DC, Tyrrell JB, Wilson CB. Pituitary tumors. Current concepts in diagnosis and management. [Review] [111 refs]. West J Med 1995;162:340–352.

Greenman Y, Melmed S. Diagnosis and management of nonfunctioning pituitary tumors [review]. Annu Rev Med 1996;47:95–106.

Melmed S. Pituitary neoplasia. [Review]. Endocrinol Metab Clin North Am 1994;23:81–92.

Klibanski A, Zervas NT. Diagnosis and management of hormone-secreting pituitary adenomas. [Review]. N Engl J Med 1991;324:822–831.

Molitch ME. Clinical review 65. Evaluation and treatment of the patient with a pituitary incidentaloma. [Review]. J Clin Endocrinol Metab 1995;80:3–6.

Hennessey JV, Jackson IM. Clinical features and differential diagnosis of pituitary tumours with emphasis on acromegaly. [Review] [211 refs]. Baillieres Clin Endocrinol Metab 1995;9:271–314.

Snyder PJ. Clinically nonfunctioning pituitary adenomas. [Review]. Metab Clin North Am 1993;22:163–175.

Young WF, Scheithauer BW, Kovacs KT, et al. Gonadotroph adenoma of the pituitary gland: a clinicopathologic analysis of 100 cases. Mayo Clin Proc 1996;71:649–656.

See Also

- Multiple endocrine neoplasia I
- Hyperprolactinemia
- Empty sella syndrome
- Hypopituitarism
- Sella turcica, enlarged

ENDOCRINOLOGY AND METABOLISM

Polycystic Ovaries

Indications and Timing for Referral

- Confirmation of etiology and diagnosis
- Assistance with management

Timing: Routine (less than 4 weeks)

Advice for Referral

- Records of all previous endocrine testing are vital.

Tests to Prepare for Consult

- Testosterone

Tests Not Useful Before Consult

- None

Tests Consultant May Need to Do

- LH, FSH
- Free testosterone
- Androstenedione
- Prolactin
- Glucose
- Lipid profile, fasting (cholesterol, HDL, TG)
- Insulin
- Free cortisol, 24-hour urine, or overnight dexamethasone suppression test, 1 mg
- Creatinine, 24-hour urine
- ACTH stimulation test (17-hydroxyprogesterone)
- Androstanediol glucuronide
- Ultrasound, ovarian
- CT scan, adrenal

Follow-up Visits Generally Required

- Two

Suggested Readings

Franks S. Medical progress: polycystic ovary syndrome. N Engl J Med 1995;333:853–861.

Hall JE. Polycystic ovarian disease as a neuroendocrine disorder of the female reproductive axis. [Review]. Endocrinol Metab Clin North Am 1993;22:75–92.

Goldzieher JW, Young RL. Selected aspects of polycystic ovarian disease. [Review]. Endocrinol Metab Clin North Am 1992;21:141–171.

Barbieri RL. Polycystic ovarian disease. [Review]. Annu Rev Med 1991;42:199–204.

See Also

- Delayed puberty, female
- Amenorrhea, secondary
- Hirsutism
- Anovulatory syndrome, chronic

THE CONSULTATION GUIDE

Sella Turcica, Enlarged

Indications and Timing for Referral

- If CT or MRI shows pituitary mass or other regional abnormality, then see *Pituitary Tumor* or *Empty Sella Syndrome*

Timing: Routine (less than 4 weeks)

Advice for Referral

- MR preferred test if available and not contraindicated.
- Visual field testing is appropriate if chiasmal region is involved or a change in vision is noted.
- Factors favoring initial referral to endocrinologist include:
  - Pituitary mass
  - Clinical or laboratory evidence of pituitary hormone excess or deficiency
- Factors favoring initial referral to neurosurgeon include:
  - Principally extra-sellar mass

Tests to Prepare for Consult

- MR, cranial with pituitary cuts

Tests Not Useful Before Consult

- ACTH level, plasma
- GH
- Arteriography
- Sellar tomograms

Tests Consultant May Need to Do

- Cortisol, 8 am
- GH
- IGF-1
- Estradiol, in women
- Testosterone, in men
- LH, FSH
- CRH stimulation test (serial for cortisol and ACTH)
- ACTH stimulation test, 1-hour (for cortisol)
- Insulin tolerance test (for cortisol and GH)

Follow-up Visits Generally Required

- One

Suggested Readings

von Werder K. Pituitary enlargement. Clin Endocrinol (Oxf) 1996;44:299–303.

Molitch ME. Clinical review 65. Evaluation and treatment of the patient with a pituitary incidentaloma. [Review]. J Clin Endocrinol Metab 1995;80:3–6.

Freda PU, Wardlaw SL, Post KD. Unusual causes of sellar/parasellar masses in a large transsphenoidal surgical series. J Clin Endocrinol Metab 1996;81:3455–3459.

Felsberg GJ, Tien RD. Sellar and parasellar lesions involving the skull base. [Review]. Neuroimaging Clin North Am 1994;4:543–560.

Chakeres DW, Curtin A, Ford G. Magnetic resonance imaging of pituitary and parasellar abnormalities. [Review]. Radiol Clin North Am 1989;27:265–281.

See Also

- Empty sella syndrome
- Pituitary tumor
- Hypopituitarism

ENDOCRINOLOGY AND METABOLISM

Thyroid Nodule

Indications and Timing for Referral

- Diagnostic uncertainty
- Assistance with management

Timing: Routine (4 weeks)

Tests to Prepare for Consult

- TSH (assay sensitivity <0.1 mU/L)

Tests Not Useful Before Consult

- CT or MR, neck

Tests Consultant May Need to Do

- TSH (assay sensitivity <0.1 mU/L)
- Free T_4
- Triiodothyronine (T_3)
- Anti-TPO antibody
- Calcitonin
- Fine needle aspiration biopsy
- Radionuclide uptake and scan, thyroid
- Sonogram, thyroid

Follow-up Visits Generally Required

- One

Suggested Readings

Ladenson PW. Optimal laboratory testing for diagnosis and monitoring of thyroid nodules, goiter, and thyroid cancer. [Review] [27 refs]. Clin Chem 1996;42:183–187.

Mazzaferri EL. Management of a solitary thyroid nodule [see comments]. [Review]. N Engl J Med 1993;328:553–559.

Goellner GH. Fine-needle aspiration biopsy of the thyroid: an appraisal. Ann Intern Med 1993;118:282–289.

Tan GH, Gharib H. Thyroid incidentalomas: management approaches to nonpalpable nodules discovered incidentally on thyroid imaging. [Review] [45 refs]. Ann Intern Med 1997;126:226–231.

Woeber KA. Cost-effective evaluation of the patient with a thyroid nodule. [Review]. Surg Clin North Am 1995;75:357–363.

Selected Guidelines

Singer PA, Cooper DS, Daniels GH, et al. Treatment guidelines for patients with thyroid nodules and well-differentiated thyroid cancer. American Thyroid Association. Arch Intern Med 1996;156:2165–2172.

Guidelines of the Papanicolaou Society of Cytopathology for the Examination of Fine-Needle Aspiration Specimens from Thyroid Nodules. The Papanicolaou Society of Cytopathology Task Force on Standards of Practice. Mod Pathol 1996;9:710–715.

See Also

- Goiter, simple/diffuse

THE CONSULTATION GUIDE

Thyroid Ophthalmopathy

Indications and Timing for Referral

- Diminished visual acuity
- Severe inflammation
- Keratitis

Timing: Urgent (less than 24 hours)

- Disabling diplopia

Timing: Expedited (less than 1 week)

- Diagnostic uncertainty
- Assistance with management

Timing: Routine (less than 4 weeks)

Advice for Referral

- Serious consideration should be given to having such patients co-managed with an endocrinologist.
- Co-management with an ophthalmologist is appropriate whenever there is a related change in visual acuity, diplopia, or severe inflammation.

Tests to Prepare for Consult

- TSH (assay sensitivity <0.1 mU/L)
- Free T_4
- Triiodothyronine (T_3)

Tests Not Useful Before Consult

- None

Tests Consultant May Need to Do

- Anti-TPO antibody
- Thyroid-stimulating immunoglobulin (TSI)
- Radionuclide iodine uptake
- MR, CT, or sonogram of orbit

Follow-up Visits Generally Required

- Co-management, see *Advice for Referral*

Suggested Readings

Yeatts RP. Graves' ophthalmopathy. [Review]. Med Clin North Am 1995;79:195–209.

Bahn RS, Heufelder AE. Pathogenesis of Graves' ophthalmopathy. [Review]. N Engl J Med 1993;329:1468–1475.

Burch HB, Wartofsky L. Graves' ophthalmopathy: current concepts regarding pathogenesis and management. [Review]. Endocrine Reviews 1993;14:747–793.

Tallstedt L, Lundell G, Torring O, et al. Occurrence of ophthalmopathy after treatment for Graves' hyperthyroidism. The Thyroid Study Group. N Engl J Med 1992;326:1733–1738.

Carter JA, Utiger RD. The ophthalmopathy of Graves' disease. [Review]. Annu Rev Med 1992;43:487–495.

See Also

- Thyrotoxicosis

ENDOCRINOLOGY AND METABOLISM

Thyroid, Painful

Indications and Timing for Referral

- Severe pain

Timing: Urgent (less than 24 hours)

- Diagnostic uncertainty
- Assistance with management
- Associated thyroid function abnormality

Timing: Expedited (less than 1 week)

Tests to Prepare for Consult

- CBC
- ESR
- TSH (assay sensitivity <0.1 mU/L)
- Free T_4

Tests Not Useful Before Consult

- None

Tests Consultant May Need to Do

- TSH (assay sensitivity <0.1 mU/L)
- Free T_4
- Sonogram, thyroid
- Radionuclide uptake and scan
- Fine needle aspiration biopsy
- CT or MR, neck

Follow-up Visits Generally Required

- One

Suggested Readings

Farwell AP, Braverman LE. Inflammatory thyroid disorders. [Review] [112 refs]. Otolaryngol Clin North Am 1996;29:541–556.

Singer PA. Thyroiditis. Acute, subacute, and chronic. [Review]. Med Clin North Am 1991;75:61–77.

Walfish PG. Thyroiditis. Curr Ther Endocrinol Metab 1997;6:117–122.

See Also

- Thyroiditis, subacute
- Thyrotoxicosis

169

THE CONSULTATION GUIDE

Thyroid Function Tests, Abnormal

Indications and Timing for Referral

- Assess clinical significance when test results are inconsistent with one another or discordant with the patient's clinical status

Timing: Expedited (less than 1 week)

Advice for Referral

- Complete medication history is vital.

Tests to Prepare for Consult

- Free T_4
- TSH (assay sensitivity <0.1 mU/L)

Tests Not Useful Before Consult

- Sonogram, thyroid

Tests Consultant May Need to Do

- TSH (assay sensitivity <0.1 mU/L)
- Free T_4, by dialysis
- Triiodothyronine (T_3)
- T_4 binding panel
- Anti-TPO antibody
- TRH test (for TSH)

Follow-up Visits Generally Required

- None

Suggested Readings

Bauer DC, Brown AN. Sensitive thyrotropin and free thyroxine testing in outpatients. Are both necessary? Arch Intern Med 1996;156:2333–2337.

Spencer CA. Clinical utility and cost-effectiveness of sensitive thyrotropin assays in ambulatory and hospitalized patients. [Review]. Mayo Clin Proc 1988;63: 1214–1222.

Cavalieri RR. The effects of nonthyroid disease and drugs on thyroid function tests. [Review]. Med Clin North Am 1991;75:27–39.

Surks MI, Sievert R. Drugs and thyroid function. [Review] [94 refs]. N Engl J Med 1995;333:1688–1694.

Chopra IJ. Clinical review 86: Euthyroid sick syndrome: is it a misnomer? J Clin Endocrinol Metab 1997;82:329–334.

Ladenson PW. Diagnosis of hypothyroidism. In: Braverman LE, Utiger RD, eds. The Thyroid: a Fundamental and Clinical Text. 7th ed. Philadelphia: JB Lippincott Co, 1996:878–882.

Ladenson PW. Diagnosis of thyrotoxicosis. In: Braverman LE, Utiger RD, eds. The Thyroid: a Fundamental and Clinical Text. 7th ed. Philadelphia: JB Lippincott Co, 1996:708–712.

See Also

- Hypothyroidism
- Thyrotoxicosis

ENDOCRINOLOGY AND METABOLISM

Thyroiditis, Subacute

Indications and Timing for Referral

- Severe pain or constitutional symptoms present
- Thyrotoxicosis present

Timing: Urgent (less than 24 hours)

- Confirm diagnosis
- Assistance with pain control, or potential use of corticosteroids

Timing: Expedited (less than 1 week)

Tests to Prepare for Consult

- Free T_4
- TSH (assay sensitivity <0.1 mU/L)
- ESR
- CBC

Tests Not Useful Before Consult

- Antithyroid antibodies

Tests Consultant May Need to Do

- TSH (assay sensitivity <0.1 mU/L)
- Free T_4
- ESR
- CBC
- Sonogram, thyroid
- Radionuclide uptake and scan
- CT or MR, neck
- Fine needle aspiration biopsy

Follow-up Visits Generally Required

- Two

Suggested Readings

Singer PA. Thyroiditis. Acute, subacute, and chronic. [Review]. Med Clin North Am 1991;75:61–77.

Farwell AP, Braverman LE. Inflammatory thyroid disorders. [Review] [112 refs]. Otolaryngol Clin North Am 1996;29:541–556.

Walfish PG. Thyroiditis. Curr Ther Endocrinol Metab 1997;6:117–122.

See Also

- Thyroid, painful

THE CONSULTATION GUIDE

Thyrotoxicosis

Indications and Timing for Referral

- Atrial fibrillation or congestive heart failure

Timing: Immediate

- Associated thyroid ophthalmopathy with change in vision

Timing: Urgent (less than 24 hours)

- Confirm diagnosis
- Determine etiology
- Assistance with management

Timing: Expedited (less than 1 week)

Advice for Referral

- Serious consideration should be given to having such patients co-managed with an endocrinologist.

Tests to Prepare for Consult

- TSH (assay sensitivity <0.1 mU/L)
- Free T_4
- CBC
- ALT, AST, alkaline phosphatase

Tests Not Useful Before Consult

- Radiocontrast studies

Tests Consultant May Need to Do

- TSH (assay sensitivity <0.1 mU/L)
- Free T_4
- Triiodothyronine (T_3)
- Thyroglobulin
- CBC
- ALT, AST, alkaline phosphatase
- ESR
- Anti-TPO antibody
- Thyroid-stimulating immunoglobulin (TSI)
- Radionuclide uptake and scan
- Radionuclide iodine uptake
- Beta HCG, serum
- ECG
- MR, CT, or sonogram of orbit

Follow-up Visits Generally Required

- Co-management, see *Advice for Referral*

Thyrotoxicosis (continued)

Suggested Readings

Franklyn JA. The management of hyperthyroidism [published erratum appears in N Engl J Med 1994;331:559]. [Review]. N Engl J Med 1994;330:1731–1738.

Sherman SI, Simonson L, Ladenson PW. Clinical and socioeconomic predispositions to complicated thyrotoxicosis: a predictable and preventable syndrome? Am J Med 1996;101:192–198.

Solomon B, Glinoer D, Lagasse R, Wartofsky L. Current trends in the management of Graves' disease. J Clin Endocrinol Metab 1990;70:1518–1524.

Braverman LE. Evaluation of thyroid status in patients with thyrotoxicosis. Clin Chem 1996;42:174–178.

Harjai KJ, Licata AA. Effects of amiodarone on thyroid function. Ann Intern Med 1997;126:63–73.

Dillmann WH. Thyroid storm. Curr Ther Endocrinol Metab 1997;6:81–85.

Wartofsky L. Treatment options for hyperthyroidism. Hosp Pract (Off Ed) 1996;31:69–85.

Wartofsky L. Radioiodine therapy for Graves' disease: case selection and restrictions recommended to patients in North America. Thyroid 1997;7:213–216.

Hung W. Graves' disease in children. Curr Ther Endocrinol Metab 1997;6:77–81.

Ladenson PW. Diagnosis of thyrotoxicosis. In: Braverman LE, Utiger RD, eds. The thyroid: a fundamental and clinical text. 7th ed. Philadelphia: JB Lippincott Co, 1996; 708–712.

Selected Guidelines

Singer PA, Cooper DS, Levy EG, et al. Treatment guidelines for patients with hyperthyroidism and hypothyroidism. Standards of Care Committee, American Thyroid Association. JAMA 1995;273:808–812.

See Also

- Goiter, simple/diffuse
- Thyroid ophthalmopathy

CHAPTER 4

Gastroenterology

Abdominal Mass
   Epigastric 177
   Left Lower Quadrant 178
   Mid-Abdominal 179
   Right Lower Quadrant 180
Abdominal Pain, Chronic 181
Alkaline Phosphatase, Elevated 182
Ascites 183
Barrett's Esophagus and Gastroesophageal Reflux 184
Chest Pain, Atypical, Possible Gastrointestinal Origin 185
Cirrhosis
   Etiology Unknown 186
   Primary Biliary 188
   with Complications 189
Colitis
   Infectious 190
   Ulcerative 191
   Ulcerative, History of, Currently Asymptomatic 192
Colon Cancer, Family History of 193
Colorectal Cancer, History of 194
Constipation 195
Crohn's Disease
   Colitis 196
   Regional Ileitis 197
Diarrhea, Chronic 198
Diverticulitis 200
Dyspepsia/Indigestion 201
Dyspepsia, Nonulcer and *Helicobacter pylori*-Positive 202
Dysphagia 203
Duodenal Ulcer, Recurrent 204
Esophagitis 205
Flatulence, Persistent or Recurrent 206
Gastric Ulcer, by Upper Gastrointestinal Series 207
Heartburn 208
Hematochezia 209
Hemochromatosis 210

(continued)

Gastroenterology (continued)

Hepatic Cyst
    Multiple 211
    Solitary 212
Hepatic Mass, Solid, on Imaging 213
Hepatitis
    Autoimmune 214
    Exposure to 215
    Hepatitis B 216
    Hepatitis C 217
    Hepatitis D 218
Hepatomegaly/Abdominal Mass, Right Upper Quadrant 219
Hyperamylasemia 220
Irritable Bowel Syndrome 221
Jaundice/Hyperbilirubinemia 222
Liver Disease in the Alcohol Drinker 223
Malabsorption 224
Melena, Tarry Stools, Recent History of 225
Nausea, Persistent or Recurrent 226
Odynophagia 227
Pancreatic Mass
    Cystic, on Radiograph 228
    Solid, on Radiograph 229
Pancreatitis, Chronic or Recurrent 230
Peptic Distress, on Nonsteroidal Anti-Inflammatory Drugs 231
Peptic Ulcer Disease
    Helicobacter pylori-Negative, Persistent Symptoms 232
    Refractory 233
Polyps, Family History of 234
Right Upper Quadrant Pain, Intermittent 235
Sclerosing Cholangitis 236
Splenomegaly, Abdominal Mass, Left Upper Quadrant 237
Steatorrhea 238
Tenesmus 239
Transaminase Elevation 240
Vomiting, Persistent or Recurrent 241
Weight Loss, Despite Good Appetite 242
Wilson's Disease, Personal or Family History 243

GASTROENTEROLOGY

Abdominal Mass, Epigastric

Indications and Timing for Referral
- Diagnostic uncertainty

Timing: Expedited (less than 1 week)

Tests to Prepare for Consult
- Amylase
- Albumin, total protein
- Bilirubin
- ALT, AST, alkaline phosphatase
- CBC with differential
- Urinalysis with microscopic
- CT scan, abdomen

Tests Not Useful Before Consult
- None

Tests Consultant May Need to Do
- Glucose
- BUN, creatinine
- Calcium
- Electrolytes (Na, K, Cl, CO_2)
- Alpha-fetoprotein (AFP)
- Echinococcal IgM
- Ultrasound, abdomen
- Barium enema
- UGIS
- Small bowel follow-through
- Upper endoscopy
- Colonoscopy
- Liver biopsy

Follow-up Visits Generally Required
- Two

Suggested Readings
Barker CS, Lindsell DR. Ultrasound of the palpable abdominal mass. Clin Radiol 1990;41:98–99.

Edoute Y, Ben-Haim SA, Malberger E. Value of direct fine needle aspirative cytology in diagnosing palpable abdominal masses [see comments]. Am J Med 1991;91:377–382.

See Also
- Abdominal mass, RLQ
- Abdominal mass, midabdominal
- Abdominal mass, LLQ

Abdominal Mass, Left Lower Quadrant

Indications and Timing for Referral

- Diagnostic uncertainty

Timing: Expedited (less than 1 week)

Advice for Referral

- Gynecological evaluation is vital to diagnostic work-up in women.

Tests to Prepare for Consult

- CBC
- Stool for occult blood
- CT scan, abdomen and pelvis

Tests Not Useful Before Consult

- None

Tests Consultant May Need to Do

- CA-125
- Sonogram, pelvic
- Barium enema
- Small bowel follow-through
- Flexible sigmoidoscopy

Follow-up Visits Generally Required

- Two

Suggested Readings

Abdomen. In: Willms JL, Schniederman H, Algranati PS, eds. Physical Diagnosis: Bedside Evaluation of Diagnosis and Function. Baltimore: Williams & Wilkins, 1994; 347–386.

See Also

- Abdominal mass, epigastric
- Abdominal mass, midabdominal
- Abdominal mass, RLQ

GASTROENTEROLOGY

Abdominal Mass, Mid-Abdominal

Indications and Timing for Referral

- Diagnostic uncertainty

Timing: Expedited (less than 4 weeks)

Tests to Prepare for Consult

- CBC with differential
- Albumin, total protein
- Amylase
- Bilirubin
- ALT, AST, alkaline phosphatase
- Urinalysis with microscopic
- Ultrasound or CT, abdomen

Tests Not Useful Before Consult

- None

Tests Consultant May Need to Do

- MR, abdomen
- UGIS
- Small bowel follow-through
- Enteroscopy
- Sonogram, pelvis
- CT scan, pelvis

Follow-up Visits Generally Required

- Two

Suggested Readings

Barker CS, Lindsell DR. Ultrasound of the palpable abdominal mass. Clin Radiol 1990;41:98–99.

Edoute Y, Ben-Haim SA, Malberger E. Value of direct fine needle aspirative cytology in diagnosing palpable abdominal masses [see comments]. Am J Med 1991;91:377–382.

See Also

- Abdominal mass, epigastric
- Abdominal mass, RLQ
- Abdominal mass, LLQ

THE CONSULTATION GUIDE

Abdominal Mass, Right Lower Quadrant

Indications and Timing for Referral

- Diagnostic uncertainty

Timing: Expedited (less than 1 week)

Advice for Referral

- Gynecological evaluation is vital to diagnostic work-up in women, including consideration of pregnancy in premenopausal patients.

Tests to Prepare for Consult

- CBC
- Stool for occult blood
- Ultrasound or CT, abdomen and pelvis

Tests Not Useful Before Consult

- None

Tests Consultant May Need to Do

- CA-125
- Sonogram, pelvic
- Barium enema
- Small bowel follow-through
- Colonoscopy

Follow-up Visits Generally Required

- Two

Suggested Readings

Sackier J. Diagnostic laparoscopy in nonmalignant disease. [Review]. Surg Clin North Am 1992;72:1033–1043.

Abdomen. In: Willms JL, Schniederman H, Algranati PS, eds. Physical Diagnosis: Bedside Evaluation of Diagnosis and Function. Baltimore: Williams & Wilkins, 1994:347–386.

See Also

- Abdominal mass, epigastric
- Abdominal mass, midabdominal
- Abdominal mass, LLQ

GASTROENTEROLOGY

Abdominal Pain, Chronic

Indications and Timing for Referral

- Etiology uncertain after initial evaluation

Timing: Routine (less than 4 weeks)

Advice for Referral

- Rule out lactose intolerance.
- Dietary history should exclude sorbitol intake in sugarless candy.

Tests to Prepare for Consult

- Amylase
- ALT, AST, alkaline phosphatase

Tests Not Useful Before Consult

- None

Tests Consultant May Need to Do

- VDRL test
- α-aminolevulinic acid
    - Plasma
    - Urine
- Porphobilinogen
    - Plasma
    - Urine
- Ultrasound, abdomen
- CT scan, abdomen
- Barium enema
- Barium swallow
- UGIS
- Small bowel follow-through
- Upper endoscopy
- Colonoscopy
- Mesenteric angiography

Follow-up Visits Generally Required

- One

Suggested Readings

Sharpstone D, Colin-Jones DG. Chronic, non-visceral abdominal pain. [Review]. Gut 1994;35:833–836.

Lynn RB, Friedman LS. Irritable bowel syndrome [published erratum appears in N Engl J Med 1994;330:228] [see comments]. [Review]. N Engl J Med 1993;329:1940–1945.

Greenbaum DS, Greenbaum RB, Joseph JG, Natale JE. Chronic abdominal wall pain. Diagnostic validity and costs. Dig Dis Sci 1994;39:1935–1941.

Miller K, Mayer E, Moritz E. The role of laparoscopy in chronic and recurrent abdominal pain. Am J Surg 1996;172:353–356.

Schuster MM. Diagnostic evaluation of the irritable bowel syndrome. [Review]. Gastroenterol Clin North Am 1991;20:269–278.

THE CONSULTATION GUIDE

Alkaline Phosphatase, Elevated

Indications and Timing for Referral

- Etiology uncertain
- Patient over age 50 years with alkaline phosphatase elevated more than twice normal with no new evidence of underlying liver disease
- Patient under age 50 years with alkaline phosphatase elevated more than two times normal

Timing: Routine (less than 4 weeks)

Advice for Referral

- If 5'-nucleotidase is normal, consider Paget's disease in individuals older than 50 years.

Tests to Prepare for Consult

- 5'-nucleotidase or GGT
- Calcium, phosphorus
- Amylase
- Albumin, total protein
- Bilirubin
- ALT, AST, alkaline phosphatase
- Antimitochondrial antibody
- Ultrasound, abdomen
- TSH (assay sensitivity <0.1 mU/L)

Tests Not Useful Before Consult

- None

Tests Consultant May Need to Do

- AFP
- CT scan, abdomen
- ERCP
- Percutaneous transhepatic cholangiogram
- Liver biopsy
- Radiographs, bone
- Hydroxyproline, urine

Follow-up Visits Generally Required

- One

Suggested Readings

Van Hoof VO, De Broe ME. Interpretation and clinical significance of alkaline phosphatase isoenzyme patterns. [Review]. Crit Rev Clin Lab Sci 1994;31:197–293.

Kamath PS. Clinical approach to the patient with abnormal liver test results. [Review] [00 refs]. Mayo Clin Proc 1996;71:1089–1094.

Griffiths J. Alkaline phosphatases. Newer concepts in isoenzymes and clinical applications. [Review]. Clin Lab Med 1989;9:717–730.

See Also

- Jaundice/hyperbilirubinemia
- Paget's disease
- Thyrotoxicosis

GASTROENTEROLOGY

Ascites

Indications and Timing for Referral

- Suspect presence of bacterial peritonitis

Timing: Urgent (less than 24 hours)

- Etiology uncertain
- Refractory to diuretic therapy

Timing: Expedited (less than 1 week)

Advice for Referral

- Before referring patients with ambiguous physical findings; the presence of ascites can be confirmed by sonography.

Tests to Prepare for Consult

- CBC
- Glucose
- Calcium
- BUN, creatinine
- Electrolytes (Na, K, Cl, CO_2)
- Albumin, total protein
- Prothrombin time
- TSH

Tests Not Useful Before Consult

- None

Tests Consultant May Need to Do

- Paracentesis
- AFB culture, ascitic fluid
- Albumin, ascitic fluid
- Amylase, ascitic fluid
- Cell count, ascitic fluid
- C&S, ascitic fluid
- Cytology, ascitic fluid
- Fungal culture, ascitic fluid
- Glucose, ascitic fluid
- Gram stain, ascitic fluid
- Protein, ascitic fluid
- pH, ascitic fluid
- Triglycerides, ascitic fluid
- CEA
- CA-125
- Radiograph, chest, PA and lateral
- Sonogram, abdomen
- CT scan, abdomen and pelvis

Follow-up Visits Generally Required

- One

Suggested Readings

Lipsky MS, Sternbach MR. Evaluation and initial management of patients with ascites. [Review] [18 refs]. Am Fam Physician 1996;54:1327–1333.

Williams JW Jr, Simel DL. Does this patient have ascites? How to divine fluid in the abdomen [see comments]. [Review]. JAMA 1992;267:2645–2648.

Parson SL, Watson SA, Steele RJC. Malignant ascites [review]. Br J Surg 1996;83:6–14.

Habeeb KS, Herrera JL. Management of ascites. Paracentesis as a guide. [Review] [15 refs]. Postgrad Med 1997;101:191–192.

Inturri P, Graziotto A, Rossaro L. Treatment of ascites—old and new remedies. Dig Dis 1996;14:145–156.

Arroyo V, Gines P, Planas R. Treatment of ascites in cirrhosis. Diuretics, peritoneovenous shunt, and large-volume paracentesis. [Review]. Gastroenterol Clin North Am 1992;21:237–256.

See Also

- Cirrhosis, etiology unknown
- Cirrhosis, with complications

Barrett's Esophagus and Gastroesophageal Reflux

Indications and Timing for Referral

- Any patient with a confirmed diagnosis

Timing: Routine (less than 4 weeks)

Advice for Referral

- Important to have copies of old biopsy and endoscopy reports when seeing consultant.
- This condition often requires co-management with gastroenterologist to assist with surveillance for esophageal malignancy.

Tests to Prepare for Consult

- None

Tests Not Useful Before Consult

- UGIS
- CT or MR, neck
- CA19-9
- Carcinoembryonic antigen (CEA)

Tests Consultant May Need to Do

- Esophageal manometry
- Esophageal pH monitoring
- Upper endoscopy

Follow-up Visits Generally Required

- Co-management, see *Advice for Referral*

Suggested Readings

Eisen GM, Sandler RS, Murray S, Gottfried M. The relationship between gastroesophageal reflux disease and its complications with Barrett's esophagus [see comments]. Am J Gastroenterol 1997;92:27–31.

DeVault KR, Castell DO. Current diagnosis and treatment of gastroesophageal reflux disease. [Review]. Mayo Clin Proc 1994;69:867–876.

Pope CE 2nd. Acid-reflux disorders [see comments]. [Review]. N Engl J Med 1994;331:656–660.

Crooks GW, Lichtenstein GR. Clinical implications of Barrett's esophagus. [Review] [63 refs]. Arch Intern Med 1996;156:2174–2180.

Falk GW. Barrett's esophagus. [Review]. Gastrointest Endosc Clin N Am 1994;4:773–789.

Phillips RW, Wong RK. Barrett's esophagus. Natural history, incidence, etiology, and complications. [Review]. Gastroenterol Clin North Am 1991;20:791–816.

Selected Guidelines

The role of endoscopy in the surveillance of premalignant conditions of the upper gastrointestinal tract. Guidelines for clinical application. Gastrointest Endosc 1988;34(3 Suppl):18S–20S.

Appropriate Use of Gastrointestinal Endoscopy: a Consensus Statement from the American Society for Gastrointestinal Endoscopy. Manchester, MA: The Society, 1989;11:1995.

A standardized protocol for the methodology of esophageal pH monitoring and interpretation of the data for the diagnosis of gastroesophageal reflux. Working Group of the European Society of Pediatric Gastroenterology and Nutrition. J Pediatr Gastroenterol Nutr 1992;14:467–471.

See Also

- Heartburn
- Chest pain, atypical, possible gastrointestinal (GI) origin
- Esophagitis
- Dyspepsia, indigestion

GASTROENTEROLOGY

Chest Pain, Atypical, Possible Gastrointestinal Origin

Indications and Timing for Referral

- Symptoms progressive
- Refractory to routine medical therapy, i.e., antacids and H2-receptor antagonists

Timing: Routine (less than 4 weeks)

Advice for Referral

- Ischemic heart disease should be considered and excluded before GI referral.

Tests to Prepare for Consult

- None

Tests Not Useful Before Consult

- UGIS
- CT or MR, chest

Tests Consultant May Need to Do

- UGIS
- Esophageal pH monitoring
- Esophageal manometry
- Upper endoscopy
- Barium swallow

Follow-up Visits Generally Required

- Two

Suggested Readings

Castell DO. Chest pain of undetermined origin: overview of pathophysiology. [Review]. Am J Med 1992;92(Suppl 5A):2S–4S.

Snape WJ Jr. Managing the patient with atypical chest pain. Hosp Pract (Off Ed) 1997;32:159–173.

Singh S, Richter JE, Hewson EG, et al. The contribution of gastroesophageal reflux to chest pain in patients with coronary artery disease. Ann Intern Med 1992;117:824–830.

Paterson WG, Abdollah H, Beck IT, Da Costa LR. Ambulatory esophageal manometry, pH-metry, and Holter ECG monitoring in patients with atypical chest pain. Dig Dis Sci 1993;38:795–802.

Richter JE. Overview of diagnostic testing for chest pain of unknown origin. [Review]. Am J Med 1992;92(Suppl 5A):41S–45S.

Rao SS, Gregersen H, Hayek B, et al. Unexplained chest pain: the hypersensitive, hyperreactive, and poorly compliant esophagus [comment] [see comments]. Ann Intern Med 1996;124:950–958.

Selected Guidelines

Browning TH. Diagnosis of chest pain of esophageal origin. A guideline of the Patient Care Committee of the American Gastroenterological Association. Dig Dis Sci 1990;35:289–293.

Appropriate Use of Gastrointestinal Endoscopy: a Consensus Statement from the American Society for Gastrointestinal Endoscopy. Manchester, MA: The Society, 1989;11:1995.

A standardized protocol for the methodology of esophageal pH monitoring and interpretation of the data for the diagnosis of gastroesophageal reflux. Working Group of the European Society of Pediatric Gastroenterology and Nutrition. J Pediatr Gastroenterol Nutr 1992;14:467–471.

An American Gastroenterological Association medical position statement on the clinical use of esophageal manometry. American Gastroenterological Association. Gastroenterology 1994;107:1865.

See Also

- Heartburn
- Barrett's esophagus and GERD
- Esophagitis
- Chest discomfort, possible angina
- Chest discomfort, nonanginal
- Dyspepsia/Indigestion

Cirrhosis, Etiology Unknown

Indications and Timing for Referral

- Massive ascites
- Renal dysfunction

Timing: Urgent (less than 24 hours)

- Severe or progressive hepatic decompensation (e.g., mental status changes or coagulopathy)

Timing: Expedited (less than 1 week)

- Etiology unclear
- Patient presenting with esophageal varices or ascites

Timing: Routine (less than 4 weeks)

Advice for Referral

- This condition often requires co-management with a gastroenterologist.

Tests to Prepare for Consult

- CBC with differential
- Platelet count
- Prothrombin time
- Activated PTT
- Albumin, total protein
- BUN, creatinine
- Bilirubin
- Calcium, phosphorus
- Glucose
- ALT, AST, alkaline phosphatase
- Ferritin
- Iron/TIBC
- Hepatitis B surface antibody
- Hepatitis B surface antigen
- Hepatitis C antibody
- Amylase

Tests Not Useful Before Consult

- None

Tests Consultant May Need to Do

- Anti-mitochondrial antibody
- Anti-smooth muscle antibody
- α_1-antitrypsin level
- AFP
- Ceruloplasmin
- Ultrasound with Doppler, liver
- CT scan, abdomen
- Upper endoscopy
- Liver biopsy
- Paracentesis
- Protein, ascitic fluid
- Glucose, ascitic fluid
- Albumin, ascitic fluid
- pH, ascitic fluid
- Cell count, ascitic fluid
- C&S, ascitic fluid
- Gram stain, ascitic fluid
- AFB culture, ascitic fluid
- Fungal culture, ascitic fluid
- Cytology, ascitic fluid
- Amylase, ascitic fluid
- Triglycerides, ascitic fluid

GASTROENTEROLOGY

Cirrhosis, Etiology Unknown (*continued*)

Follow-up Visits Generally Required

- Co-management, see *Advice for Referral*

Suggested Readings

Greeve M, Ferrell L, Kim M, et al. Cirrhosis of undefined pathogenesis: absence of evidence for unknown viruses or autoimmune processes. Hepatology 1993;17:593–598.

Podolsky DK, Isselbacher KJ. Cirrhosis and alcoholic liver disease. In: Fauci AS, Braunwald E, Isselbacher KJ, et al., eds. Harrison's Principles of Internal Medicine. 14th ed. New York: McGraw Hill, 1998:1704–1710.

See Also

- Cirrhosis with complications
- Ascites
- Liver disease in the alcohol drinker

Cirrhosis, Primary Biliary

Indications and Timing for Referral

- Diagnostic uncertainty
- Assistance with management
- Decision-making about liver transplant

Timing: Routine (less than 4 weeks)

Advice for Referral

- This condition often requires co-management with a gastroenterologist.

Tests to Prepare for Consult

- CBC
- Platelet count
- Prothrombin time
- Amylase
- Albumin, total protein
- Bilirubin
- ALT, AST, alkaline phosphatase
- ANA
- Anti-mitochondrial antibody
- TSH

Tests Not Useful Before Consult

- None

Tests Consultant May Need to Do

- ERCP
- Liver biopsy

Follow-up Visits Generally Required

- Co-management, see *Advice for Referral*

Suggested Readings

Kaplan MM. Primary biliary cirrhosis. [Review] [153 refs]. N Engl J Med 1996;335:1570–1580.

Sherlock S. Primary biliary cirrhosis: clarifying the issues. [Review]. Am J Med 1994;96(Suppl 1A):27S–33S.

Khandelwal M, Malet PF. Pruritus associated with cholestasis. A review of pathogenesis and management. [Review]. Dig Dis Sci 1994;39:1–8.

Poupon RE, Poupon R, Balkau B. Ursodiol for the long-term treatment of primary biliary cirrhosis. The UDCA-PBC Study Group [see comments]. N Engl J Med 1994;330:1342–1347.

Laurin JM, DeSotel CK, Jorgensen RA, et al. The natural history of abdominal pain associated with primary biliary cirrhosis. Am J Gastroenterol 1994;89:1840–1843.

See Also

- Cirrhosis, etiology unknown
- Cirrhosis, with complications

GASTROENTEROLOGY

Cirrhosis, with Complications

Indications and Timing for Referral

- Ascites with fever
- Encephalopathy

Timing: Urgent (less than 24 hours)

- Assistance with management of complications (e.g., ascites or esophageal varices)

Timing: Expedited (less than 1 week)

Advice for Referral

- This condition often requires co-management with a gastroenterologist.

Tests to Prepare for Consult

- Glucose
- Albumin, total protein
- Amylase
- BUN, creatinine
- Calcium, phosphorus
- Electrolytes (Na, K, Cl, CO_2)
- Bilirubin
- ALT, AST, alkaline phosphatase
- CBC with differential
- Platelet count
- Prothrombin time

Tests Not Useful Before Consult

- None

Tests Consultant May Need to Do

- Ultrasound with Doppler, liver
- CT scan, abdomen
- Upper endoscopy
- Liver biopsy
- Paracentesis
- Albumin, ascitic fluid
- Cell count, ascitic fluid
- C&S, ascitic fluid
- AFB culture, ascitic fluid
- Amylase, ascitic fluid
- Cytology, ascitic fluid
- Glucose, ascitic fluid
- Fungal culture, ascitic fluid
- Protein, ascitic fluid
- Triglycerides, ascitic fluid
- pH, ascitic fluid
- Gram stain, ascitic fluid

Follow-up Visits Generally Required

- Co-management, see *Advice for Referral*

Suggested Readings

Gannecarrie N, Chastang C, Chapel F, et al. Predictive score for the development of hepatocellular carcinoma and additional value of liver large cell dysplasia in western patients with cirrhosis. Hepatology 1996;23:1112–1118.

Podolsky DK, Isselbacher KJ. Major complications of cirrhosis. In: Fauci AS, Braunwald E, Isselbacher KJ, et al., eds. Harrison's Principles of Internal Medicine. 14th ed. New York: McGraw Hill, 1998:1710–1717.

Selected Guidelines

Consensus statement on indications for liver transplantation: Paris, June 22–23, 1993. Hepatology 1994;20:63S–68S.

See Also

- Cirrhosis, etiology unknown
- Liver disease in the alcohol drinker
- Ascites

THE CONSULTATION GUIDE

Colitis, Infectious

Indications and Timing for Referral

- Diagnostic uncertainty

Timing: Expedited (less than 1 week)

Advice for Referral

- *Clostridium difficile* stool toxin necessary if there has been previous antibiotic use.

Tests to Prepare for Consult

- CBC with differential
- Glucose
- Electrolytes (Na, K, Cl, CO_2)
- BUN, creatinine
- Calcium
- *C. difficile* stool toxin
- Stool O&P
- Stool C&S
- Stool WBC

Tests Not Useful Before Consult

- None

Tests Consultant May Need to Do

- Plain film, abdomen
- Barium enema
- Colonoscopy
- Flexible sigmoidoscopy

Follow-up Visits Generally Required

- One

Suggested Readings

Kelly CP, Pothoulakis C, LaMont JT. *Clostridium difficile* colitis [see comments]. [Review]. N Engl J Med 1994;330:257–262.

Fekety R, Shah AB. Diagnosis and treatment of *Clostridium difficile* colitis [see comments]. [Review]. JAMA 1993;269:71–75.

Pothoulakis C, LaMont JT. *Clostridium difficile* colitis and diarrhea. [Review]. Gastroenterol Clin North Am 1993;22:623–637.

Gerding DN, Brazier JS. Optimal methods for identifying *Clostridium difficile* infections. Clin Infect Dis 1993;16(Suppl 4):S439–S442.

Ramaswamy R, Grover H, Corpuz M, et al. Prognostic criteria in *Clostridium difficile* colitis. Am J Gastroenterol 1996;91:460–464.

Fekety R, DuPont HL, Cooperstock M, et al. Evaluation of new anti-infective drugs for the treatment of antibiotic-associated colitis. Infectious Diseases Society of America and the Food and Drug Administration. Clin Infect Dis 1992;15(Suppl 1):S263–S267.

GASTROENTEROLOGY

Colitis, Ulcerative

Indications and Timing for Referral

- Patients with an initial confirmed diagnosis often benefit from seeing a gastroenterologist for evaluation to develop a long-term management plan
- Diagnostic uncertainty
- Assistance with management

Timing: Routine (less than 4 weeks)

Advice for Referral

- Condition often requires co-management with a gastroenterologist.

Tests to Prepare for Consult

- CBC
- Glucose
- Electrolytes (Na, K, Cl, CO_2)
- Albumin, total protein
- Amylase
- BUN, creatinine
- Calcium, phosphorus
- Bilirubin
- ALT, AST, alkaline phosphatase

Tests Not Useful Before Consult

- None

Tests Consultant May Need to Do

- CBC
- Glucose
- Electrolytes (Na, K, Cl, CO_2)
- Amylase
- Albumin, total protein
- Bilirubin
- BUN, creatinine
- Calcium, phosphorus
- ALT, AST, alkaline phosphatase
- *C. difficile* stool toxin
- Stool C&S
- Stool O&P
- Plain film, abdomen
- Barium enema
- Small bowel follow-through
- Colonoscopy
- Flexible sigmoidoscopy

Follow-up Visits Generally Required

- Co-management, see *Advice for Referral*

Suggested Readings

Hanauer SB. Inflammatory bowel disease [published erratum appears in N Engl J Med 1996;335:143]. [Review] [111 refs]. N Engl J Med 1996;334:841–848.

Cohen RD, Hanauer SB. Surveillance colonoscopy in ulcerative colitis—is the message loud and clear? Am J Gastroenterol 1995;90:2090–2092.

Danzi JT. Extraintestinal manifestations of idiopathic inflammatory bowel disease. [Review]. Arch Intern Med 1988;148:297–302.

Selected Guidelines

Kornbluth A, Sachar DB. Ulcerative colitis practice guidelines in adults. American College of Gastroenterology, Practice Parameters Committee. [Review] [119 refs]. Am J Gastroenterol 1997;92:204–211.

The role of colonoscopy in the management of patients with inflammatory bowel disease. Guidelines for clinical application. Gastrointest Endosc 1988;34(3 Suppl):10S–11S.

See Also

- Crohn's disease, regional ileitis
- Crohn's disease, colitis

Colitis, Ulcerative, History of, Currently Asymptomatic

Indications and Timing for Referral

- Assistance with management

Timing: Routine (less than 4 weeks)

Advice for Referral

- Records of histologic and/or radiologic studies establishing diagnoses are essential.

Tests to Prepare for Consult

- None

Tests Not Useful Before Consult

- None

Tests Consultant May Need to Do

- Glucose
- Albumin, total protein
- Amylase
- Bilirubin
- BUN, creatinine
- Calcium, phosphorus
- ALT, AST, alkaline phosphatase
- CBC
- Barium enema
- Colonoscopy
- Flexible sigmoidoscopy

Follow-up Visits Generally Required

- One

Suggested Readings

Cohen RD, Hanauer SB. Surveillance colonoscopy in ulcerative colitis—is the message loud and clear. Am J Gastroenterol 1995;90:2090–2092.

Bachwich DR, Lichtenstein GR, Traber PG. Cancer in inflammatory bowel disease. [Review]. Med Clin North Am 1994;78:1399–1412.

Hanauer SB. Inflammatory bowel disease [published erratum appears in N Engl J Med 1996;335:143]. [Review] [111 refs]. N Engl J Med 1996;334:841–848.

Selected Guidelines

Practice parameters for the detection of colorectal neoplasms. The American Society of Colon and Rectal Surgeons. Dis Colon Rectum 1992;35:389–390.

GASTROENTEROLOGY

Colon Cancer, Family History of

Indications and Timing for Referral

- All patients should be periodically monitored by colonoscopy for evidence of malignancy, particularly if two first-degree relatives developed cancer before age 50 years

Timing: Routine (less than 4 weeks)

Advice for Referral

- If history of associated polyposis, see *Familial Polyposis*.
- Consideration should be given to having such patients referred to a specialist familiar with estimating genetic risk for colon cancer.

Tests to Prepare for Consult

- CBC
- Stool occult blood ×3

Tests Not Useful Before Consult

- None

Tests Consultant May Need to Do

- Colonoscopy
- Flexible sigmoidoscopy
- Barium enema

Follow-up Visits Generally Required

- One

Suggested Readings

Brewer DA, Fung CL, Chapuis PH, Bokey EL. Should relatives of patients with colorectal cancer be screened? A critical review of the literature. [Review]. Dis Colon Rectum 1994;37:1328–1338.

Fuchs CS, Giovannucci EL, Colditz GA, et al. A prospective study of family history and the risk of colorectal cancer. N Engl J Med 1994;331:1669–1674.

Stephenson BM, Murday VA, Finan PJ, et al. Feasibility of family based screening for colorectal neoplasia: experience in one general surgical practice. Gut 1993;34:96–100.

Rhodes M, Bradburn DM. Overview of screening and management of familial adenomatous polyposis [see comments]. [Review]. Gut 1992;33:125–131.

Fleischer DE, Goldberg SB, Browning TH. Detection and surveillance of colorectal cancer. JAMA 1989;261:580–585.

Selected Guidelines

U. S. Preventive Services Task Force. Screening for colorectal cancer. In: DiGuiseppi C, Atkins D, Woolf S, eds. Guide to Clinical Preventive Services. 2nd ed. Baltimore: Williams & Wilkins, 1996:89–104.

Practice parameters for the detection of colorectal neoplasms. The American Society of Colon and Rectal Surgeons. Dis Colon Rectum 1992;35:389–390.

See Also

- Colorectal cancer, history of
- Polyps, family history of

Colorectal Cancer, History of

Indications and Timing for Referral

- All patients should be periodically monitored by colonoscopy for recurrence

Timing: Routine (less than 4 weeks)

Advice for Referral

- Optimal plan for oncology follow-up is best defined by preliminary discussion with the consultant considering the type and initial stage of disease; time since completion of anti-tumor treatment(s); and potential late complications of therapy.

Tests to Prepare for Consult

- Stool for occult blood
- Carcinoembryonic antigen (CEA)
- Bilirubin
- ALT, AST, alkaline phosphatase
- Chest radiograph
- CBC

Tests Not Useful Before Consult

- None

Tests Consultant May Need to Do

- Barium enema
- Colonoscopy
- Flexible sigmoidoscopy
- CT scan, abdomen

Follow-up Visits Generally Required

- One

Suggested Readings

Toribara NW, Sleisenger MH. Screening for colorectal cancer. [Review]. N Engl J Med 1995;332:861–867.

Vignati PV, Roberts PL. Preoperative evaluation and postoperative surveillance for patients with colorectal carcinoma. [Review]. Surg Clin North Am 1993;73:67–84.

Solomon MJ, McLeod RS. Screening strategies for colorectal cancer. [Review]. Surg Clin North Am 1993;73:31–45.

Fleischer DE, Goldberg SB, Browning TH. Detection and surveillance of colorectal cancer. JAMA 1989;261:580–585.

Selected Guidelines

U. S. Preventive Services Task Force. Screening for colorectal cancer. In: DiGuiseppi C, Atkins D, Woolf S, eds. Guide to Clinical Preventive Services. 2nd ed. Baltimore: Williams & Wilkins, 1996:89–104.

Practice parameters for the detection of colorectal neoplasms. The American Society of Colon and Rectal Surgeons. Dis Colon Rectum 1992;35:389–390.

See Also

- Colon cancer, family history of
- Polyps, family history of

GASTROENTEROLOGY

Constipation

Indications and Timing for Referral

- Recent onset or progressive with unclear etiology

Timing: Routine (less than 4 weeks)

Advice for Referral

- A careful medication history is vital (e.g., calcium channel blockers, laxatives, narcotics, iron supplements, antacids).

Tests to Prepare for Consult

- CBC
- Glucose
- Electrolytes (Na, K, Cl, CO_2)
- Calcium
- TSH
- Stool for occult blood

Tests Not Useful Before Consult

- CT scan, abdomen

Tests Consultant May Need to Do

- Barium enema
- Colonoscopy
- Flexible sigmoidoscopy

Follow-up Visits Generally Required

- One

Suggested Readings

Velio P, Bassotti G. Chronic idiopathic constipation: pathophysiology and treatment. [Review] [92 refs]. J Clin Gastroenterol 1996;22:190–196.

Camilleri M, Thompson WG, Fleshman JW, Pemberton JH. Clinical management of intractable constipation. [Review]. Ann Intern Med 1994;121:520–528.

Moriarty KJ, Irving MH. ABC of colorectal disease. Constipation. [Review]. Br Med J 1992;304:1237–1240.

Wrenn K. Fecal impaction [see comments]. [Review]. N Engl J Med 1989;321:658–662.

See Also

- Tenesmus

Crohn's Disease, Colitis

Indications and Timing for Referral

- Patients with a suspected or confirmed diagnosis often benefit from seeing a gastroenterologist for baseline evaluation

Timing: Routine (less than 4 weeks)

Advice for Referral

- This condition often requires co-management with a gastroenterologist.
- Before consult, old records confirming diagnosis and treatment should be available, including biopsies, radiographic studies, and surgical records.

Tests to Prepare for Consult

- CBC
- Glucose
- Electrolytes (Na, K, Cl, CO_2)
- Amylase
- Albumin, total protein
- BUN, creatinine
- Calcium, phosphorus
- Bilirubin
- ALT, AST, alkaline phosphatase
- Stool C&S
- Stool O&P
- *C. difficile* stool toxin

Tests Not Useful Before Consult

- None

Tests Consultant May Need to Do

- CBC
- Glucose
- Electrolytes (Na, K, Cl, CO_2)
- BUN, creatinine
- Calcium
- *C. difficile* stool toxin
- Stool C&S
- Stool O&P
- Plain film, abdomen
- Ultrasound, abdomen
- CT scan, abdomen
- UGIS
- Small bowel follow-through
- Barium enema
- Colonoscopy
- Flexible sigmoidoscopy

Follow-up Visits Generally Required

- Co-management, see *Advice for Referral*

Suggested Readings

Barnett JL. Medical management of colorectal Crohn's disease. Curr Opin Gastroenterol 1996;12:26–31.

Hanauer SB, Meyers S. Management of Crohn's disease in adults. [Review] [105 refs]. Am J Gastroenterol 1997;92:559–566.

Danzi JT. Extraintestinal manifestations of idiopathic inflammatory bowel disease. [Review]. Arch Intern Med 1988;148:297–302.

Connell WR, Sheffield JP, Kamm MA, et al. Lower gastrointestinal malignancy in Crohn's disease. [Review]. Gut 1994;35:347–352.

Bayless TM. Maintenance therapy for Crohn's disease. Gastroenterology 1996;110:299–302.

See Also

- Crohn's disease, regional ileitis
- Colitis, ulcerative

GASTROENTEROLOGY

Crohn's Disease, Regional Ileitis

Indications and Timing for Referral

- Fever and severe abdominal pain or tender abdominal mass
- Recurrent vomiting with dehydration

Timing: Urgent (less than 24 hours)

- Patients with a suspected or confirmed diagnosis often benefit from seeing a gastroenterologist for baseline evaluation

Timing: Routine (less than 4 weeks)

Advice for Referral

- This condition often requires co-management with a gastroenterologist.
- Before consult, old records confirming diagnosis and treatment should be available, including biopsies, radiographic studies, and surgical records.

Tests to Prepare for Consult

- CBC
- Glucose
- Electrolytes (Na, K, Cl, CO_2)
- Amylase
- Albumin, total protein
- BUN, creatinine
- Calcium, phosphorus
- Bilirubin
- ALT, AST, alkaline phosphatase

Tests Not Useful Before Consult

- None

Tests Consultant May Need to Do

- CBC
- Glucose
- Electrolytes (Na, K, Cl, CO_2)
- BUN, creatinine
- Calcium
- Plain film, abdomen
- Ultrasound, abdomen
- CT scan, abdomen
- UGIS
- Small bowel follow through
- Barium enema
- Colonoscopy

Follow-up Visits Generally Required

- Co-management, see *Advice for Referral*

Suggested Readings

Hanauer SB, Meyers S. Management of Crohn's disease in adults. [Review] [105 refs]. Am J Gastroenterol 1997;92:559–566.

Barnett JL. Medical management of colorectal Crohn's disease. Curr Opin Gastroenterol 1996;12:26–31.

Bayless TM. Maintenance therapy for Crohn's disease. Gastroenterology 1996;110:299–302.

Bernstein D, Rogers A. Malignancy in Crohn's disease [review]. Am J Gastroenterol 1996;91:434–440.

Danzi JT. Extraintestinal manifestations of idiopathic inflammatory bowel disease. [Review]. Arch Intern Med 1988;148:297–302.

Selected Guidelines

The role of colonoscopy in the management of patients with inflammatory bowel disease. Guidelines for clinical application. Gastrointest Endosc 1988;34(3 Suppl):10S–11S.

See Also

- Colitis, ulcerative
- Crohn's disease, colitis

Diarrhea, Chronic

Indications and Timing for Referral

- Blood present in stool
- Persists for more than 10 days
- More than 10 stools per day in frequency

Timing: Expedited (less than 1 week)

Advice for Referral

- Fresh stool specimen needed to assess stool for C&S and O&P.
- *C. difficile* stool toxin required in setting of previous antibiotic use.
- Consultation with a gastroenterologist should generally precede infectious disease consult in the absence of fever or other clinical findings suggesting infection.

Tests to Prepare for Consult

- CBC
- Electrolytes (Na, K, Cl, CO_2)
- Glucose
- BUN, creatinine
- Calcium, phosphorus
- Albumin, total protein
- Stool for occult blood
- Stool C&S
- Stool O&P
- Stool WBC
- *C. difficile* stool toxin
- TSH (assay sensitivity <0.1 mU/L)

Tests Not Useful Before Consult

- Plain film, abdomen
- CT scan, abdomen
- Barium enema
- Small bowel series
- UGIS

Tests Consultant May Need to Do

- CBC
- Electrolytes (Na, K, Cl, CO_2)
- Glucose
- Albumin, total protein
- BUN, creatinine
- Calcium, phosphorus
- Prothrombin time
- *Giardia* antigen
- Stool O&P
- Stool C&S
- Qualitative fecal fat and fiber
- CT scan, abdomen
- UGIS
- Barium enema
- Small bowel follow-through
- Upper endoscopy
- Colonoscopy
- Flexible sigmoidoscopy

GASTROENTEROLOGY

Diarrhea, Chronic (*continued*)

Follow-up Visits Generally Required
- One

Suggested Readings

Donowitz M, Kokke FT, Saidi R. Evaluation of patients with chronic diarrhea. [Review]. N Engl J Med 1995;332:725–729.

Cook GC. Persisting diarrhoea and malabsorption. [Review]. Gut 1994;35:582–586.

Blanshard C, Gazzard BG. Natural history and prognosis of diarrhoea of unknown cause in patients with acquired immunodeficiency syndrome (AIDS). Gut 1995;36:283–286.

Valdovinos MA, Camilleri M, Zimmerman BR. Chronic diarrhea in diabetes mellitus: mechanisms and an approach to diagnosis and treatment. [Review]. Mayo Clin Proc 1993;68:691–702.

Trier JS. Celiac sprue. [Review]. N Engl J Med 1991;325:1709–1719.

Friedman LS, Isselbacher KJ. Diarrhea and constipation. In: Fauci AS, Braunwald E, Isselbacher KJ, et al., eds. Harrison's Principles of Internal Medicine. 14th ed. New York: McGraw Hill, 1998:236–244.

See Also
- Malabsorption
- Steatorrhea

Diverticulitis

Indications and Timing for Referral

- Multiple flares of disease

Timing: Routine (less than 4 weeks)

- Symptoms persist despite medical therapy
- Assistance with management

Timing: Urgent (less than 24 hours)

Advice for Referral

- Old records confirming diagnosis and previous treatment including biopsies, radiographic studies, and surgical records are vital.

Tests to Prepare for Consult

- CBC with differential
- Urinalysis with microscopic

Tests Not Useful Before Consult

- None

Tests Consultant May Need to Do

- CBC with differential
- Urinalysis with microscopic
- Stool C&S
- Plain film, abdomen
- CT scan, abdomen
- Sonogram, abdomen
- Barium enema
- Flexible sigmoidoscopy

Follow-up Visits Generally Required

- Two

Suggested Readings

Jones DJ. ABC of colorectal diseases. Diverticular disease. [Review]. Br Med J 1992;304:1435–1437.

Pohlman T. Diverticulitis. [Review]. Gastroenterol Clin North Am 1988;17:357–385.

Cheskin LJ, Bohlman M, Schuster MM. Diverticular disease in the elderly. [Review]. Gastroenterol Clin North Am 1990;19:391–403.

Smith TR, Cho KC, Morehouse HT, Kratka PS. Comparison of computed tomography and contrast enema evaluation of diverticulitis. Dis Colon Rectum 1990;33:1–6.

Selected Guidelines

Roberts P, Abel M, Rosen L, et al. Practice parameters for sigmoid diverticulitis. The Standards Task Force American Society of Colon and Rectal Surgeons. Dis Colon Rectum 1995;38:125–132.

GASTROENTEROLOGY

Dyspepsia/Indigestion

Indications and Timing for Referral
- Persistent for longer than 8 weeks
- Refractory to routine medical therapy, i.e., antacids and H2-receptor antagonists
- Positive stool occult blood

Timing: Routine (less than 4 weeks)

Advice for Referral
- Ischemic heart disease should be excluded before referral
- Careful medication history is vital (e.g., nonsteroidal anti-inflammatory drugs [NSAIDs], theophylline use)
- In the absence of right upper quadrant pain, ultrasound is unlikely to be helpful

Tests to Prepare for Consult
- CBC
- Electrolytes (Na, K, Cl, CO_2)
- Glucose
- BUN, creatinine
- Albumin, total protein
- Bilirubin
- Calcium, phosphorus
- ALT, AST, alkaline phosphatase
- Amylase

Tests Not Useful Before Consult
- *Helicobacter pylori* serology
- Barium enema
- UGIS
- CT scan, abdomen

Tests Consultant May Need to Do
- UGIS
- Gastric emptying study
- Upper endoscopy

Follow-up Visits Generally Required
- Two

Suggested Readings
Thomson AB. A suggested approach to patients with dyspepsia. [Review] [59 refs]. Can J Gastroenterol 1997;11:135–140.

Camilleri M. Nonulcer dyspepsia: a look into the future. [Review] [75 refs]. Mayo Clin Proc 1996;71:614–622.

Ofman JJ, Etchason J, Fullerton S, et al. Management strategies for *Helicobacter pylori*-seropositive patients with dyspepsia: clinical and economic consequences [see comments]. [Review] [69 refs]. Ann Intern Med 1997;126:280–291.

Schwartz LM, Woloshin S, Welch HG. Trends in diagnostic testing following a national guideline for evaluation of dyspepsia. Arch Intern Med 1996;156:873–875.

Barbara L, Camilleri M, Corinaldesi R, et al. Definition and investigation of dyspepsia. Consensus of an international ad hoc working party [see comments]. [Review]. Dig Dis Sci 1989;34:1272–1276.

Jones R, Lydeard S. Prevalence of symptoms of dyspepsia in the community. Br Med J 1989;298:30–32.

Selected Guidelines
Appropriate Use of Gastrointestinal Endoscopy: a Consensus Statement from the American Society for Gastrointestinal Endoscopy. Manchester, MA: The Society, 1989;11:1995.

See Also
- Esophagitis
- Barrett's esophagus & GERD
- Atypical chest pain, possible GI origin
- Heartburn
- Irritable bowel syndrome

THE CONSULTATION GUIDE

Dyspepsia, Nonulcer and *Helicobacter pylori*-Positive

Indications and Timing for Referral

- Symptoms persist on medical therapy for more than 4 weeks, including antibiotic therapy for *H. pylori*

Timing: Routine (less than 4 weeks)

Tests to Prepare for Consult

- *H. pylori* serology

Tests Not Useful Before Consult

- None

Tests Consultant May Need to Do

- Upper endoscopy

Follow-up Visits Generally Required

- One

Suggested Readings

Lambert JR. The role of *Helicobacter pylori* in nonulcer dyspepsia. A debate—for. [Review]. Gastroenterol Clin North Am 1993;22:141–151.

Talley NJ. The role of *Helicobacter pylori* in nonulcer dyspepsia. A debate—against. [Review]. Gastroenterol Clin North Am 1993;22:153–167.

Ofman JJ, Etchason J, Fullerton S, et al. Management strategies for *Helicobacter pylori*-seropositive patients with dyspepsia: clinical and economic consequences [see comments]. [Review] [69 refs]. Ann Intern Med 1997;126:280–291.

Sheu BS, Lin CY, Lin XZ, et al. Long-term outcome of triple therapy in *Helicobacter pylori*-related nonulcer dyspepsia: a prospective controlled assessment [see comments]. Am J Gastroenterol 1996;91:441–447.

Patchett S, Beattie S, Leen E, et al. Eradicating *Helicobacter pylori* and symptoms of non-ulcer dyspepsia. Br Med J 1991;303:1238–1240.

Selected Guidelines

NIH Consensus Conference. *Helicobacter pylori* in peptic ulcer disease. NIH Consensus Development Panel on *Helicobacter pylori* in Peptic Ulcer Disease [see comments]. JAMA 1994;272:65–69.

See Also

- Peptic ulcer disease, refractory
- Gastric ulcer, by UGIS
- Duodenal ulcer, recurrent
- Peptic ulcer disease, *H. pylori*-negative, persistent symptoms
- Peptic distress, on NSAIDs

GASTROENTEROLOGY

Dysphagia

Indications and Timing for Referral

- Dysphagia associated with solids, particularly if severe and progressive
- Concern about previous episode of acute obstruction
- Rule out esophageal cancer

Timing: Expedited (less than 1 week)

Advice for Referral

- Lower threshold for referral if dysphagia is clinically characterized as proximal (upper) versus distal (lower).
- Lower threshold for referral of dysphagia if symptom is significant and sustained.

Tests to Prepare for Consult

- Barium swallow

Tests Not Useful Before Consult

- Esophageal pH monitoring
- CT or MR, chest

Tests Consultant May Need to Do

- Radiograph, chest, PA and lateral
- Barium swallow
- Cine esophagogram
- Esophageal manometry
- Upper endoscopy

Follow-up Visits Generally Required

- One

Suggested Readings

Hendrix TR. Art and science of history taking in the patient with difficulty swallowing. [Review]. Dysphagia 1993;8:69–73.

Rothstein RD. A systematic approach to the patient with dysphagia. [Review] [9 refs]. Hosp Pract (Off Ed) 1997;32:169–175.

Buchholz DW. Neurogenic dysphagia: what is the cause when the cause is not obvious?. [Review]. Dysphagia 1994;9:245–255.

Logemann JA. Role of the modified barium swallow in management of patients with dysphagia. Otolaryngol Head Neck Surg 1997;116:335–338.

Selected Guidelines

Appropriate Use of Gastrointestinal Endoscopy: a Consensus Statement from the American Society for Gastrointestinal Endoscopy. Manchester, MA: The Society, 1989;11:1995.

An American Gastroenterological Association medical position statement on the clinical use of esophageal manometry. American Gastroenterological Association. Gastroenterology 1994;107:1865.

See Also

- Synonym: difficulty swallowing
- Odynophagia
- Dysphagia or odynophagia in HIV-positive patient

Duodenal Ulcer, Recurrent

Indications and Timing for Referral

- Symptoms refractory to medical therapy, e.g., antacids and H2-receptor antagonists
- *H. pylori* serology negative with recurrent symptoms
- History of treated *H. pylori* in patient with recurrent symptoms
- Assistance with management

Timing: Routine (less than 4 weeks)

Advice for Referral

- *H. pylori* serology not useful for follow-up of previously positive patients.
- Gastrin level should only be obtained after temporary discontinuation of H2 blockers.

Tests to Prepare for Consult

- *H. pylori* serology
- Gastrin

Tests Not Useful Before Consult

- None

Tests Consultant May Need to Do

- Upper endoscopy

Follow-up Visits Generally Required

- One

Suggested Readings

Peura DA. Ulcerogenesis: integrating the roles of *Helicobacter pylori* and acid secretion in duodenal ulcer. [Review] [63 refs]. Am J Gastroenterol 997;92(4:Suppl):8S–13S.

Neil GA. Do ulcers burn out or burn on? Managing duodenal ulcer diathesis in the *Helicobacter pylori* era. Ad Hoc Committee on FDA-Related Matters. [Review] [59 refs]. Am J Gastroenterol 1997;92:387–393.

Armstrong D, Arnold R, Classen M, et al. RUDER—a prospective, two-year, multicenter study of risk factors for duodenal ulcer relapse during maintenance therapy with ranitidine. RUDER Study Group. Dig Dis Sci 1994;39:1425–1433.

Hansson LE, Nyren O, Hsing AW, et al. The risk of stomach cancer in patients with gastric or duodenal ulcer disease [see comments]. N Engl J Med 1996;335:242–249.

Graham DY, Lew GM, Klein PD, et al. Effect of treatment of *Helicobacter pylori* infection on the long-term recurrence of gastric or duodenal ulcer. A randomized, controlled study [see comments]. Ann Intern Med 1992;116:705–708.

Walsh JH, Peterson WL. Drug therapy: The treatment of *Helicobacter pylori* infection in the management of peptic ulcer disease. N Engl J Med 1995;333:984–991.

Selected Guidelines

NIH Consensus Conference. *Helicobacter pylori* in peptic ulcer disease. NIH Consensus Development Panel on *Helicobacter pylori* in Peptic Ulcer Disease [see comments]. JAMA 1994;272:65–69.

Appropriate Use of Gastrointestinal Endoscopy: a Consensus Statement from the American Society for Gastrointestinal Endoscopy. Manchester, MA: The Society, 1989;11:1995.

See Also

- Peptic ulcer disease, *H. pylori*-negative, persistent symptoms
- Peptic distress, on NSAIDs
- Peptic ulcer disease, refractory
- Dyspepsia, nonulcer and *H. pylori*-positive
- Gastric ulcer, by UGIS

GASTROENTEROLOGY

Esophagitis

Indications and Timing for Referral

- Immunosuppressed patient refractory to medical therapy
- Dysphagia to solids

Timing: Expedited (less than 1 week)

- Refractory to primary medical therapy

Timing: Routine (less than 4 weeks)

Advice for Referral

- Careful medication history is vital (e.g., NSAIDs).

Tests to Prepare for Consult

- None

Tests Not Useful Before Consult

- None

Tests Consultant May Need to Do

- UGIS
- Esophageal pH monitoring
- Esophageal manometry
- Upper endoscopy

Follow-up Visits Generally Required

- One

Suggested Readings

Richter JE. Severe reflux esophagitis. [Review]. Gastrointest Endosc Clin N Am 1994;4:677–698.

Boyce HW. Therapeutic approaches to healing esophagitis. [Review] [37 refs]. Am J Gastroenterol 1997;92(4 Suppl):22S–27S.

Heudebert GR, Marks R, Wilcox CM, Centor RM. Choice of long-term strategy for the management of patients with severe esophagitis: a cost-utility analysis. Gastroenterology 1997;112:1078–1086.

Wu WC. Ancillary tests in the diagnosis of gastroesophageal reflux disease. [Review]. Gastrointest Endosc Clin N Am 1990;19:671–682.

Trowers E, Thomas C Jr, Silverstein FE. Chemical- and radiation-induced esophageal injury. [Review]. Gastrointest Endosc Clin N Am 1994;4:657–675.

Sutton FM, Graham DY, Goodgame RW. Infectious esophagitis. [Review]. Gastrointest Endosc Clin N Am 1994;4:713–729.

Dachman AH, Levine MS. Radiology of the esophagus. [Review]. Gastroenterol Clin North Am 1991;20:635–658.

de Caestecker JS, Heading RC. Esophageal pH monitoring. [Review]. Gastroenterol Clin North Am 1990;19:645–669.

Selected Guidelines

The role of endoscopy in the management of esophagitis. Guidelines for clinical application. Gastrointest Endosc 1988;34(3 Suppl):9S.

A standardized protocol for the methodology of esophageal pH monitoring and interpretation of the data for the diagnosis of gastroesophageal reflux. Working Group of the European Society of Pediatric Gastroenterology and Nutrition. J Pediatr Gastroenterol Nutr 1992;14:467–471.

See Also

- Heartburn
- Atypical chest pain, possible GI origin
- Dyspepsia, indigestion
- Barrett's esophagus and GERD

Flatulence, Persistent or Recurrent

Indications and Timing for Referral

- Presents with associated symptoms

Timing: Routine (less than 4 weeks)

Advice for Referral

- Rule out lactose intolerance before referral.
- Careful dietary history is important to exclude sorbitol intake in sugarless candy, heavy bran ingestion, or very high fiber diet.

Tests to Prepare for Consult

- None

Tests Not Useful Before Consult

- Ultrasound, abdomen
- UGIS
- Barium enema
- CT scan, abdomen
- Colonoscopy

Tests Consultant May Need to Do

- Lactose breath test

Follow-up Visits Generally Required

- None

Suggested Readings

Fardy J, Sullivan S. Gastrointestinal gas. [Review]. Can Med Assoc J 1988;139:1137–1142.

Suarez FL, Savaiano DA, Levitt MD. A comparison of symptoms after the consumption of milk or lactose-hydrolyzed milk by people with self-reported severe lactose intolerance [see comments]. N Engl J Med 1995;333:1–4.

Lynn RB, Friedman LS. Irritable bowel syndrome [published erratum appears in N Engl J Med 1994;;330:228] [see comments]. [Review]. N Engl J Med 1993;329:1940–1945.

GASTROENTEROLOGY

Gastric Ulcer, by Upper Gastrointestinal Series

Indications and Timing for Referral

- Patients with a diagnosis of gastric ulcer by UGIS should see a gastroenterologist at least once for baseline evaluation to exclude malignancy

Timing: Routine (less than 4 weeks)

Advice for Referral

- Ascertain history of NSAID use

Tests to Prepare for Consult

- None

Tests Not Useful Before Consult

- Activated PTT
- Prothrombin time
- Platelet count

Tests Consultant May Need to Do

- Upper endoscopy

Follow-up Visits Generally Required

- One

Suggested Readings

Levine MS. Erosive gastritis and gastric ulcers. [Review]. Radiol Clin North Am 1994;32:1203–1214.

Hunt RH. Peptic ulcer disease: defining the treatment strategies in the era of *Helicobacter pylori.* [Review] [56 refs]. Am J Gastroenterol 1997;92(4:Suppl): 36S–40S.

Ott DJ, Chen YM, Gelfand DW, Wu WC. Radiographic efficacy in gastric ulcer: comparison of single-contrast and multiphasic examinations. AJR 1994:697–700.

Koch M, Dezi A, Ferrario F, Capurso I. Prevention of nonsteroidal anti-inflammatory drug-induced gastrointestinal mucosal injury. A meta-analysis of randomized controlled clinical trials [see comments]. Arch Intern Med 1996;156:2321–2332.

Hansson LE, Nyren O, Hsing AW, et al. The risk of stomach cancer in patients with gastric or duodenal ulcer disease [see comments]. N Engl J Med 1996;335:242–249.

Walsh JH, Peterson WL. Drug therapy: The treatment of *Helicobacter pylori* infection in the management of peptic ulcer disease. N Engl J Med 1995;333:984–991.

Selected Guidelines

NIH Consensus Conference. *Helicobacter pylori* in peptic ulcer disease. NIH Consensus Development Panel on *Helicobacter pylori* in Peptic Ulcer Disease [see comments]. JAMA 1994;272:65–69.

Appropriate Use of Gastrointestinal Endoscopy: a Consensus Statement from the American Society for Gastrointestinal Endoscopy. Manchester, MA: The Society, 1989;11:1995.

See Also

- Peptic ulcer disease, refractory
- Duodenal ulcer, recurrent
- Peptic ulcer disease, H. pylori-negative, persistent symptoms
- Peptic distress, on NSAIDs
- Dyspepsia, nonulcer and *H. pylori*-positive

Heartburn

Indications and Timing for Referral

- Immunocompromised patient

Timing: Expedited (less than 1 week)

- Patient has history of collagen vascular disease
- Refractory to routine medical therapy, i.e., antacids and H2-receptor antagonists

Timing: Routine (less than 4 weeks)

Advice for Referral

- Careful medication history is vital (e.g., NSAIDs).

Tests to Prepare for Consult

- None

Tests Not Useful Before Consult

- None

Tests Consultant May Need to Do

- UGIS
- Esophageal pH monitoring
- Upper endoscopy
- Barium swallow

Follow-up Visits Generally Required

- Two

Suggested Readings

Allen ML, Castell JA, DiMarino AJ Jr. Mechanisms of gastroesophageal acid reflux and esophageal acid clearance in heartburn patients. Am J Gastroenterol 1996;91:1739–1744.

DeVault KR, Castell DO. Current diagnosis and treatment of gastroesophageal reflux disease. [Review]. Mayo Clinic Proc 1994;69:867–876.

Howard PJ, Maher L, Pryde A, Heading RC. Symptomatic gastro-oesophageal reflux, abnormal oesophageal acid exposure, and mucosal acid sensitivity are three separate, though related, aspects of gastro-oesophageal reflux disease. Gut 1991;32:128–132.

Wu WC. Ancillary tests in the diagnosis of gastroesophageal reflux disease. [Review]. Gastroenterol Clin North Am 1990;19:671–682.

de Caestecker JS, Heading RC. Esophageal pH monitoring. [Review]. Gastroenterol Clin North Am 1990;19:645–669.

Selected Guidelines

Browning TH. Diagnosis of chest pain of esophageal origin. A guideline of the Patient Care Committee of the American Gastroenterological Association. Dig Dis Sci 1990;35:289–293.

The role of endoscopy in the management of esophagitis. Guidelines for clinical application. Gastrointest Endosc 1988;34(3 Suppl):9S.

A standardized protocol for the methodology of esophageal pH monitoring and interpretation of the data for the diagnosis of gastroesophageal reflux. Working Group of the European Society of Pediatric Gastroenterology and Nutrition. J Pediatr Gastroenterol Nutr 1992;14:467–471.

See Also

- Atypical chest pain, possible GI origin
- Esophagitis
- Dyspepsia, indigestion
- Barrett's esophagus and GERD

GASTROENTEROLOGY

Hematochezia

Indications and Timing for Referral

- No identified benign source of bleeding can be observed
- Concurrent anemia exists
- Family history or past personal history of colon cancer
- Duration of bleeding is greater than 2 months
- Lower threshold to refer patients over age 45 years

Timing: Routine (less than 4 weeks)

Tests to Prepare for Consult

- CBC

Tests Not Useful Before Consult

- None

Tests Consultant May Need to Do

- CBC
- Barium enema
- Colonoscopy
- Flexible sigmoidoscopy
- Proctoscopy

Follow-up Visits Generally Required

- One

Suggested Readings

Friedman LS, Martin P. The problem of gastrointestinal bleeding. [Review]. Gastroenterol Clin North Am 1993;22:717–721.

Wilcox CM, Alexander LN, Cotsonis G. A prospective characterization of upper gastrointestinal hemorrhage presenting with hematochezia. Am J Gastroenterol 1997;92:231–235.

Miller LS, Barbarevech C, Friedman LS. Less frequent causes of lower gastrointestinal bleeding. [Review]. Gastroenterol Clin North Am 1994;23:21–52.

Lewis BS. Small intestinal bleeding. [Review]. Gastroenterol Clin North Am 1994;23:67–91.

Selected Guidelines

The role of endoscopy in the patient with lower gastrointestinal bleeding. Guidelines for clinical application. Gastrointest Endosc 1988;34(3 Suppl):23S–25S.

Appropriate Use of Gastrointestinal Endoscopy: a Consensus Statement from the American Society for Gastrointestinal Endoscopy. Manchester, MA: The Society, 1989;11:1995.

See Also

- Melena, tarry stools, recent history of

THE CONSULTATION GUIDE

Hemochromatosis

Indications and Timing for Referral

- Diagnostic uncertainty in patients and family members
- Initial evaluation of all affected patients
- Assistance with management
- Decision-making about liver transplantation

Timing: Routine (less than 4 weeks)

Advice for Referral

- Diagnosis based on iron binding saturation greater than 60% in males or greater than 50% in females.
- Careful history of previous alcohol intake is important.
- Consideration should be given to human lymphocyte antigen (HLA) typing of patient and family members.
- This condition often requires co-management with a gastroenterologist.

Tests to Prepare for Consult

- CBC
- Prothrombin time
- Platelet count
- Amylase
- Albumin, total protein
- Bilirubin
- ALT, AST, alkaline phosphatase
- Ferritin
- Iron/TIBC
- Glucose

Tests Not Useful Before Consult

- None

Tests Consultant May Need to Do

- LH, FSH
- Testosterone or estradiol
- AFP
- HLA haplotyping
- MR, liver with quantitative iron
- Liver biopsy with iron analysis
- ECG
- Echocardiogram

Follow-up Visits Generally Required

- Co-management, see *Advice for Referral*

Suggested Readings

Bacon BR, Sadiq SA. Hereditary hemochromatosis: presentation and diagnosis in the 1990s. Am J Gastroenterol 1997;92:784–789.

Edwards CQ, Kushner JP. Screening for hemochromatosis [see comments]. [Review]. N Engl J Med 1993;328:1616–1620.

Rouault TA. Hereditary hemochromatosis [clinical conference]. JAMA 1993;269:3152–3154.

Phatak PD, Guzman G, Woll JE, et al. Cost-effectiveness of screening for hereditary hemochromatosis. Arch Intern Med 1994;154:769–776.

Little DR. Hemochromatosis: diagnosis and management [see comments]. [Review] [20 refs]. Am Fam Physician 1996;53:2623–2628.

GASTROENTEROLOGY

Hepatic Cyst, Multiple

Indications and Timing for Referral

- Diagnostic uncertainty

Timing: Routine (less than 4 weeks)

Tests to Prepare for Consult

- Amebic serology

Tests Not Useful Before Consult

- None

Tests Consultant May Need to Do

- ERCP

Follow-up Visits Generally Required

- One

Suggested Readings

Forbes A, Murray-Lyon IM. Cystic disease of the liver and biliary tract. [Review]. Gut 1991;Suppl:S116–S122.

Vauthey JN, Maddern GJ, Blumgart LH. Adult polycystic disease of the liver. [Review]. Br J Surg 1991;78:524–527.

Doty JE, Tompkins RK. Management of cystic disease of the liver. [Review]. Surg Clin North Am 1989;69:285–295.

Everson GT. Hepatic cysts in autosomal dominant polycystic kidney disease [comment]. [Review]. Mayo Clinic Proc 1990;65:1020–1025.

Murphy BJ, Casillas J, Ros PR, Morillo G, et al. The CT appearance of cystic masses of the liver. [Review]. Radiographics 1989;9:307–322.

See Also

- Hepatic mass, solid, on imaging
- Hepatic cyst, solitary

Hepatic Cyst, Solitary

Indications and Timing for Referral

- Cyst is complex with a solid component
- Patient with history of travel to endemic areas for amebiasis

Timing: Routine (less than 4 weeks)

Advice for Referral

- Simple hepatic cysts do not usually require consultation
- AFP only helpful if cyst is solid or complex

Tests to Prepare for Consult

- CBC
- Alpha-fetoprotein (AFP)
- Amebic serology

Tests Not Useful Before Consult

- None

Tests Consultant May Need to Do

- Tagged red cell scan
- MR, liver
- ERCP
- Liver biopsy

Follow-up Visits Generally Required

- One

Suggested Readings

Barreda R, Ros PR. Diagnostic imaging of liver abscess. [Review]. Crit Rev Diagnostic Imaging 1992;33:29–58.

Forbes A, Murray-Lyon IM. Cystic disease of the liver and biliary tract. [Review]. Gut 1991;Suppl:S116–S122.

Doty JE, Tompkins RK. Management of cystic disease of the liver. [Review]. Surg Clin North Am 1989;69:285–295.

Murphy BJ, Casillas J, Ros PR, et al. The CT appearance of cystic masses of the liver. [Review]. Radiographics 1989;9:307–322.

Selected Guidelines

Jacobs WH, Goldberg SB. Statement on outpatient percutaneous liver biopsy. Dig Dis Sci 1989;34:322–323.

See Also

- Hepatomegaly, abdominal mass, RUQ
- Hepatic mass, solid, on imaging
- Hepatic cysts, multiple

GASTROENTEROLOGY

Hepatic Mass, Solid, on Imaging

Indications and Timing for Referral

- Most patients should be seen by a gastroenterologist for consideration of liver biopsy

Timing: Expedited (less than 1 week)

Tests to Prepare for Consult

- AFP
- CBC
- Glucose
- BUN, creatinine
- Calcium
- Electrolytes (Na, K, Cl, CO_2)
- CEA

Tests Not Useful Before Consult

- None

Tests Consultant May Need to Do

- 5′-HIAA, 24-hour urine
- Tagged red cell scan
- Hepatitis B surface antibody
- Hepatitis B surface antigen
- Hepatitis C antibody
- MR, liver
- Liver biopsy

Follow-up Visits Generally Required

- One

Suggested Readings

Rubin RA, Mitchell DG. Evaluation of the solid hepatic mass. [Review] [114 refs]. Med Clin North Am 1996;80:907–928.

Reddy KR, Schiff ER. Approach to a liver mass. [Review]. Semin Liver Dis 1993;13:423–435.

Houn HY, Sanders MM, Walker EM Jr, Pappas AA. Fine needle aspiration in the diagnosis of liver neoplasms: a review. [Review]. Ann Clin Lab Sci 1991;21:2–11.

Halvorsen RA Jr, Thompson WM. Imaging primary and metastatic cancer of the liver. [Review]. Semin Oncol 1991;18:111–122.

Drane WE. Nuclear medicine techniques for the liver and biliary system. Update for the 1990s. [Review]. Radiol Clin North Am 1991;29:1129–1150.

Selected Guidelines

Jacobs WH, Goldberg SB. Statement on outpatient percutaneous liver biopsy. Dig Dis Sci 1989;34:322–323.

See Also

- Hepatomegaly, abdominal mass, RUQ
- Hepatic cysts, solitary
- Hepatic cysts, multiple

THE CONSULTATION GUIDE

Hepatitis, Autoimmune

Indications and Timing for Referral

- Diagnostic uncertainty
- Assistance with management
- Decision-making about liver transplant

Timing: Routine (less than 4 weeks)

Advice for Referral

- This condition often requires co-management with a gastroenterologist.

Tests to Prepare for Consult

- CBC
- Platelet count
- Prothrombin time
- Albumin, total protein
- Amylase
- Bilirubin
- ALT, AST, alkaline phosphatase
- Antismooth muscle antibody
- ANA
- TSH (assay sensitivity <0.1 mU/L)

Tests Not Useful Before Consult

- None

Tests Consultant May Need to Do

- Anti-LKM antibody
- Quantitative immunoglobulins
- Liver biopsy

Follow-up Visits Generally Required

- Co-management, see *Advice for Referral*

Suggested Readings

Krawitt EL. Autoimmune hepatitis. [Review] [79 refs]. N Engl J Med 1996;334:897–903.

Czaja AJ. Diagnosis and therapy of autoimmune liver disease. [Review] [100 refs]. Med Clin North Am 1996;80:973–994.

Krawitt EL. Autoimmune hepatitis: classification, heterogeneity, and treatment. [Review]. Am J Med 1994;96(Suppl 1A):23S–26S.

Czaja AJ. Autoimmune hepatitis. Evolving concepts and treatment strategies. [Review]. Dig Dis Sci 1995;40:435–456.

214

GASTROENTEROLOGY

Hepatitis, Exposure to

Indications and Timing for Referral

- Assistance with decisions regarding prophylaxis

Timing: Urgent (less than 24 hours)

Advice for Referral

- Status of the exposer's HB$_s$Ag and HB$_s$Ab need to be available before consultant visit.
- It is also important to determine the status of the exposer's hepatitis C antibody.

Tests to Prepare for Consult

- None

Tests Not Useful Before Consult

- None

Tests Consultant May Need to Do

- Albumin, total protein
- Amylase
- Bilirubin
- ALT, AST, alkaline phosphatase
- Hepatitis B surface antigen
- Hepatitis B surface antibody

Follow-up Visits Generally Required

- Two

Suggested Readings

Delamothe T. Hepatitis B and exposure prone procedures [editorial]. Br Med J 1994;309:73–74.

Strader DB, Seeff LB. New hepatitis a vaccines and their role in prevention [review]. Drugs 1996;51:359–366.

Selected Guidelines

Hepatitis C virus: guidance on the risks and current management of occupational exposure. PHLS Hepatitis Subcommittee. [Review]. Communicable Disease Report 1994;CDR(10):R135–R139.

See Also

- Hepatitis B
- Hepatitis C
- Hepatitis D

THE CONSULTATION GUIDE

Hepatitis B

Indications and Timing for Referral

- Evidence of severe or progressive hepatic decompensation (e.g., recent onset of mental status change, ascites, coagulopathy, or transaminase level higher than 1000)

Timing: Urgent (less than 24 hours) or Expedited (less than 1 week)

- Diagnostic uncertainty
- Management of chronic active hepatitis
- Decision-making about liver transplantation
- Assistance with contact management

Timing: Routine (less than 4 weeks)

Tests to Prepare for Consult

- CBC
- Platelet count
- Prothrombin time
- Amylase
- Albumin, total protein
- Bilirubin
- ALT, AST, alkaline phosphatase
- Hepatitis B surface antigen
- Hepatitis E antigen
- Hepatitis E antibody

Tests Not Useful Before Consult

- Hepatitis B core antibody

Tests Consultant May Need to Do

- Hepatitis B core antibody
- Hepatitis D antibody
- Alpha-fetoprotein
- Liver biopsy

Follow-up Visits Generally Required

- Two

Suggested Readings

Trepo C, Zoulim F, Alonso C, et al. Diagnostic markers of viral hepatitis B and C. [Review]. Gut 1993;34(2:Suppl):S20–S25.

Perrillo RP. The management of chronic hepatitis B. [Review]. Am J Med 1994;96(Suppl 1A):34S–39S.

Schmilovitz-Weiss H, Levy M, Thompson N, Dusheiko G. Viral markers in the treatment of hepatitis B and C. [Review]. Gut 1993;34(2:Suppl):S26–S35.

Sherlock S. Viruses and hepatocellular carcinoma. [Review]. Gut 1994;35:828–832.

Selected Guidelines

Screening for hepatitis B. In: U. S. Preventive Services Task Force Guide to Clinical Preventive Services: An Assessment of the Effectiveness of 169 Interventions: Report of the U. S. Preventive Services Task Force. Baltimore: Williams & Wilkins, 1989: 121–124; 1995; U. S. Preventive Serv-4.

See Also

- Hepatitis D
- Jaundice/hyperbilirubinemia
- Transaminase elevation
- Hepatitis C

Hepatitis C

Indications and Timing for Referral

- Evidence of severe or progressive hepatic decompensation (e.g., mental status change, ascites, coagulopathy, or transaminase elevation higher than 1000)

Timing: Urgent (less than 24 hours) or Expedited (less than 1 week)

- Diagnostic uncertainty
- Assistance with contact management
- Management of chronic hepatitis C
- Decision-making about liver transplantation

Timing: Routine (less than 4 weeks)

Tests to Prepare for Consult

- CBC
- Platelet count
- Prothrombin time
- Albumin, total protein
- Amylase
- Bilirubin
- ALT, AST, alkaline phosphatase
- Hepatitis C antibody

Tests Not Useful Before Consult

- None

Tests Consultant May Need to Do

- Hepatitis C, PCR
- Hepatitis C genotype
- Liver biopsy

Follow-up Visits Generally Required

- Two

Suggested Readings

Weiss JB Jr, Persing DH. Hepatitis C: advances in diagnosis. [Review]. Mayo Clin Proc 1995;70:296–297.

Gumber SC, Chopra S. Hepatitis C: A multifaceted disease. Review of extrahepatic manifestations. Ann Intern Med 1995;123:615–620.

Roggendorf M, Lu M, Meisel H, et al. Rational use of diagnostic tools in hepatitis C. [Review] [68 refs]. J Hepatol 1996;24(2:Suppl):26–34.

Neiblum DR, Boynton RF. Evaluation and treatment of chronic hepatitis C infection. [Review] [65 refs]. Prim Care 1996;23:535–549.

Rubin RA, Falestiny M, Malet PF. Chronic hepatitis C. Advances in diagnostic testing and therapy. [Review]. Arch Intern Med 1994;154:387–392.

Trepo C, Zoulim F, Alonso C, et al. Diagnostic markers of viral hepatitis B and C. [Review]. Gut 1993;34(2:Suppl):S20–S25.

Selected Guidelines

Hepatitis C virus: guidance on the risks and current management of occupational exposure. PHLS Hepatitis Subcommittee. [Review]. Communicable Disease Report 1994;CDR(10):R135–R139.

See Also

- Hepatitis D
- Hepatitis B
- Transaminase elevation
- Jaundice/hyperbilirubinemia

Hepatitis D

Indications and Timing for Referral

- Evidence of severe or progressive hepatic decompensation (e.g., mental status change, ascites, coagulopathy, or transaminase elevation higher than 1000)

Timing: Urgent (less than 24 hours) or Expedited (less than 1 week)

- Diagnostic uncertainty
- Assistance with management
- Decision-making about liver transplantation

Timing: Routine (less than 4 weeks)

Tests to Prepare for Consult

- CBC
- Platelet count
- Prothrombin time
- Albumin, total protein
- Amylase
- Bilirubin
- ALT, AST, alkaline phosphatase
- Hepatitis B surface antigen
- Hepatitis B surface antibody
- Hepatitis D antibody
- Hepatitis E antibody
- Hepatitis E antigen

Tests Not Useful Before Consult

- None

Tests Consultant May Need to Do

- Liver biopsy

Follow-up Visits Generally Required

- Two

Suggested Readings

Keitel W. Hepatitis delta virus—an important human pathogen. Clin Infect Dis 1996;22:605.

Polish LB, Gallagher M, Fields HA, Hadler SC. Delta hepatitis: molecular biology and clinical and epidemiological features. [Review]. Clinical Microbiol Rev 1993;6:211–229.

Wu JC, Chen CM, Chen TZ, et al. Prevalence and type of precore hepatitis b virus mutants in hepatitis d virus superinfection and its clinical implications. J Infect Dis 1996;173:457–459.

See Also

- Jaundice/hyperbilirubinemia
- Transaminase elevation
- Hepatitis B
- Hepatitis C

GASTROENTEROLOGY

Hepatomegaly/Abdominal Mass, Right Upper Quadrant

Indications and Timing for Referral

- Diagnostic uncertainty

Timing: Expedited (less than 1 week)

Tests to Prepare for Consult

- Amylase
- Albumin, total protein
- Bilirubin
- ALT, AST, alkaline phosphatase
- CBC
- Urinalysis with microscopic
- Ultrasound or CT, abdomen

Tests Not Useful Before Consult

- None

Tests Consultant May Need to Do

- Glucose
- Calcium
- BUN, creatinine
- Electrolytes (Na, K, Cl, CO_2)
- Alpha-fetoprotein (AFP)
- Echinococcal IgM
- Ultrasound, abdomen
- MR, abdomen
- Barium enema
- Colonoscopy
- ERCP
- Liver biopsy

Follow-up Visits Generally Required

- Two

Suggested Readings

Naylor CD. Physical examination of the liver. JAMA 1994;271:1859–1865.

Barker CS, Lindsell DR. Ultrasound of the palpable abdominal mass. Clin Radiol 1990;41:98–99.

Meidl EJ, Ende J. Evaluation of liver size by physical examination. J Gen Intern Med 1993;8:635–637.

Abdomen. In: Willms JL, Schniederman H, Algranati PS, eds. Physical Diagnosis: Bedside Evaluation of Diagnosis and Function. Baltimore: Williams & Wilkins, 1994:347–386.

See Also

- Right upper quadrant pain, intermittent
- Hepatic mass, solid, on imaging
- Hepatic cyst, solitary

Hyperamylasemia

Indications and Timing for Referral

- Clinical evidence of possible bowel ischemia

Timing: Urgent (less than 24 hours)

- Other evidence of intra-abdominal disease
- Evidence of chronic pancreatitis of uncertain etiology, such as
  - Urine amylase also abnormal
  - Amylase elevated twice normal level in patients with normal renal function
  - Lipase level concurrently elevated

Timing: Routine (less than 4 weeks)

Advice for Referral

- Consider salivary gland disease

Tests to Prepare for Consult

- Amylase
- Amylase, urine
- Glucose
- Lipase
- Bilirubin
- Albumin, total protein
- ALT, AST, alkaline phosphatase
- Creatinine

Tests Not Useful Before Consult

- None

Tests Consultant May Need to Do

- None

Follow-up Visits Generally Required

- None

Suggested Readings

Panteghini M, Pagani F. Clinical evaluation of an algorithm for the interpretation of hyperamylasemia. Arch Pathol Lab Med 1991;115(4):355–358.

Pieper-Bigelow C, Strocchi A, Levitt MD. Where does serum amylase come from and where does it go?. [Review]. Gastroenterol Clin North Am 1990;19:793–810.

Winslet M, Hall C, London NJ, Neoptolemos JP. Relation of diagnostic serum amylase levels to aetiology and severity of acute pancreatitis [see comments]. Gut 1992;33:982–986.

See Also

- Pancreatitis, chronic or recurrent

GASTROENTEROLOGY

Irritable Bowel Syndrome

Indications and Timing for Referral

- Diagnostic uncertainty
- Symptoms uncontrolled by previous medical therapy
- Progression of symptoms
- Associated weight loss
- Presence of occult stool blood

Timing: Routine (less than 4 weeks)

Advice for Referral

- *C. difficile* stool toxin necessary only if there is previous antibiotic use.
- Ascertain lactose, sorbitol intake.

Tests to Prepare for Consult

- CBC
- Calcium
- TSH (assay sensitivity <0.1 mU/L)
- Stool for occult blood
- Stool O&P
- *C. difficile* stool toxin

Tests Not Useful Before Consult

- None

Tests Consultant May Need to Do

- Lactose breath test
- Barium enema
- Small bowel follow through
- UGIS
- Colonoscopy
- Flexible sigmoidoscopy

Follow-up Visits Generally Required

- One

Suggested Readings

Lynn RB, Friedman LS. Irritable bowel syndrome [published erratum appears in N Engl J Med 1994;330:228] [see comments]. [Review]. N Engl J Med 1993;329:1940–1945.

Thompson WG, Gick M. Irritable bowel syndrome. [Review] [142 refs]. Semin Gastrointest Dis 1996;7:217–229.

Schuster MM. Diagnostic evaluation of the irritable bowel syndrome. [Review]. Gastroenterol Clin North Am 1991;20:269–278.

Camilleri M, Prather CM. The irritable bowel syndrome: mechanisms and a practical approach to management [see comments]. [Review]. Ann Intern Med 1992;116:1001–1008.

Drossman DA, Thompson WG. The irritable bowel syndrome: review and a graduated multicomponent treatment approach [see comments]. [Review]. Ann Intern Med 1992;116:1009–1016.

Friedman G. Diet and the irritable bowel syndrome. [Review]. Gastroenterol Clin North Am 1991;20:313–324.

Whitehead WE, Crowell MD. Psychologic considerations in the irritable bowel syndrome. [Review]. Gastroenterol Clin North Am 1991;20:249–267.

See Also

- Dyspepsia, indigestion

THE CONSULTATION GUIDE

Jaundice/Hyperbilirubinemia

Indications and Timing for Referral

- Severe RUQ pain
- Associated fever
- Bilirubin greater than 10 mg/dL
- Elevated prothrombin time

Timing: Urgent (less than 24 hours)

- Diagnostic uncertainty after initial testing

Timing: Routine (less than 4 weeks)

Advice for Referral

- Complete medication history is vital.

Tests to Prepare for Consult

- CBC
- Prothrombin time
- Glucose
- Electrolytes (Na, K, Cl, CO_2)
- BUN, creatinine
- Albumin, total protein
- Calcium, phosphorus
- Amylase
- Bilirubin
- ALT, AST, alkaline phosphatase

Tests Not Useful Before Consult

- None

Tests Consultant May Need to Do

- Amylase
- Albumin, total protein
- Bilirubin
- ALT, AST, alkaline phosphatase
- Iron/TIBC
- Ferritin
- Acetaminophen level
- Ceruloplasmin
- Antismooth muscle antibody

- Antimitochondrial antibody
- ANA
- Hepatitis A antibody, IgM specific
- Hepatitis B surface antigen
- Hepatitis B surface antibody
- Hepatitis C, PCR
- Hepatitis C antibody
- Ultrasound, abdomen
- Ultrasound, liver and pancreas
- Percutaneous transhepatic cholangiogram
- ERCP

Follow-up Visits Generally Required

- Two

Suggested Readings

Kaplan LM, Isselbacher KJ. Jaundice. In: Fauci AS, Braunwald E, Isselbacher KJ, et al., eds. Harrison's Principles of Internal Medicine. 14th ed. New York: McGraw Hill, 1998:249–255.

Selected Guidelines

Frank BB. Clinical evaluation of jaundice. A guideline of the Patient Care Committee of the American Gastroenterological Association [see comments]. [Review]. JAMA 1989;262:3031–3034.

See Also

- Hepatitis B
- Hepatitis C
- Alkaline phosphatase, elevated
- Hepatitis D
- Transaminase elevation

GASTROENTEROLOGY

Liver Disease in the Alcohol Drinker

Indications and Timing for Referral

- Evidence of severe or progressive hepatic decompensation (e.g., recent onset of mental status change, ascites, coagulopathy, or transaminase level greater than 1000)

Timing: Urgent (less than 24 hours) or Expedited (less than 1 week)

- Etiology of hepatic dysfunction uncertain

Timing: Routine (less than 4 weeks)

Tests to Prepare for Consult

- CBC
- Glucose
- Amylase
- Albumin, total protein
- Bilirubin
- BUN, creatinine
- Calcium, phosphorus
- Electrolytes (Na, K, Cl, CO_2)
- ALT, AST, alkaline phosphatase
- Iron/TIBC
- Ferritin
- 5'-nucleotidase or GGT
- Prothrombin time
- Platelet count

Tests Not Useful Before Consult

- None

Tests Consultant May Need to Do

- Anti-smooth muscle antibody
- Hepatitis B surface antibody
- Hepatitis B surface antigen
- Hepatitis C antibody
- Liver biopsy

Follow-up Visits Generally Required

- One

Suggested Readings

Lieber CS. Alcohol and the liver: 1994 update. [Review]. Gastroenterology 1994;106:1085–1105.

Day CP, Bassendine MF. Genetic predisposition to alcoholic liver disease. [Review]. Gut 1992;33:1444–1447.

Lucey MR. Liver transplantation for the alcoholic patient. [Review]. Gastroenterologist 1993;22:243–256.

Kamath PS. Clinical approach to the patient with abnormal liver test results. [Review]. Mayo Clin Proc 1996;71:1089–1094.

See Also

- Cirrhosis, etiology unknown
- Cirrhosis with complications

Malabsorption

Indications and Timing for Referral

- Etiology uncertain after initial testing

Timing: Routine (less than 4 weeks)

Tests to Prepare for Consult

- CBC
- Electrolytes (Na, K, Cl, CO_2)
- Glucose
- Albumin, total protein
- BUN, creatinine
- Amylase
- Bilirubin
- ALT, AST, alkaline phosphatase
- Prothrombin time
- Calcium
- Qualitative fecal fat and fiber
- D-xylose test

Tests Not Useful Before Consult

- Small bowel series

Tests Consultant May Need to Do

- Plain film, abdomen
- CT scan, abdomen
- Lactulose breath test
- Ultrasound, pancreas
- Small bowel series
- Upper endoscopy
- ERCP

Follow-up Visits Generally Required

- Two

Suggested Readings

Cook GC. Persisting diarrhoea and malabsorption. [Review]. Gut 1994;35:582–586.

Brasitus TA, Sitrin MD. Intestinal malabsorption syndromes. [Review]. Annu Rev Med 1990;41:339–347.

Misra S, Ament ME. Diagnosis of coeliac sprue in 1994. [Review]. Gastroenterol Clin North Am 1995;24:133–143.

Trier JS. Celiac sprue. [Review]. N Engl J Med 1991;325:1709–1719.

Greenberger MJ, Isselbacher KJ. Disorders of absorption. In: Fauci AS, Braunwald E, Isselbacher KJ, et al., eds. Harrison's Principles of Internal Medicine. 14th ed. New York: McGraw Hill, 1998:1616–1633.

See Also

- Diarrhea, chronic
- Steatorrhea

GASTROENTEROLOGY

Melena, Tarry Stools, Recent History of

Indications and Timing for Referral

- Evidence of significant blood loss

Timing: Immediate

- Patients who have no established diagnosis
- Patients with known peptic ulcer or liver disease

Timing: Urgent (less than 24 hours)

Advice for Referral

- Ascertain history of NSAID use.

Tests to Prepare for Consult

- CBC
- BUN, creatinine

Tests Not Useful Before Consult

- None

Tests Consultant May Need to Do

- Barium enema
- Colonoscopy
- Upper endoscopy

Follow-up Visits Generally Required

- One

Suggested Readings

Richter JM. Occult gastrointestinal bleeding. [Review]. Gastroenterol Clin North Am 1994;23:53–66.

Selected Guidelines

The role of endoscopy in the patient with lower gastrointestinal bleeding. Guidelines for clinical application. Gastrointest Endosc 1988;34(3 Suppl):23S–25S.

Rosen L, Abel ME, Gordon PH, et al. Practice parameters for the detection of colorectal neoplasms—supporting documentation. The Standards Task Force. American Society of Colon and Rectal Surgeons. Dis Colon Rectum 1992;35:391–394.

Appropriate Use of Gastrointestinal Endoscopy: a Consensus Statement from the American Society for Gastrointestinal Endoscopy. Manchester, MA: The Society, 1989;11:1995.

See Also

- Hematochezia

THE CONSULTATION GUIDE

Nausea, Persistent or Recurrent

Indications and Timing for Referral

- Diagnosis uncertain after initial evaluation
- Presentation with associated clinical manifestations of systemic disease
- Multiple flares that require unscheduled office visits
- Nausea persisting for longer than 4 weeks

Timing: Routine (less than 4 weeks)

Advice for Referral

- Careful medication history is vital, e.g., NSAIDs, theophylline, digoxin, opiates.
- Rule out pregnancy if appropriate.

Tests to Prepare for Consult

- CBC
- Electrolytes (Na, K, Cl, CO_2)
- Glucose
- BUN, creatinine
- Amylase
- ALT, AST, alkaline phosphatase
- Albumin, total protein
- Bilirubin
- Calcium, phosphorus

Tests Not Useful Before Consult

- CT scan, abdomen
- MR, abdomen
- Ultrasound, abdomen
- Ultrasound, biliary

Tests Consultant May Need to Do

- Ultrasound, abdomen
- Ultrasound, biliary
- UGIS
- CT scan, abdomen
- Gastric emptying study
- Upper endoscopy

Follow-up Visits Generally Required

- One

Suggested Readings

Katelaris PH, Jones DB. Chronic nausea and vomiting. [Review]. Dig Dis 1989;7:324–333.

Brzana RJ, Koch KL. Gastroesophageal reflux disease presenting with intractable nausea. Ann Intern Med 1997;126:704–707.

Kerlin P. Postprandial antral hypomotility in patients with idiopathic nausea and vomiting. Gut 1989;30:54–59.

Friedman LS, Isselbacher KJ. Nausea, vomiting, and indigestion. In: Fauci AS, Braunwald E, Isselbacher KJ, et al., eds. Harrison's Principles of Internal Medicine. 14th ed. New York: McGraw Hill, 1998:230–236.

Selected Guidelines

Appropriate Use of Gastrointestinal Endoscopy: a Consensus Statement from the American Society for Gastrointestinal Endoscopy. Manchester, MA: The Society, 1989;11:1995.

See Also

- Vomiting, persistent or recurrent

GASTROENTEROLOGY

Odynophagia

Indications and Timing for Referral

- Clinical suspicion of presence of foreign body

Timing: Immediate

- Immunocompromised patient

Timing: Expedited (less than 1 week)

- Failure of H2-blocker therapy
- Sustained symptoms
- Primary complaint without other symptoms of reflux

Timing: Routine (less than 4 weeks)

Advice for Referral

- If patient immunocompromised, perform pharyngeal swab for potassium hydroxide (KOH) prep.
- If patient immunocompromised and KOH-positive, refer if empiric therapy unsuccessful.

Tests to Prepare for Consult

- None

Tests Not Useful Before Consult

- CT or MR, chest
- CT or MR, neck

Tests Consultant May Need to Do

- Radiograph, chest, PA and lateral
- Barium swallow
- Cine esophagogram
- Esophageal manometry
- Upper endoscopy

Follow-up Visits Generally Required

- One

Suggested Readings

Cooper GS. Indications and contraindications for upper gastrointestinal endoscopy. [Review]. Gastrointest Endosc Clin N Am 1994;4:439–454.

Brady PG. Esophageal foreign bodies. [Review]. Gastroenterol Clin North Am 1991;20:691–701.

Frantz TD, Rasgon BM, Quesenberry CP Jr. Acute epiglottitis in adults. Analysis of 129 cases. JAMA 1994;272:1358–1360.

Wilcox CM. Esophageal disease in the acquired immunodeficiency syndrome: etiology, diagnosis, and management [see comments]. [Review]. Am J Med 1992;92:412–421.

Selected Guidelines

Browning TH. Diagnosis of chest pain of esophageal origin. A guideline of the Patient Care Committee of the American Gastroenterological Association. Dig Dis Sci 1990;35:289–293.

An American Gastroenterological Association medical position statement on the clinical use of esophageal manometry. American Gastroenterological Association. Gastroenterology 1994;107:1865.

Appropriate Use of Gastrointestinal Endoscopy: a Consensus Statement from the American Society for Gastrointestinal Endoscopy. Manchester, MA: The Society, 1989;11:1995.

Goyal RK. Dysphagia. In: Fauci AS, Braunwald E, Isselbacher KJ, et al., eds. Harrison's Principles of Internal Medicine. 14th ed. New York: McGraw Hill, 1998: 228–230.

See Also

- Dysphagia
- Dysphagia or odynophagia in HIV-positive patient
- Synonym: painful swallowing

THE CONSULTATION GUIDE

Pancreatic Mass, Cystic, on Radiograph

Indications and Timing for Referral

- Diagnostic uncertainty
- Assistance with selection of optimal procedure(s) for diagnosis

Timing: Expedited (less than 1 week)

Tests to Prepare for Consult

- Ultrasound or CT, abdomen

Tests Not Useful Before Consult

- None

Tests Consultant May Need to Do

- Amylase
- CA19-9
- CT scan, abdomen
- Endoscopic ultrasound
- ERCP
- Needle biopsy

Follow-up Visits Generally Required

- One

Suggested Readings

Yeo CJ, Sarr MG. Cystic and pseudocystic diseases of the pancreas. [Review]. Curr Probl Surg 1994;31:165–243.

Adler J, Barkin JS. Management of pseudocysts, inflammatory masses, and pancreatic ascites. [Review]. Gastroenterol Clin North Am 1990;19:863–871.

Yang EY, Joehl RJ, Talamonti MS. Cystic neoplasms of the pancreas. [Review]. J Am College Surg 1994;179:747–757.

Ros PR, Hamrick-Turner JE, Chiechi MV, et al. Cystic masses of the pancreas. [Review]. Radiographics 1992;12:673–686.

See Also

- Pancreatitis, chronic or recurrent
- Transaminase elevation
- Pancreatic mass, solid, on radiograph

GASTROENTEROLOGY

Pancreatic Mass, Solid, on Radiograph

Indications and Timing for Referral

- Diagnostic uncertainty
- Assistance with selection of optimal procedure(s) for diagnosis

Timing: Expedited (less than 1 week)

Tests to Prepare for Consult

- Ultrasound or CT, abdomen

Tests Not Useful Before Consult

- None

Tests Consultant May Need to Do

- Needle biopsy
- Insulin
- Glucose
- Gastrin
- Pancreatic polypeptide
- Vasoactive intestinal peptide (VIP)
- CA19-9
- CT scan, abdomen
- Endoscopic ultrasound
- ERCP

Follow-up Visits Generally Required

- One

Suggested Readings

Nakaizumi A, Uehara H, Iishi H, et al. Endoscopic ultrasonography in diagnosis and staging of pancreatic cancer. Dig Dis Sci 1995;40:696–700.

Brandt KR, Charboneau JW, Stephens DH, et al. CT- and US-guided biopsy of the pancreas [see comments]. Radiology 1993;187:99–104.

Freeny PC. Radiologic diagnosis and staging of pancreatic ductal adenocarcinoma. [Review]. Radiol Clin North Am 1989;27:121–128.

Selected Guidelines

Screening for pancreatic cancer. In: U. S. Preventive Services Task Force Guide to Clinical Preventive Services: An Assessment of the Effectiveness of 169 Interventions: Report of the U. S. Preventive Services Task Force. Baltimore: Williams & Wilkins, 1989:87–89; 1995; U. S. Preventive Serv-9.

See Also

- Pancreatic mass, cystic, on radiograph
- Transaminase elevation

THE CONSULTATION GUIDE

Pancreatitis, Chronic or Recurrent

Indications and Timing for Referral

- Etiology unclear
- Assistance with management

Timing: Routine (less than 4 weeks)

Advice for Referral

- This condition may require co-management with a gastroenterologist.

Tests to Prepare for Consult

- CBC with differential
- Electrolytes (Na, K, Cl, CO_2)
- Albumin, total protein
- BUN, creatinine
- Calcium, phosphorus
- Glucose
- Bilirubin
- ALT, AST, alkaline phosphatase
- Amylase
- Lipase
- Triglycerides
- Iron/TIBC
- Prothrombin time
- Qualitative fecal fat and fiber
- Plain film, abdomen
- Ultrasound, abdomen

Tests Not Useful Before Consult

- None

Tests Consultant May Need to Do

- Amylase
- Lipase
- Ultrasound, abdomen
- CT scan, abdomen
- Endoscopic ultrasound
- ERCP

Follow-up Visits Generally Required

- Co-management, see *Advice for Referral*

Suggested Readings

Bank S, Chow KW. Diagnostic tests in chronic pancreatitis. [Review]. Gastroenterologist 1994;2:224–232.

Gullo L. Chronic pancreatitis and pancreatic cancer. Gastroenterology 1996;110:968–969.

Pedersen NT, Worning H. Chronic pancreatitis. Scan J Gastroenterol 1996;31(Suppl 216):52–58.

Ammann RW. Chronic pancreatitis in the elderly. [Review]. Gastroenterol Clin North Am 1990;19:905–914.

Panteghini M, Pagani F. Clinical evaluation of an algorithm for the interpretation of hyperamylasemia. Arch Pathol Lab Med 1991;115:355–358.

Greenberger MJ, Toskes PP, Isselbacher KJ. Acute and chronic pancreatitis. In: Fauci AS, Braunwald E, Isselbacher KJ, et al., eds. Harrison's Principles of Internal Medicine. 14th ed. New York: McGraw Hill, 1998:1741–1752.

See Also

- Hyperamylasemia
- Abdominal mass, epigastric

GASTROENTEROLOGY

Peptic Distress, on Nonsteroidal Anti-Inflammatory Drugs

Indications and Timing for Referral

- Symptoms persistent for longer than 4 weeks and patient unable to discontinue NSAIDs

Timing: Routine (less than 4 weeks)

Tests to Prepare for Consult

- None

Tests Not Useful Before Consult

- UGIS

Tests Consultant May Need to Do

- Upper endoscopy

Follow-up Visits Generally Required

- None

Suggested Readings

Kurata JH, Nogawa AN. Meta-analysis of risk factors for peptic ulcer. Nonsteroidal antiinflammatory drugs, *Helicobacter pylori*, and smoking. J Clin Gastroenterol 1997;24:2–17.

Graham DY. Nonsteroidal anti-inflammatory drugs, *Helicobacter pylori*, and ulcers: where we stand. [Review] [92 refs]. Am J Gastroenterol 1996;91:2080–2086.

Pearson SP, Kelberman I. Gastrointestinal effects of NSAIDs. Difficulties in detection and management. [Review] [20 refs]. Postgrad Med 1996;100:131–132.

Soll AH, Weinstein WM, Kurata J, McCarthy D. Nonsteroidal anti-inflammatory drugs and peptic ulcer disease. [Review]. Ann Intern Med 1991;114:307–319.

Loeb DS, Ahlquist DA, Talley NJ. Management of gastroduodenopathy associated with use of nonsteroidal anti-inflammatory drugs. [Review]. Mayo Clin Proc 1992;67:354–364.

Taha AS, Hudson N, Hawkey CJ, et al. Famotidine for the prevention of gastric and duodenal ulcers caused by nonsteroidal antiinflammatory drugs [see comments]. N Engl J Med 1996;334:1435–1439.

Selected Guidelines

Appropriate Use of Gastrointestinal Endoscopy: a Consensus Statement from the American Society for Gastrointestinal Endoscopy. Manchester, MA: The Society, 1989;11:1995.

See Also

- Duodenal ulcer, recurrent
- Peptic ulcer disease, *H. pylori*-negative, persistent symptoms
- Gastric ulcer, by UGIS
- Peptic ulcer disease, refractory
- Dyspepsia, nonulcer and *H. pylori*-positive

THE CONSULTATION GUIDE

Peptic Ulcer Disease, *Helicobactor pylori*-Negative, Persistent Symptoms

Indications and Timing for Referral

- Symptoms persist on medical therapy

Timing: Routine (less than 4 weeks)

Advice for Referral

- Patient should be off anti-secretory medications when gastrin level done.
- Ascertain history of NSAID use.

Tests to Prepare for Consult

- Gastrin

Tests Not Useful Before Consult

- None

Tests Consultant May Need to Do

- Upper endoscopy

Follow-up Visits Generally Required

- One

Suggested Readings

Kurata JH, Nogawa AN. Meta-analysis of risk factors for peptic ulcer. Nonsteroidal antiinflammatory drugs, *Helicobacter pylori*, and smoking. J Clin Gastroenterol 1997;24:2–17.

Hui WM, Lam SK, Lok AS, et al. Maintenance therapy for duodenal ulcer: a randomized controlled comparison of seven forms of treatment. Am J Med 1992;92:265–274.

Armstrong D, Arnold R, Classen M, et al. RUDER—a prospective, two-year, multicenter study of risk factors for duodenal ulcer relapse during maintenance therapy with ranitidine. RUDER Study Group. Dig Dis Sci 1994;39:1425–1433.

Selected Guidelines

Soll AH. Consensus conference. Medical treatment of peptic ulcer disease. Practice guidelines. Practice Parameters Committee of the American College of Gastroenterology [published erratum appears in JAMA 1996;275:1314]. [Review] [99 refs]. JAMA 1996;275:622–629.

Appropriate Use of Gastrointestinal Endoscopy: a Consensus Statement from the American Society for Gastrointestinal Endoscopy. Manchester, MA: The Society, 1989;11:1995.

The role of endoscopy in the management of the patient with peptic ulcer disease. Guidelines for clinical application. Gastrointest Endosc 1988;34(3 Suppl):21S–22S.

See Also

- Peptic ulcer disease, refractory
- Gastric ulcer, by UGIS
- Duodenal ulcer, recurrent
- Peptic distress, on NSAIDs
- Dyspepsia, nonulcer and *H. pylori*-positive

GASTROENTEROLOGY

Peptic Ulcer Disease, Refractory

Indications and Timing for Referral

- Symptoms persistent for more than 4 weeks despite medical therapy

Timing: Routine (less than 4 weeks)

Advice for Referral

- Careful medication history is vital (e.g., NSAIDs).
- If possible, patient should be off NSAIDs before referral.

Tests to Prepare for Consult

- Calcium
- Gastrin

Tests Not Useful Before Consult

- *H. pylori* serology
- UGIS

Tests Consultant May Need to Do

- Gastrin
- Upper endoscopy

Follow-up Visits Generally Required

- Two

Suggested Readings

Hunt RH. Peptic ulcer disease: defining the treatment strategies in the era of *Helicobacter pylori*. [Review] [56 refs]. Am J Gastroenterol 1997;92(4:Suppl): 36S–40S.

Kurata JH, Nogawa AN. Meta-analysis of risk factors for peptic ulcer. Nonsteroidal antiinflammatory drugs, *Helicobacter pylori*, and smoking. J Clin Gastroenterol 1997;24:2–17.

Walsh JH, Peterson WL. Drug therapy: The treatment of *Helicobacter pylori* infection in the management of peptic ulcer disease. N Engl J Med 1995;333:984–991.

Armstrong D, Arnold R, Classen M, et al. RUDER—a prospective, two-year, multicenter study of risk factors for duodenal ulcer relapse during maintenance therapy with ranitidine. RUDER Study Group. Dig Dis Sci 1994;39:1425–1433.

Selected Guidelines

Soll AH. Consensus conference. Medical treatment of peptic ulcer disease. Practice guidelines. Practice Parameters Committee of the American College of Gastroenterology [published erratum appears in JAMA 1996;275:1314]. [Review] [99 refs]. JAMA 1996;275:622–629.

Appropriate Use of Gastrointestinal Endoscopy: a Consensus Statement from the American Society for Gastrointestinal Endoscopy. Manchester, MA: The Society, 1989;11:1995.

NIH Consensus Conference. *Helicobacter pylori* in peptic ulcer disease. NIH Consensus Development Panel on *Helicobacter pylori* in Peptic Ulcer Disease [see comments]. JAMA 1994;272:65–69.

See Also

- Peptic ulcer disease, *H. pylori*-negative, persistent symptoms
- Peptic distress, on NSAIDs
- Duodenal ulcer, recurrent
- Gastric ulcer, by UGIS
- Dyspepsia, nonulcer and *H. pylori*-positive

Polyps, Family History of

Indications and Timing for Referral

- Patients with a significant family history of polyps (defined below) should be periodically monitored by colonoscopy for evidence of malignancy

Timing: Routine (less than 4 weeks)

Advice for Referral

- Family history is significant if there is a history of multiple polyps at an early age associated with colon cancer. Individuals lacking these features should only have routinely recommended screening for colon cancer.
- Consideration should be given to having such patients co-managed with a specialist who is expert in familial polyposis.

Tests to Prepare for Consult

- None

Tests Not Useful Before Consult

- None

Tests Consultant May Need to Do

- Barium enema
- Colonoscopy
- Flexible sigmoidoscopy
- APC gene analysis

Follow-up Visits Generally Required

- One

Suggested Readings

Rustgi AK. Hereditary gastrointestinal polyposis and nonpolyposis syndromes. N Engl J Med 1994;331:1694–1702.

Powell SM, Petersen GM, Krush AJ, et al. Molecular diagnosis of familial adenomatous polyposis [see comments]. N Engl J Med 1993;329:1982–1987.

Offerhaus GJ, Giardiello FM, Krush AJ, et al. The risk of upper gastrointestinal cancer in familial adenomatous polyposis [see comments]. Gastroenterology 1992;102:1980–1982.

Rhodes M, Bradburn DM. Overview of screening and management of familial adenomatous polyposis [see comments]. [Review]. Gut 1992;33:125–131.

Bond JH. Colorectal cancer and polyps: clinical decisions for screening, early diagnosis, and surveillance of high-risk groups. [Review] [47 refs]. Compr Ther 1996;22:100–106.

Lefton HB, Pilchman J, Harmatz A. Colon cancer screening and the evaluation and follow-up of colonic polyps. [Review] [15 refs]. Prim Care 1996;23:515–523.

Selected Guidelines

The role of colonoscopy in the management of patients with colonic polyps. Guidelines for clinical application. Gastrointest Endosc 1988;34(3 Suppl):6S–7S.

See Also

- Colon cancer, family history of
- Colorectal cancer, history of

GASTROENTEROLOGY

Right Upper Quadrant Pain, Intermittent

Indications and Timing for Referral

- Clinical, laboratory, or sonographic evidence of biliary tract obstruction or infection

Timing: Expedited (less than 1 week)

- Diagnostic uncertainty

Timing: Routine (less than 4 weeks)

Tests to Prepare for Consult

- CBC with differential
- Amylase
- Albumin, total protein
- Bilirubin
- ALT, AST, alkaline phosphatase
- Ultrasound, abdomen

Tests Not Useful Before Consult

- None

Tests Consultant May Need to Do

- CBC with differential
- Amylase
- Albumin, total protein
- Bilirubin
- ALT, AST, alkaline phosphatase
- CT scan, abdomen
- Barium enema
- Tc-HIDA scan
- ERCP
- Percutaneous transhepatic cholangiogram

Follow-up Visits Generally Required

- One

Suggested Readings

Rathgaber S, Rex DK. Right upper quadrant abdominal pain. Diagnosis in patients without evident gallstones [published erratum appears in Postgrad Med 1993;94:45]. Postgrad Med 1993;94:153–156.

Kang JY, Tay HH, Guan R. Chronic upper abdominal pain: site and radiation in various structural and functional disorders and the effect of various foods. Gut 1992;33:743–748.

Sharpstone D, Colin-Jones DG. Chronic, non-visceral abdominal pain. [Review]. Gut 1994;35:833–836.

Laurin JM, DeSotel CK, Jorgensen RA, et al. The natural history of abdominal pain associated with primary biliary cirrhosis. Am J Gastroenterol 1994;89:1840–1843.

See Also

- Hepatomegaly, abdominal mass, RUQ
- Jaundice/hyperbilirubinemia
- Alkaline phosphatase, elevated

Sclerosing Cholangitis

Indications and Timing for Referral

- Clinical findings suggesting acute cholangitis

Timing: Urgent (less than 24 hours)

- Diagnostic uncertainty
- Assistance with management
- Decision-making about liver transplantation

Timing: Routine (less than 4 weeks)

Advice for Referral

- This condition often requires co-management with a gastroenterologist.

Tests to Prepare for Consult

- CBC
- Prothrombin time
- Amylase
- Albumin, total protein
- Bilirubin
- ALT, AST, alkaline phosphatase
- Ultrasound, biliary

Tests Not Useful Before Consult

- None

Tests Consultant May Need to Do

- ANCA
- ERCP
- Percutaneous transhepatic cholangiogram
- Liver biopsy

Follow-up Visits Generally Required

- Co-management, see *Advice for Referral*

Suggested Readings

Lee YM, Kaplan MM. Primary sclerosing cholangitis. [Review]. N Engl J Med 1995;332:924–933.

Wiesner RH. Current concepts in primary sclerosing cholangitis. [Review]. Mayo Clinic Proc 1994;69:969–982.

Harnois DM, Lindor KD. Primary sclerosing cholangitis: evolving concepts in diagnosis and treatment. [Review] [155 refs]. Dig Dis 1997;15:23–41.

Brentnall TA, Haggitt RC, Rabinovitch PS, et al. Risk and natural history of colonic neoplasia in patients with primacy sclerosing cholangitis and ulcerative colitis. Gastroenterology 1996;110:331–338.

GASTROENTEROLOGY

Splenomegaly, Abdominal Mass, Left Upper Quadrant

Indications and Timing for Referral

- Diagnostic uncertainty

Timing: Expedited (less than 1 week)

Tests to Prepare for Consult

- CBC with differential
- Platelet count
- Urinalysis with microscopic
- CT scan, abdomen

Tests Not Useful Before Consult

- None

Tests Consultant May Need to Do

- Radiograph, chest
- Ultrasound with Doppler, abdomen
- Barium enema
- Colonoscopy
- Upper endoscopy
- ERCP

Follow-up Visits Generally Required

- Two

Suggested Readings

Grover SA, Barkun AN, Sackett DL. Does this patient have splenomegaly? [see comments]. JAMA 1993;270:2218–2221.

Barkun AN, Camus M, Green L, et al. The bedside assessment of splenic enlargement. Am J Med 1991;91:512–518.

Haynes BF. Enlargement of lymph nodes and spleen. In: Isselbacher KJ, Braunwald E, Wilson JD, et al., eds. Harrison's Principles of Internal Medicine. 13th ed. NY: McGraw-Hill, 1994:323–329.

Kurtz AB. The spleen. [Review]. Clinics in Diagnostic Ultrasound 1988;23:139–164.

THE CONSULTATION GUIDE

Steatorrhea

Indications and Timing for Referral

- Etiology uncertain after initial testing

Timing: Routine (less than 4 weeks)

Tests to Prepare for Consult

- CBC
- Electrolytes (Na, K, Cl, CO_2)
- Glucose
- Albumin, total protein
- BUN, creatinine
- Amylase
- Bilirubin
- ALT, AST, alkaline phosphatase
- Prothrombin time
- Calcium
- Qualitative fecal fat and fiber
- D-xylose test

Tests Not Useful Before Consult

- Small bowel series

Tests Consultant May Need to Do

- Plain film, abdomen
- CT scan, abdomen
- Lactulose breath test
- Small bowel series
- Upper endoscopy

Follow-up Visits Generally Required

- Two

Suggested Readings

Brasitus TA, Sitrin MD. Intestinal malabsorption syndromes. [Review]. Annu Rev Med 1990;41:339–347.

Misra S, Ament ME. Diagnosis of coeliac sprue in 1994. [Review]. Gastroenterol Clin North Am 1995;24:133–143.

Cook GC. Persisting diarrhoea and malabsorption. [Review]. Gut 1994;35:582–586.

Donowitz M, Kokke FT, Saidi R. Evaluation of patients with chronic diarrhea. [Review]. N Engl J Med 1995;332:725–729.

Greenberger MJ, Isselbacher KJ. Disorders of absorption. In: Fauci AS, Braunwald E, Isselbacher KJ, et al., eds. Harrison's Principles of Internal Medicine. 14th ed. New York: McGraw Hill, 1998:1616–1633.

See Also

- Malabsorption
- Diarrhea, chronic

GASTROENTEROLOGY

Tenesmus

Indications and Timing for Referral

- Clinical findings suggesting perirectal abscess

Timing: Expedited (less than 1 week)

- Symptoms persist for 2 weeks
- Unclear etiology
- Unassociated with a local acute disease process

Timing: Routine (less than 4 weeks)

Tests to Prepare for Consult

- None

Tests Not Useful Before Consult

- Barium enema
- CT scan, abdomen

Tests Consultant May Need to Do

- Stool C&S
- Stool O&P
- Stool WBC
- Barium enema
- Colonoscopy
- Flexible sigmoidoscopy
- Proctoscopy

Follow-up Visits Generally Required

- One

Suggested Readings

Janicke DM, Pundt MR. Anorectal disorders. Emerg Med Clin North Am 1996;14:757–788.

Fred HL. Diagnostic and therapeutic tenesmus. South Med J 1978;71:617–618.

Shrock TR. Diseases of the rectum and anus. In: Bennett JC, Plum F, eds. Cecil Textbook of Medicine. 20th ed. Philadelphia: WB Saunders, 1998:740–743.

Selected Guidelines

The role of colonoscopy in the management of patients with colonic polyps. Guidelines for clinical application. Gastrointest Endosc 1988;34(3 Suppl):6S–7S.

See Also

- Constipation

THE CONSULTATION GUIDE

Transaminase Elevation

Indications and Timing for Referral

- Evidence of severe or progressive hepatic decompensation (e.g., mental status change, ascites, or coagulopathy)

Timing: Urgent (less than 24 hours) or Expedited (less than 1 week)

- Persistently elevated for over 2 months
- Transaminase elevation is 1.5 × baseline at 2 separate readings more than 2 weeks apart

Timing: Routine (less than 4 weeks)

Advice for Referral

- A careful history of medication, alcohol intake, and industrial exposure is vital.

Tests to Prepare for Consult

- CBC
- Lipid profile, fasting (cholesterol, HDL, TG)
- Amylase
- Albumin, total protein
- Bilirubin
- ALT, AST, alkaline phosphatase
- Glucose
- Iron/TIBC
- Hepatitis B surface antigen
- Hepatitis C antibody

Tests Not Useful Before Consult

- Hepatitis A IgG antibody

Tests Consultant May Need to Do

- ANA
- Antismooth muscle antibody
- Anti-LKM antibody
- Ceruloplasmin
- Ferritin
- Hepatitis B core antibody
- Hepatitis D antibody
- Hepatitis E antibody
- Liver biopsy

Follow-up Visits Generally Required

- One

Suggested Readings

Kundrotas LW, Clement DJ. Serum alanine aminotransferase (ALT) elevation in asymptomatic US Air Force basic trainee blood donors. Dig Dis Sci 1993;38:2145–2150.

Sherman KE. Alanine aminotransferase in clinical practice. A review [see comments]. [Review]. Arch Intern Med 1991;151:260–265.

Kamath PS. Clinical approach to the patient with abnormal liver test results. [Review] [00 refs]. Mayo Clin Proc 1996;71:1089–1094.

See Also

- Jaundice/hyperbilirubinemia
- Hepatitis B
- Hepatitis C
- Hepatitis D

GASTROENTEROLOGY

Vomiting, Persistent or Recurrent

Indications and Timing for Referral

- Vomiting blood of more than 1 tsp (in absence of epistaxis)
- Electrolyte imbalance present
- Dehydration present
- Patient in great discomfort

Timing: Urgent (less than 24 hours)

- Vomiting present intermittently for more than 2 weeks

Timing: Expedited (greater than 1 week)

- Diagnosis uncertain after initial evaluation

Timing: Routine (less than 4 weeks)

Advice for Referral

- Careful medication history is vital, e.g., NSAIDs, theophylline, digoxin, opiates.
- Rule out pregnancy if appropriate.

Tests to Prepare for Consult

- CBC
- Electrolytes (Na, K, Cl, CO_2)
- Glucose
- BUN, creatinine
- Amylase
- ALT, AST, alkaline phosphatase
- Albumin, total protein
- Bilirubin
- Calcium, phosphorus

Tests Not Useful Before Consult

- CT scan, abdomen
- MR, abdomen
- Ultrasound, abdomen
- Ultrasound, biliary

Tests Consultant May Need to Do

- Ultrasound, abdomen
- Ultrasound, biliary
- UGIS
- CT scan, abdomen
- Gastric emptying study
- Upper endoscopy

Follow-up Visits Generally Required

- One

Suggested Readings

Katelaris PH, Jones DB. Chronic nausea and vomiting. [Review]. Dig Dis 1989;7:324–333.

Friedman LS, Isselbacher KJ. Nausea, vomiting, and indigestion. In: Fauci AS, Braunwald E, Isselbacher KJ, et al., eds. Harrison's Principles of Internal Medicine. 14th ed. New York: McGraw Hill, 1998:230–236.

Selected Guidelines

Appropriate Use of Gastrointestinal Endoscopy: a Consensus Statement from the American Society for Gastrointestinal Endoscopy. Manchester, MA: The Society, 1989;11:1995.

The role of endoscopy in the management of the patient with peptic ulcer disease. Guidelines for clinical application. Gastrointest Endosc 1988;34(3 Suppl):21S–22S.

See Also

- Nausea, persistent or recurrent

THE CONSULTATION GUIDE

Weight Loss, Despite Good Appetite

Indications and Timing for Referral

- Diagnostic uncertainty

Timing: Routine (less than 4 weeks)

Advice for Referral

- Defined as greater than 10% loss in total body weight within 1 year.
- Preliminary testing described should assist the primary care physician in determining which consultant will be most appropriate: gastroenterology, oncology, or endocrinology.

Tests to Prepare for Consult

- Glucose
- Electrolytes (Na, K, Cl, CO_2)
- Amylase
- Albumin, total protein
- Bilirubin
- BUN, creatinine
- Calcium, phosphorus
- ALT, AST, alkaline phosphatase
- TSH (assay sensitivity <0.1 mU/L)
- CBC with differential
- Stool for occult blood
- Stool O&P
- Qualitative fecal fat and fiber
- Radiograph, chest
- Urinalysis with microscopic

Tests Not Useful Before Consult

- None

Tests Consultant May Need to Do

- CBC
- Glucose
- Electrolytes (Na, K, Cl, CO_2)
- Albumin, total protein
- Amylase
- BUN, creatinine
- Bilirubin
- Calcium, phosphorus
- ALT, AST, alkaline phosphatase
- 72-hour fecal fat
- Glycohemoglobin
- TSH (assay sensitivity <0.1 mU/L)
- Free T_4
- Triiodothyronine (T_3)
- Metanephrines, 24-hour urine
- CT scan, abdomen
- Colonoscopy
- Upper endoscopy

Follow-up Visits Generally Required

- Two

Suggested Readings

Reife CM. Involuntary weight loss. [Review]. Med Clin North Am 1995;79:299–313.

Wise GR, Craig D. Evaluation of involuntary weight loss. Where do you start?. [Review]. Postgrad Med J 1994;95:143–146.

Thompson MP, Morris LK. Unexplained weight loss in the ambulatory elderly. J Am Geriatr Soc 1991;39:497–500.

GASTROENTEROLOGY

Wilson's Disease, Personal or Family History

Indications and Timing for Referral

- Diagnostic uncertainty in patients and family members
- Initial evaluation of all affected patients
- Assistance with management
- Decision-making about liver transplantation

Timing: Routine (less than 4 weeks)

Advice for Referral

- Ophthlamologic evaluation is useful.
- This condition often requires co-management with gastroenterologist.

Tests to Prepare for Consult

- Ceruloplasmin
- Prothrombin time
- Albumin, total protein
- Amylase
- Bilirubin
- ALT, AST, alkaline phosphatase

Tests Not Useful Before Consult

- Hepatic imaging

Tests Consultant May Need to Do

- Ceruloplasmin
- Quantitative copper analysis of histology
- Urinary copper excretion
- Liver biopsy

Follow-up Visits Generally Required

- Co-management, see *Advice for Referral*

Suggested Readings

Yarze JC, Martin P, Munoz SJ, Friedman LS. Wilson's disease: current status. [Review]. Am J Med 1992;92:643–654.

Yarze JC, Munoz SJ, Friedman LS. Diagnosing Wilson disease [letter; comment]. Ann Intern Med 1992;117:91.

Stremmel W, Meyerrose KW, Niederau C, et al. Wilson disease: clinical presentation, treatment, and survival [see comments]. Ann Intern Med 1991;115:720–726.

Berman DH, Leventhal RI, Gavaler JS, et al. Clinical differentiation of fulminant Wilsonian hepatitis from other causes of hepatic failure. Gastroenterology 1991;100:1129–1134.

CHAPTER 5

Hematology

Anemia 247
    Aplastic 248
    Hemolytic 249
    Hemolytic, Hereditary 250
    in Chronic Renal Failure 251
    in Pregnancy 252
    Macrocytic 253
    Microcytic 255
    Normocytic, Elevated Corrected Reticulocyte Count 257
    Normocytic, Normal or Low Corrected Reticulocyte Count 258
    Sickle Cell, Management 259
Bleeding Disorder 260
Eosinophilia 261
Folate Deficiency 263
Glucose-6-phosphate Dehydrogenase (G6PD) Deficiency 264
Hematocrit, Elevated 265
Hypercoagulable State 266
Hyperglobulinemia 267
Hypersplenism 268
Iron Deficiency 269
Leukemia
    Acute Lymphocytic, History of 270
    Acute Myelogenous, History of 271
Leukocytosis 272
Leukocytosis in Pregnancy 273
Lupus Anticoagulant, in Nonpregnant Patient 274
Lymphocytosis 275
Lymphoma 276
Monocytosis 277
Myelodysplastic Syndromes 278
Myeloma, Multiple, Management 279
Neutropenia 280
Pancytopenia
    Elevated Reticulocyte Count 281
    Normal or Low Reticulocyte Count 282
Paroxysmal Nocturnal Hemoglobinuria 283

(continued)

Hematology (continued)

Polycythemia Vera 284
Porphyria, Acute, Intermittent 285
Splenomegaly 286
Thalassemia 287
Thrombocytopenia 288
Thrombocytosis 290
Vitamin B_{12} Deficiency 291

HEMATOLOGY

Anemia

Indications and Timing for Referral
- Severe or rapidly progressive anemia
- Patient has co-existing medical condition that could be adversely affected by anemia

Timing: Expedited (less than 1 week)

- Unresponsive to conventional therapy for apparent problem
- Anemia unexplained and confirmed on second CBC

Timing: Routine (less than 4 weeks)

Advice for Referral
- Even mild anemia requires explanation.
- Anemia should be categorized based on mean corpuscular volume (MCV) and reticulocyte count
- Based on MCV and reticulocyte count, see recommendations for
  - Anemia, microcytic
  - Anemia, normocytic, normal or low corrected reticulocyte count
  - Anemia, normocytic, elevated corrected reticulocyte count
  - Anemia, macrocytic
- Records of previous blood counts are vital.
- Complete medication history is vital.
- Important to ascertain if family history of anemia is present.

Tests to Prepare for Consult
- CBC × 2
- Reticulocyte count

Tests Not Useful Before Consult
- Bone marrow aspirate and biopsy

Tests Consultant May Need to Do
- None

Follow-up Visits Generally Required
- One

Suggested Readings
Nardone DA, Roth KM, Mazur DJ, McAfee JH. Usefulness of physical examination in detecting the presence or absence of anemia [see comments]. Arch Intern Med 1990;150:201–204.

Mansouri A, Lipschitz DA. Anemia in the elderly patient. [Review]. Med Clin North Am 1992;76:619–630.

Sears DA. Anemia of chronic disease. [Review]. Med Clin North Am 1992;76:567–579.

Moliterno AR, Spivak JL. Anemia of cancer. Hematol Oncol Clin North Am 1996;10:345.

Doukas MA. Human immunodeficiency virus associated anemia. [Review]. Med Clin North Am 1992;76:699–709.

Beutler E. The common anemias. [Review]. JAMA 1988;259:2433–2437.

See Also
- Anemia, microcytic
- Anemia, aplastic
- Anemia, hemolytic
- Anemia, in chronic renal failure
- Anemia, in pregnancy
- Anemia, normocytic, elevated corrected reticulocyte count
- Anemia, normocytic, normal or low corrected reticulocyte count
- Anemia, macrocytic

Anemia, Aplastic

Indications and Timing for Referral

- Confirmed diagnosis requires referral to facility capable of bone marrow transplantation

Timing: Urgent (less than 24 hours)

Advice for Referral

- Presence of fever or bleeding requires immediate medical care.
- Serious consideration should be given to HLA typing of parents, siblings, and children.
- Complete medication history is vital.
- Serious consideration should be given to having such patients co-managed by a hematologist.

Tests to Prepare for Consult

- CBC with differential
- Reticulocyte count
- Blood, type and cross

Tests Not Useful Before Consult

- None

Tests Consultant May Need to Do

- CBC with blood smear
- Reticulocyte count
- Urine hemosiderin
- Bilirubin
- ALT, AST, alkaline phosphatase
- Bone marrow aspirate and biopsy
- Cytogenetics on marrow aspirate
- Flow cytometry on marrow aspirate
- HIV antibody testing
- EBV antibody
- CMV antibody
- Hepatitis A antibody
- HB_sAb
- HB_sAg
- Hepatitis C antibody

Follow-up Visits Generally Required

- Co-management, see *Advice for Referral*

Suggested Readings

Young NS, Maciejewski J. The pathophysiology of acquired aplastic anemia. [Review] [72 refs]. N Engl J Med 1997;336:1365–1372.

Keisu M, Ost A. Diagnoses in patients with severe pancytopenia suspected of having aplastic anemia. Eur J Haematol 1990;45:11–14.

Nissen C, Gratwohl A, Speck B. Management of aplastic anemia. [Review]. Eur J Haematol 1991;46:193–197.

Selected Guidelines

Bacigalupo A. Guidelines for the treatment of severe aplastic anemia. Working Party on Severe Aplastic Anemia (WPSAA) of the European Group of Bone Marrow Transplantation (EBMT). Haematologica 1994;79:438–444.

Anemia, Hemolytic

Indications and Timing for Referral
- Rapidly progressive

Timing: Urgent (less than 24 hours)

- Severe anemia
- Patient has co-existing medical condition that could be adversely affected by anemia

Timing: Expedited (less than 1 week)

- Diagnostic uncertainty
- Assistance with management

Timing: Routine (less than 4 weeks)

Advice for Referral
- Complete medication history is vital.
- Important to ascertain if family history of anemia is present.

Tests to Prepare for Consult
- CBC × 2
- Reticulocyte count
- RDW
- Coombs' test

Tests Not Useful Before Consult
- Bone marrow aspirate and biopsy

Tests Consultant May Need to Do
- CBC with blood smear
- Reticulocyte count
- Coombs' test with elution
- Coombs', by ELISA
- Cold agglutinins
- Osmotic fragility
- Haptoglobin
- Urine hemosiderin
- RBC G6PD level
- Heinz body assay
- Hb electrophoresis
- HAM test
- Bone marrow aspirate and biopsy

Follow-up Visits Generally Required
- One

Suggested Readings
Tabbara IA. Hemolytic anemias. Diagnosis and management. [Review]. Med Clin North Am 1992;76:649–668.

Petz LD. Drug-induced autoimmune hemolytic anemia. [Review]. Transfus Med Rev 1993;7:242–254.

Rose W, Bunn HF. Hemolytic anemias and acute blood loss. In: Fauci AS, Braunwald E, Isselbacher KJ, et al., eds. Harrison's Principles of Internal Medicine. 14th ed. New York: McGraw Hill, 1998:659–671.

See Also
- Anemia
- Anemia, aplastic
- Anemia, in chronic renal failure
- Anemia, hemolytic, hereditary
- Anemia, macrocytic
- Anemia, in pregnancy
- Anemia, microcytic
- Anemia, normocytic, normal or low corrected reticulocyte count
- G6PD deficiency
- Paroxysmal nocturnal hemoglobinuria
- Anemia, normocytic, elevated corrected reticulocyte count

Anemia, Hemolytic, Hereditary

Indications and Timing for Referral

- Assistance with management and/or counseling

Timing: Routine (less than 4 weeks)

Advice for Referral

- Records documenting putative cause of hemolysis are vital.
- Studies listed under *Tests Consultant May Need to Do* may also be appropriate for family members.

Tests to Prepare for Consult

- CBC
- Reticulocyte count

Tests Not Useful Before Consult

- Bone marrow aspirate and biopsy

Tests Consultant May Need to Do

- CBC with blood smear
- Reticulocyte count
- Osmotic fragility
- Hb electrophoresis
- Heinz body assay
- RBC enzyme studies
- Ultrasound, abdomen

Follow-up Visits Generally Required

- One

Suggested Readings

Tabbara IA. Hemolytic anemias. Diagnosis and management. [Review]. Med Clin North Am 1992;76:649–668.

Lux SE. Hereditary defects in the membrane or metabolism of the red cells. In: Bennett JC, Plum F, eds. Cecil Textbook of Medicine. 20th ed. Philadelphia: WB Saunders, 1996:851–859.

See Also

- G6PD deficiency
- Anemia, hemolytic

HEMATOLOGY

Anemia, in Chronic Renal Failure

Indications and Timing for Referral
- Assistance with management of symptomatic anemia refractory to conventional therapy

Timing: Routine (less than 4 weeks)

Advice for Referral
- A complete medication history is vital.

Tests to Prepare for Consult
- CBC with differential
- Reticulocyte count
- Erythropoietin level
- Ferritin
- Iron/TIBC
- Folate, red cell level
- Creatinine

Tests Not Useful Before Consult
- Bone marrow aspirate and biopsy

Tests Consultant May Need to Do
- CBC with blood smear
- Reticulocyte count
- Coombs', direct and indirect
- IEP
  - Serum
  - Urine
- Bone marrow aspirate and biopsy

Follow-up Visits Generally Required
- One

Suggested Readings

Beusterien KM, Nissenson AR, Port FK, et al. The effects of recombinant human erythropoietin on functional health and well-being in chronic dialysis patients. J Am Soc Nephrol 1996;7:763–773.

Humphries JE. Anemia of renal failure. Use of erythropoietin. [Review]. Med Clin North Am 1992;76:711–725.

Klahr S. Anemia, dialysis, and dollars. N Engl J Med 1996;334:461–463.

Besarab A. Anemia in renal disease. In: Schrier RW, Gottschalk CW, eds. Diseases of the Kidney. 6th ed. Boston: Little Brown, 1996:2581–2596.

See Also
- Anemia, hemolytic
- Anemia, aplastic
- Anemia
- Anemia, normocytic, normal or low corrected reticulocyte count
- Anemia, normocytic, elevated corrected reticulocyte count
- Anemia, microcytic
- Anemia, in pregnancy
- Anemia, macrocytic

Anemia, in Pregnancy

Indications and Timing for Referral
- Diagnostic uncertainty
- Assistance with management

Timing: Expedited (less than 1 week)

Advice for Referral
- Anemia defined as a hemoglobin level less than 10 grams.
- Complete dietary, medication, and vitamin history are important.

Tests to Prepare for Consult
- CBC × 2
- Reticulocyte count
- RDW
- Red cell folate level
- Ferritin
- Creatinine
- Bilirubin
- ALT, AST, alkaline phosphatase

Tests Not Useful Before Consult
- Bone marrow aspirate and biopsy

Tests Consultant May Need to Do
- CBC with blood smear
- Reticulocyte count
- Hb electrophoresis
- Coombs', direct and indirect
- Bone marrow aspirate and biopsy

Follow-up Visits Generally Required
- One

Suggested Readings
Williams MD, Wheby MS. Anemia in pregnancy. [Review]. Med Clin North Am 1992;76:631–647.

Lops VR, Hunter LP, Dixon LR. Anemia in pregnancy. [Review]. Am Fam Physician 1995;51:1189–1197.

Selected Guidelines
Routine iron supplementation during pregnancy. Policy statement. U. S. Preventive Services Task Force. JAMA 1993;270:2846–2848.

See Also
- Anemia, microcytic
- Anemia, aplastic
- Anemia, in chronic renal failure
- Anemia, macrocytic
- Anemia, normocytic, elevated corrected reticulocyte count
- Anemia, normocytic, normal or low corrected reticulocyte count
- Anemia
- Anemia, hemolytic

Anemia, Macrocytic

Indications and Timing for Referral

- Unresponsive to conventional therapy for apparent condition
- Unexplained
- Assistance with management

Timing: Routine (less than 4 weeks)

Timing of referral may be Urgent (less than 24 hours) or Expedited (less than 1 week) if anemia is severe or if evidence of hemolysis is present

Advice for Referral

- Clinical evidence of alcohol and drug intake is vital.

Tests to Prepare for Consult

- CBC with differential
- Reticulocyte count
- Vitamin B_{12}, serum
- Red cell folate level
- RDW
- LDH
- ALT, AST, alkaline phosphatase
- Bilirubin
- TSH

Tests Not Useful Before Consult

- Serum folate level
- Bone marrow aspirate and biopsy

Tests Consultant May Need to Do

- CBC with blood smear
- Reticulocyte count
- Cold agglutinins
- Coombs' test
- Schilling test ± intrinsic factor
- TSH (assay sensitivity <0.1 mU/L)
- Bone marrow aspirate and biopsy
- Cytogenetics on marrow aspirate
- Flow cytometry on marrow aspirate

Follow-up Visits Generally Required

- One

Suggested Readings

Hoffbrand V, Provan D. ABC of clinical haematology. Macrocytic anaemias. [Review] [0 refs]. Br Med J 1997;314: 430–433.

Colon-Otero G, Menke D, Hook CC. A practical approach to the differential diagnosis and evaluation of the adult patient with macrocytic anemia. [Review]. Med Clin North Am 1992;76:581–597.

Beck WS. Diagnosis of megaloblastic anemia. [Review]. Annu Rev Med 1991;42:311–322.

Davenport J. Macrocytic anemia. Am Fam Physician 1996;53:155–162.

Pruthi RK, Tefferi A. Pernicious anemia revisited. [Review]. Mayo Clin Proc 1994;69:144–150.

Savage DG, Lindenbaum J, Stabler SP, Allen RH. Sensitivity of serum methylmalonic acid and total homocysteine determinations for diagnosing cobalamin and folate deficiencies. Am J Med 1994;96:239–246.

Selected Guidelines

Guidelines on the investigation and diagnosis of cobalamin and folate deficiencies. A publication of the British Committee for Standards in Haematology. BCSH General Haematology Test Force. Clin Lab Haematol 1994;16:101–115.

Anemia, Macrocytic (continued)

See Also
- Vitamin B$_{12}$ deficiency
- Anemia, aplastic
- Anemia, chronic renal failure
- Anemia, hemolytic
- Folate deficiency
- Anemia, normocytic, elevated corrected reticulocyte count
- Anemia, microcytic
- Iron deficiency
- Anemia, normocytic, normal or low corrected reticulocyte count
- Anemia
- Anemia, in pregnancy

HEMATOLOGY

Anemia, Microcytic

Indications and Timing for Referral
- Severe anemia
- Patient has co-existing medical condition that could be adversely affected by anemia
- Suspicion of unidentified chronic disease causing anemia

Timing: Expedited (less than 1 week)

- Unexplained
- Unresponsive to conventional therapy for apparent problem (i.e., iron)
- Family history of anemia

Timing: Routine (less than 4 weeks)

Advice for Referral
- Records of previous blood counts are vital.

Tests to Prepare for Consult
- CBC × 2
- Reticulocyte count
- Iron/TIBC and/or ferritin
- ESR
- RDW
- Stool occult blood × 3

Tests Not Useful Before Consult
- None

Tests Consultant May Need to Do
- CBC with blood smear
- Reticulocyte count
- Ferritin
- Hb electrophoresis
- Hb F level
- Hb H level
- Hb A2 level
- Urine hemosiderin
- Osmotic fragility
- IEP, serum
- Bone marrow aspirate and biopsy

Follow-up Visits Generally Required
- One

Suggested Readings

Massey AC. Microcytic anemia. Differential diagnosis and management of iron deficiency anemia. [Review]. Med Clin North Am 1992;76:549–566.

van Zeben D, Bieger R, van Wermeskerken RK, et al. Evaluation of microcytosis using serum ferritin and red blood cell distribution width. Eur J Haematol 1990;44:106–109.

Rockey DC, Cello JP. Evaluation of the gastrointestinal tract in patients with iron-deficiency anemia [see comments]. N Engl J Med 1993;329:1691–1695.

Gordon S, Bensen S, Smith R. Long term Follow-up of older patients with iron deficiency anemia after a negative gi evaluation. Am J Gastroenterol 1996;91:885–889.

THE CONSULTATION GUIDE

Anemia, Microcytic (continued)

Selected Guidelines

Routine iron supplementation during pregnancy. Policy statement. U. S. Preventive Services Task Force. JAMA 1993;270:2846–2848.

See Also

- Anemia, macrocytic
- Anemia, in pregnancy
- Anemia, aplastic
- Anemia, hemolytic
- Anemia, normocytic, elevated corrected reticulocyte count
- Anemia, normocytic, normal or low corrected reticulocyte count
- Anemia
- Melena, tarry stools, recent history of
- Anemia, in chronic renal failure
- Iron deficiency

HEMATOLOGY

Anemia, Normocytic, Elevated Corrected Reticulocyte Count

Indications and Timing for Referral
- Severe anemia
- Patient has co-existing medical condition that could be adversely affected by anemia

Timing: Expedited (less than 1 week)

- Unexplained

Timing: Routine (less than 4 weeks)

Tests to Prepare for Consult
- CBC with differential
- Reticulocyte count
- Iron/TIBC and/or ferritin
- ESR
- BUN, creatinine
- Stool occult blood × 3
- Bilirubin
- ALT, AST, alkaline phosphatase
- Coombs', direct and indirect

Tests Not Useful Before Consult
- Bone marrow aspirate and biopsy

Tests Consultant May Need to Do
- CBC with blood smear
- Reticulocyte count
- Cold agglutinins
- Osmotic fragility
- HAM test
- RBC G6PD level
- Erythropoietin level
- Heinz body assay
- Haptoglobin
- LDH
- Hb electrophoresis
- Bone marrow aspirate and biopsy

Follow-up Visits Generally Required
- One

Suggested Readings
Tabbara IA. Hemolytic anemias. Diagnosis and management. [Review]. Med Clin North Am 1992;76:649–668.

Petz LD. Drug-induced autoimmune hemolytic anemia. [Review]. Transfus Med Rev 1993;7:242–254.

Rose W, Bunn HF. Hemolytic anemias and acute blood loss. In: Fauci AS, Braunwald E, Isselbacher KJ, et al., eds. Harrison's Principles of Internal Medicine. 14th ed. New York: McGraw Hill, 1998:659–671.

See Also
- Anemia, in pregnancy
- Anemia, aplastic
- Anemia, in chronic renal failure
- Anemia, macrocytic
- Anemia, microcytic
- Pancytopenia, elevated reticulocyte count
- Anemia, normocytic, normal or low corrected reticulocyte count
- Anemia
- Anemia, hemolytic
- Anemia, in pregnancy
- Anemia, hemolytic
- Anemia
- Melena, tarry stools, recent history of
- Iron deficiency

Anemia, Normocytic, Normal or Low Corrected Reticulocyte Count

Indications and Timing for Referral

- Severe anemia
- Patient has co-existing medical condition that could be adversely affected by anemia

Timing: Expedited (less than 1 week)

- Unexplained

Timing: Routine (less than 4 weeks)

Tests to Prepare for Consult

- CBC with differential
- Reticulocyte count
- Iron/TIBC and/or ferritin
- ESR
- BUN, creatinine
- Stool occult blood × 3
- TSH
- Free T_4
- Bilirubin
- ALT, AST, alkaline phosphatase

Tests Not Useful Before Consult

- Bone marrow aspirate and biopsy

Tests Consultant May Need to Do

- CBC with blood smear
- Reticulocyte count
- IEP
    - Serum
    - Urine
- Bone marrow aspirate and biopsy

Follow-up Visits Generally Required

- One

Suggested Readings

Sears DA. Anemia of chronic disease. [Review]. Med Clin North Am 1992;76:567–579.

Mansouri A, Lipschitz DA. Anemia in the elderly patient. [Review]. Med Clin North Am 1992;76:619–630.

Moliterno AR, Spivak JL. Anemia of cancer. Hematol Oncol Clin North Am 1996;10:345.

Doukas MA. Human immunodeficiency virus associated anemia. [Review]. Med Clin North Am 1992;76:699–709.

See Also

- Anemia, normocytic, elevated corrected reticulocyte count
- Anemia, macrocytic
- Anemia, aplastic
- Anemia, in chronic renal failure
- Anemia, hemolytic
- Anemia, microcytic
- Anemia
- Pancytopenia, normal or low reticulocyte count
- Anemia, in pregnancy

HEMATOLOGY

Anemia, Sickle Cell, Management

Indications and Timing for Referral
- Assistance with management of acute crisis
- Assistance with long-term management and counseling

Timing: Routine (less than 4 weeks)

Advice for Referral
- Serious consideration should be given to having such patients co-managed by a hematologist or specialized clinic.
- Records documenting disease course and management are vital (e.g., ferritin levels, immunization and transfusion records).
- Tests listed under *Tests Consultant May Need to Do* may be appropriate for genetic counseling of family members.

Tests to Prepare for Consult
- CBC with differential
- Reticulocyte count
- Ferritin
- Iron/TIBC
- ALT, AST, alkaline phosphatase
- Creatinine
- Urinalysis with microscopic
- Bilirubin
- ECG
- Chest radiograph

Tests Not Useful Before Consult
- None

Tests Consultant May Need to Do
- CBC with blood smear
- Oxygen saturation level
- Detailed red cell phenotyping
- Hb electrophoresis
- Hb F level

Follow-up Visits Generally Required
- Co-management, see *Advice for Referral*

Suggested Readings
Bookchin RM, Lew VL. Pathophysiology of sickle cell anemia. [Review] [61 refs]. Hematol Oncol Clin North Am 1996;10:1241–1253.

Steingart R. Management of patients with sickle cell disease. [Review]. Med Clin North Am 1992;76:669–682.

Pollack CV Jr. Emergencies in sickle cell disease. [Review]. Emerg Med Clin North Am 1993;11:365–378.

Charache S, Terrin ML, Moore RD, et al. Effect of hydroxyurea on the frequency of painful crises in sickle cell anemia. Investigators of the Multicenter Study of Hydroxyurea in Sickle Cell Anemia [see comments]. N Engl J Med 1995;332:1317–1322.

Vichinsky EP, Haberkern CM, Neumayr L, et al. A comparison of conservative and aggressive transfusion regimens in the perioperative management of sickle cell disease. The Preoperative Transfusion in Sickle Cell Disease Study Group [see comments]. N Engl J Med 1995;333:206–213.

Bellet PS, Kalinyak KA, Shukla R, et al. Incentive spirometry to prevent acute pulmonary complications in sickle cell diseases [see comments]. N Engl J Med 1995;333:699–703.

Samuels-Reid JH. Common problems in sickle cell disease [see comments]. [Review]. Am Fam Physician 1994;49:1477–80.

THE CONSULTATION GUIDE

Bleeding Disorder

Indications and Timing for Referral
- Diagnostic uncertainty

Timing: Routine (less than 4 weeks)

Advice for Referral
- Acute bleeding (e.g., hematoma, mucosal bleeding) requires immediate medical attention.
- Complete medication history is vital.
- Records of personal and family medical history, type of bleeding disorder, and past challenges to coagulation system (e.g., surgery) are vital.

Tests to Prepare for Consult
- CBC with differential
- Prothrombin time
- PTT
- Thrombin time
- Albumin, total protein
- Creatinine
- ALT, AST, alkaline phosphatase

Tests Not Useful Before Consult
- None

Tests Consultant May Need to Do
- CBC with blood smear
- Prothrombin time
- PTT
- Thrombin time
- Bleeding time
- IEP, serum
- Anticoagulant mixing study
- Specific coagulation factor levels
- Platelet aggregometry
- Fibrin degradation products

Follow-up Visits Generally Required
- One

Suggested Readings
Sham RL, Francis CW. Evaluation of mild bleeding disorders and easy bruising. [Review]. Blood Rev 1994;8:98–104.

Hassouna HI. Laboratory evaluation of hemostatic disorders. [Review]. Hematol Oncol Clin North Am 1993;7:1161–1249.

Handin RI. Disorders of coagulation and thrombosis. In: Fauci AS, Braunwald E, Isselbacher KJ, et al., eds. Harrison's Principles of Internal Medicine. 14th ed. New York: McGraw Hill, 1998:736–743.

See Also
- Hypercoagulable state
- Lupus anticoagulant, in nonpregnant patient

HEMATOLOGY

Eosinophilia

Indications and Timing for Referral

- Diagnostic uncertainty in patient with greater than 1,000 eosinophils/mm²
- Persistent for more than 4 weeks without obvious cause

Timing: Routine (less than 4 weeks)

Advice for Referral

- If eosinophils are greater than 10% on CBC at 2 separate readings, obtain absolute count.
- Complete medication history is vital.
- Complete travel history is important.
- Complete history of animals in household is important.
- Associated household members should be examined for eosinophilia.
- Factors favoring referral to infectious disease include:
    - Presence of fever or systemic illness
- Factors favoring referral to hematology include:
    - Eosinophilia unexplained
    - Evidence of organ involvement
    - Absolute eosinophil count higher than 50,000
- Factors favoring referral to allergy/immunology include:
    - Clinical suspicion of allergic diathesis

Tests to Prepare for Consult

- CBC with differential
- Eosinophil count, total
- Sodium
- Potassium
- Bilirubin
- ALT, AST, alkaline phosphatase
- Creatinine
- Albumin, total protein
- LDH
- Urinalysis with microscopic
- Stool O&P
- Radiograph, chest

Tests Not Useful Before Consult

- None

Tests Consultant May Need to Do

- CBC with differential
- ESR
- Nasal swab for eosinophils
- IgE, quantitative
- IEP, serum
- ACTH stimulation test, 1-hour
- Parasitic serologies for suspected agents
- Fungal serology for suspected agents
- *Aspergillus* serology
- Spirometry, before and after bronchodilator
- Echocardiogram
- CT scan, abdomen
- Bone marrow aspirate and biopsy
- Cytogenetics on marrow aspirate

Follow-up Visits Generally Required

- One

Eosinophilia (*continued*)

Suggested Readings

Liesveld JL, Abboud CN. State of the art; the hypereosinophilic syndromes. [Review]. Blood Rev 1991;5:29–37.

Weller PF. Eosinophilia in travelers. [Review]. Med Clin North Am 1992;76:1413–1432.

Marcy TW. Eosinophilia in patients presenting with pulmonary infiltrates and fever. [Review]. Semin Respir Infect 1988;3:247–257.

Varga J, Uitto J, Jimenez SA. The cause and pathogenesis of the eosinophilia-myalgia syndrome [see comments]. [Review]. Ann Intern Med 1992;116:140–147.

Wardlaw AJ, Kay AB. Eosinophilia. In: Beutler E, Lichtman MA, Coller BS, eds. Williams hematology. 5th ed. New York: McGraw Hill, 1995;844–852.

Weller PF. Eosinophilic syndromes. In: Bennett JC, Plum F, eds. Cecil textbook of medicine. 20th ed. Philadelphia: WB Saunders, 1996;956–958.

HEMATOLOGY

Folate Deficiency

Indications and Timing for Referral

- Unresponsive to folate therapy

Timing: Routine (less than 4 weeks)

Advice for Referral

- History of phenytoin or methotrexate administration is relevant.

Tests to Prepare for Consult

- CBC × 2
- Reticulocyte count
- RDW
- Red cell folate level
- Vitamin B_{12}, serum
- ALT, AST, alkaline phosphatase
- Bilirubin

Tests Not Useful Before Consult

- Serum folate level

Tests Consultant May Need to Do

- CBC with blood smear
- Schilling test ± intrinsic factor
- Bone marrow aspirate and biopsy

Follow-up Visits Generally Required

- One

Suggested Readings

Savage DG, Lindenbaum J, Stabler SP, Allen RH. Sensitivity of serum methylmalonic acid and total homocysteine determinations for diagnosing cobalamin and folate deficiencies. Am J Med 1994;96:239–246.

Hoffbrand V, Provan D. ABC of clinical haematology. Macrocytic anaemias. [Review] [0 refs]. Br Med J 1997;314:430–433.

Selected Guidelines

Guidelines on the investigation and diagnosis of cobalamin and folate deficiencies. A publication of the British Committee for Standards in Haematology. BCSH General Haematology Test Force. Clin Lab Haematol 1994;16:101–115.

See Also

- Anemia, macrocytic
- Vitamin B_{12} deficiency

Glucose-6-phosphate Dehydrogenase (G6PD) Deficiency

Indications and Timing for Referral

- Diagnostic uncertainty
- Assistance with management and/or counseling

Timing: Routine (less than 4 weeks)

Timing of referral may be Urgent (less than 24 hours) or Expedited (less than 1 week) if anemia is severe

Advice for Referral

- Records of drug exposure, CBC, and G6PD level during previous acute hemolytic episodes are vital.
- A complete medication history is vital.
- Important to ascertain if family history of anemia is present.

Tests to Prepare for Consult

- CBC
- Reticulocyte count
- RBC G6PD level

Tests Not Useful Before Consult

- None

Tests Consultant May Need to Do

- CBC with blood smear
- Reticulocyte count
- RBC G6PD level
- Heinz body assay

Follow-up Visits Generally Required

- One

Suggested Readings

Beutler E. Glucose-6-phosphate dehydrogenase deficiency [see comments]. [Review]. N Engl J Med 1991;324:169–174.

Beutler E. The molecular biology of G6PD variants and other red cell enzyme defects. [Review]. Annu Rev Med 1992;43:47–59.

See Also

- Anemia, hemolytic
- Anemia, hemolytic, hereditary

HEMATOLOGY

Hematocrit, Elevated

Indications and Timing for Referral

- Diagnostic uncertainty

Timing: Routine (less than 4 weeks)

Advice for Referral

- Old medical records and blood counts are helpful.

Tests to Prepare for Consult

- CBC with differential × 2
- Oxygen saturation

Tests Not Useful Before Consult

- Bone marrow aspirate and biopsy

Tests Consultant May Need to Do

- CBC with blood smear
- Reticulocyte count
- Red cell mass
- Erythropoietin level
- Carboxyhemoglobin
- Urinalysis with microscopic
- CT scan, abdomen
- CT scan, liver and spleen
- Bone marrow aspirate and biopsy

Follow-up Visits Generally Required

- Zero

Suggested Readings

Landaw SA, Williams WJ. Deciphering polycythemia. Hosp Pract (Off Ed) 1996;31:155.

Green AR. Pathogenesis of polycythaemia vera. Lancet 1996;347:844–845.

Landaw SA. Polycythemia vera and other polycythemic states. [Review]. Clin Lab Med 1990;10:857–871.

See Also

- Polycythemia vera

265

Hypercoagulable State

Indications and Timing for Referral

- Etiology unclear
- Assistance with management

Timing: Routine (less than 4 weeks)

Advice for Referral

- Defined as recurrent, unexplained thromboses; or if first episode occurs in patient younger than 30 years old with a family history; or affects an unusual vessel.
- Personal and family history of thromboses is vital.
- Whenever possible, obtain blood for anticoagulant testing before starting anticoagulant therapy.
- Serious consideration should be given to having such patients co-managed by a hematologist.

Tests to Prepare for Consult

- CBC
- Prothrombin time
- PTT

Tests Not Useful Before Consult

- None

Tests Consultant May Need to Do

- Fibrin split products
- Protein C, protein S
- Antithrombin III
- Factor 5 Leiden
- Lupus anticoagulant
- Sucrose hemolysis
- Homocystine level, urine
- Anticardiolipin antibody

Follow-up Visits Generally Required

- Co-management, see *Advice for Referral*

Suggested Readings

Brigden ML. The hypercoagulable state. Who, how, and when to test and treat. [Review] [24 refs]. Postgrad Med 1997;101:249–252.

Nachman RL, Silverstein R. Hypercoagulable states [see comments]. [Review]. Ann Intern Med 1993;119:819–827.

Green KB, Silverstein RL. Hypercoagulability in cancer [review]. Hematol Oncol Clin North Am 1996;10:499.

Bauer KA. Hypercoagulable state. In: Beutler E, Lichtman MA, Coller BS, eds. Williams Hematology. 5th ed. New York: McGraw Hill, 1995:1531–1550.

See Also

- Lupus anticoagulant, in nonpregnant patient
- Bleeding disorder

Hyperglobulinemia

Indications and Timing for Referral

- Diagnostic uncertainty

Timing: Routine (less than 4 weeks)

Advice for Referral

- Records of past globulin levels important

Tests to Prepare for Consult

- CBC
- ESR
- Albumin, total protein
- Calcium
- Globulin
- ALT, AST, alkaline phosphatase
- BUN, Creatinine
- Urinalysis with microscopic
- IEP, serum

Tests Not Useful Before Consult

- Bone marrow aspirate and biopsy

Tests Consultant May Need to Do

- CBC with blood smear
- ANA
- RF
- IEP, urine
- Cryoglobulins
- Viscosity, serum
- 24-hour urine protein
- Bone marrow aspirate and biopsy
- Immunophenotyping

Follow-up Visits Generally Required

- One

Suggested Readings

Kyle RA. Monoclonal gammopathy of undetermined significance. [Review]. Blood Rev 1994;8:135–141.

Longo DL. Plasma cell disorders. In: Fauci AS, Braunwald E, Isselbacher KJ, et al., eds. Harrison's Principles of Internal Medicine. 14th ed. New York: McGraw Hill, 1998:712–718.

Lee-Lewandrowski E, Lewandrowski K. The plasma proteins. In: McClatchey KD, ed. Clinical Laboratory Medicine. Baltimore: Williams & Wilkins, 1994:239–258.

See Also

- Myeloma, multiple, management

Hypersplenism

Indications and Timing for Referral
- Etiology unclear
- Diagnostic uncertainty
- Assistance with management

Timing: Routine (less than 4 weeks)

Tests to Prepare for Consult
- CBC
- Reticulocyte count
- Bilirubin
- Globulin
- ALT, AST, alkaline phosphatase

Tests Not Useful Before Consult
- Bone marrow aspirate and biopsy

Tests Consultant May Need to Do
- CBC with blood smear
- IEP, serum
- ANA
- RF
- Antineutrophil antibody
- Antiplatelet antibody
- Bone marrow aspirate and biopsy
- Coombs' test
- Haptoglobin
- Flow cytometry on marrow aspirate
- CT scan, liver and spleen

Follow-up Visits Generally Required
- One

Suggested Readings
Erslev AJ. Hypersplenism. In: Beutler E, Lichtman MA, Coller BS, eds. Williams Hematology. 5th ed. New York: McGraw Hill, 1995:709–714.

See Also
- Splenomegaly

HEMATOLOGY

Iron Deficiency

Indications and Timing for Referral

- Severe anemia
- Patient has co-existing medical condition that could be adversely affected by anemia

Timing: Expedited less than 1 week)

- Unexplained
- Unresponsive to iron therapy

Timing: Routine (less than 4 weeks)

Advice for Referral

- Ideally, reticulocyte count should be done before and after 14 to 21 days of iron therapy.

Tests to Prepare for Consult

- CBC × 2
- Reticulocyte count
- RDW
- Iron/TIBC and/or ferritin
- Stool occult blood × 3
- Creatinine
- TSH

Tests Not Useful Before Consult

- None

Tests Consultant May Need to Do

- CBC with blood smear
- Reticulocyte count
- ESR
- Ferritin
- RDW
- Urine hemosiderin
- Haptoglobin
- Stool O&P
- Bone marrow aspirate and biopsy

Follow-up Visits Generally Required

- One

Suggested Readings

Looker AC, Dallman PR, Carroll MD, et al. Prevalence of iron deficiency in the United States. JAMA 1997;277:973–976.

Massey AC. Microcytic anemia. Differential diagnosis and management of iron deficiency anemia. [Review]. Med Clin North Am 1992;76:549–566.

Rockey DC, Cello JP. Evaluation of the gastrointestinal tract in patients with iron-deficiency anemia [see comments]. N Engl J Med 1993;329:1691–1695.

Gordon S, Bensen S, Smith R. Long term Follow-up of older patients with iron deficiency anemia after a negative GI evaluation. Am J Gastroenterol 1996;91:885–889.

Selected Guidelines

Routine iron supplementation during pregnancy. Policy statement. U. S. Preventive Services Task Force. JAMA 1993;270:2846–2848.

See Also

- Anemia, microcytic
- Melena, tarry stools, recent history of

Leukemia, Acute Lymphocytic, History of

Indications and Timing for Referral

- Immature or neoplastic cells are present
- Any abnormal CBC with differential (e.g., decreased WBC, RBC, or platelets) that persists for longer than 1 week without apparent cause

Timing: Expedited (less than 1 week)

Advice for Referral

- If patient is less than 5 years in remission, patient should be generally co-managed with a hematologist-oncologist.
- If patient is more than 5 years in remission, co-management may still be appropriate.
- A complete history of previous chemotherapy is vital.

Tests to Prepare for Consult

- CBC with differential × 2

Tests Not Useful Before Consult

- None

Tests Consultant May Need to Do

- CBC with blood smear
- Bone marrow aspirate and biopsy
- Cytogenetics on marrow aspirate
- Flow cytometry on marrow aspirate
- Immunophenotyping

Follow-up Visits Generally Required

- Co-management, see *Advice for Referral*

Suggested Readings

Kantarjian HM. Adult acute lymphocytic leukemia: critical review of current knowledge. [Review]. Am J Med 1994;97:176–184.

Mauer AM. Acute lymphocytic leukemia. In: Beutler E, Lichtman MA, Coller BS, eds. Williams Hematology. 5th ed. New York: McGraw Hill, 1995:1004–1017.

See Also

- Leukemia, acute myelogenous, history of
- Myelodysplastic syndromes

HEMATOLOGY

Leukemia, Acute Myelogenous, History of

Indications and Timing for Referral

- Immature or neoplastic cells present
- Abnormal CBC with differential (e.g., decreased WBC, RBC, or platelets) that persists for more than 1 week without apparent cause

Timing: Expedited (less than 1 week)

Advice for Referral

- If patient is less than 5 years in remission, patient should be generally co-managed with a hematologist-oncologist.
- If patient is more than 5 years in remission, co-management may still be appropriate
- A complete history of previous chemotherapy is vital.

Tests to Prepare for Consult

- CBC with differential × 2

Tests Not Useful Before Consult

- None

Tests Consultant May Need to Do

- CBC with blood smear
- Bone marrow aspirate and biopsy
- Cytogenetics on marrow aspirate
- Flow cytometry on marrow aspirate

Follow-up Visits Generally Required

- Co-management, see *Advice for Referral*

Suggested Readings

Beguin Y, Sautois B, Forget P, et al. Long term Follow-up of patients with acute myelogenous leukemia who received the daunorubicin, vincristine, and cytosine arabinoside regimen. Cancer 1997;79:1351–1354.

Duque RE, Andreeff M, Braylan RC, et al. Consensus review of the clinical utility of DNA flow cytometry in neoplastic hematopathology. Cytometry 1993;14:492–496.

See Also

- Leukemia, acute lymphocytic, history of
- Myelodysplastic syndromes

Leukocytosis

Indications and Timing for Referral
- Explanation unclear (e.g., patient not infected)

Timing: Routine (less than 4 weeks)

Advice for Referral
- Consider history of recent corticosteroid use.
- Consider possible Cushing's syndrome.
- Records of old blood counts are helpful.
- Smoking history is helpful.

Tests to Prepare for Consult
- CBC with differential × 2
- Uric acid

Tests Not Useful Before Consult
- Bone marrow aspirate and biopsy

Tests Consultant May Need to Do
- CBC with blood smear
- Leukocyte alkaline phosphatase
- Bone marrow aspirate and biopsy
- Cytogenetics on marrow aspirate

Follow-up Visits Generally Required
- One

Suggested Readings
Peterson L, Hrisinko MA. Benign lymphocytosis and reactive neutrophilia. Laboratory features provide diagnostic clues. [Review] [62 refs]. Clin Lab Med 1993;13:863–877.

Dall DC. Neutrophilia. In: Beutler E, Lichtman MA, Coller BS, eds. Williams Hematology. 5th ed. New York: McGraw Hill, 1995:824–828.

See Also
- Synonym: neutrophilia
- Leukocytosis, in pregnancy
- Lymphocytosis
- Monocytosis

HEMATOLOGY

Leukocytosis in Pregnancy

Indications and Timing for Referral

- Explanation unclear (e.g., patient not infected)

Timing: Expedited (less than 1 week)

Advice for Referral

- Differential WBC critical for diagnosis.
- Presence of blasts suggests possible leukemia.

Tests to Prepare for Consult

- CBC with differential × 2

Tests Not Useful Before Consult

- Bone marrow aspirate and biopsy

Tests Consultant May Need to Do

- CBC with blood smear
- Leukocyte alkaline phosphatase
- Bone marrow aspirate and biopsy
- Cytogenetics on marrow aspirate
- Immunophenotyping

Follow-up Visits Generally Required

- None

Suggested Readings

Delgado I, Neubert R, Dudenhausen JW. Changes in white blood cells during parturition in mothers and newborn. Gynecol Abstet Invest 1994;38:227–235.

Mercelina-Roumans PE, Ubachs JM, van Wersch JW. Leucocyte count and leucocyte differential in smoking and non-smoking females during pregnancy. Eur J Obstet Gynecol Reprod Biol 1994;55:169–173.

Lupus Anticoagulant, in Nonpregnant Patient

Indications and Timing for Referral

- Assistance with management

Timing: Routine (less than 4 weeks)

Advice for Referral

- Assistance with management.
- Record of test establishing diagnosis is vital.
- History of thromboses is vital.

Tests to Prepare for Consult

- Prothrombin time
- PTT

Tests Not Useful Before Consult

- None

Tests Consultant May Need to Do

- Anticardiolipin antibody
- RVVT

Follow-up Visits Generally Required

- None

Suggested Readings

Shapiro SS. The lupus anticoagulant/antiphospholipid syndrome. [Review] [182 refs]. Annu Rev Med 1996;47:533–553.

Creagh MD, Greaves M. Lupus anticoagulant. [Review]. Blood Rev 1991;5:162–167.

Rauch J. Platelet phospholipid antigen-antibody interactions: detection and biological relevance. [Review]. Transfus Med Rev 1990;4:110–114.

See Also

- Bleeding disorder
- Hypercoagulable state

HEMATOLOGY

Lymphocytosis

Indications and Timing for Referral

- Persistent for longer than 4 weeks
- Diagnostic uncertainty

Timing: Routine (less than 4 weeks)

Advice for Referral

- Lymphocytosis defined as greater than 5,000 lymphocytes/mm^2.
- Records of past blood counts are helpful.
- Complete medication history is vital.

Tests to Prepare for Consult

- CBC
- ALT, AST, alkaline phosphatase

Tests Not Useful Before Consult

- Bone marrow aspirate and biopsy

Tests Consultant May Need to Do

- CBC with blood smear
- Immunophenotyping of lymphocytes
- ACTH stimulation test, 1-hour
- TSH (assay sensitivity <0.1 mU/L)
- Toxicology screen
- CMV antibody
- EBV antibody
- HIV antibody testing
- Hepatitis A antibody
- HB$_s$Ab
- Hepatitis C antibody
- Toxoplasma serology
- Bone marrow aspirate and biopsy

Follow-up Visits Generally Required

- One

Suggested Readings

Peterson L, Hrisinko MA. Benign lymphocytosis and reactive neutrophilia. Laboratory features provide diagnostic clues. [Review]. Clin Lab Med 1993;13:863–877.

Kipps TJ. Lymphocytosis and Lymphopenia. In: Beutler E, Lichtman MA, Coller BS, eds. Williams Hematology. 5th ed. New York: McGraw Hill, 1995:963–968.

See Also

- Monocytosis
- Leukocytosis
- Leukocytosis, in pregnancy

Lymphoma

Indications and Timing for Referral

- Confirm diagnosis
- Assistance with management

Timing: Expedited (less than 1 week)

Advice for Referral

- Records of all imaging studies and pathological reports are vital.
- Serious consideration should be given to having such patients co-managed by a hematologist-oncologist.

Tests to Prepare for Consult

- CBC
- ESR
- ALT, AST, alkaline phosphatase
- Bilirubin
- Calcium
- LDH

Tests Not Useful Before Consult

- Bone marrow aspirate and biopsy

Tests Consultant May Need to Do

- CBC with blood smear
- Gallium scan
- CT scan, thorax
- CT or MR
    - Pelvis
    - Neck
    - Abdomen
- Bone marrow aspirate and biopsy
- Cytogenetics on marrow aspirate
- Flow cytometry on marrow aspirate
- Immunoglobulin gene rearrangements
- HIV antibody testing

Follow-up Visits Generally Required

- Co-management, see *Advice for Referral*

Suggested Readings

Freedman AS, Nadler LM. Malignancies of lymphoid cells. In: Fauci AS, Braunwald E, Isselbacher KJ, et al., eds. Harrison's Principles of Internal Medicine. 14th ed. New York: McGraw Hill, 1998:695–712.

See Also

- Lymphoma, history of

HEMATOLOGY

Monocytosis

Indications and Timing for Referral

- Unexplained for more than 4 weeks

Timing: Routine (less than 4 weeks)

Advice for Referral

- Monocytosis defined as an absolute monocyte count higher than 1500.

Tests to Prepare for Consult

- CBC × 2

Tests Not Useful Before Consult

- Bone marrow aspirate and biopsy

Tests Consultant May Need to Do

- CBC with blood smear
- Muramidase
- Blood smear with peroxidase and esterase stains
- PPD
- Bone marrow aspirate and biopsy
- Cytogenetics on marrow aspirate

Follow-up Visits Generally Required

- One

Suggested Readings

Lichtman MA. Monocytosis and monocytopenia. In: Beutler E, Lichtman MA, Coller BS, eds. Williams Hematology. 5th ed. New York: McGraw Hill, 1995:881–884.

THE CONSULTATION GUIDE

Myelodysplastic Syndromes

Indications and Timing for Referral

- Diagnostic uncertainty
- Assistance with management

Timing: Routine (less than 4 weeks)

Advice for Referral

- Presence of infection or hemorrhage requires immediate consultation and medical care.
- Past medical records and medication history are vital.

Tests to Prepare for Consult

- CBC with differential
- Reticulocyte count

Tests Not Useful Before Consult

- Bone marrow aspirate and biopsy

Tests Consultant May Need to Do

- CBC with blood smear
- Ferritin
- Antineutrophil antibody
- Antiplatelet antibody
- Erythropoietin level
- Bone marrow aspirate and biopsy
- Cytogenetics on marrow aspirate
- Flow cytometry on marrow aspirate

Follow-up Visits Generally Required

- One

Suggested Readings

Ohyashiki K, Ohyashiki JH, Iwabuchi A, Toyama K. Clinical aspects, cytogenetics and disease evolution in myelodysplastic syndromes. [Review] [75 refs]. Leuk Lymphoma 1996;23:409–415.

Noel P, Solberg LA Jr. Myelodysplastic syndromes. Pathogenesis, diagnosis and treatment. [Review]. Crit Rev Oncol Hematol 1992;12:193–215.

Ganser A, Hoelzer D. Clinical course of myelodysplastic syndromes. [Review]. Hematol Oncol Clin North Am 1992;6:607–618.

McKenna RW, Allison PM. Diagnosis, classification, and course of myelodysplastic syndromes. [Review]. Clin Lab Med 1990;10:683–706.

Duque RE, Andreeff M, Braylan RC, et al. Consensus review of the clinical utility of DNA flow cytometry in neoplastic hematopathology. Cytometry 1993;14:492–496.

See Also

- Leukemia, acute lymphocytic, history of
- Leukemia, acute myelogenous, history of

HEMATOLOGY

Myeloma, Multiple, Management

Indications and Timing for Referral

- Assistance with management

Timing: Expedited (less than 1 week)

Advice for Referral

- Serious consideration should be given to having such patients co-managed by a hematologist-oncologist.

Tests to Prepare for Consult

- CBC
- Calcium, phosphorus
- Creatinine
- Uric acid
- IEP
  - Serum
  - Urine
- Skeletal survey

Tests Not Useful Before Consult

- Bone scan

Tests Consultant May Need to Do

- CBC with blood smear
- β_2-microglobulin
- 24-hour urine protein
- Serum viscosity
- Immunoglobulins, quantitative
- Bone marrow aspirate and biopsy

Follow-up Visits Generally Required

- Co-management, see *Advice for Referral*

Suggested Readings

Alexanian R, Dimopoulos M. The treatment of multiple myeloma. [Review]. N Engl J Med 1994;330:484–489.

Oken MM. Standard treatment of multiple myeloma. [Review]. Mayo Clin Proc 1994;69:781–786.

MacLennan IC, Drayson M, Dunn J. Multiple myeloma [see comments]. [Review]. Br Med J 1994;308:1033–1036.

Kyle RA. Diagnostic criteria of multiple myeloma. [Review]. Hematol Oncol Clin North Am 1992;6:347–358.

Greipp PR. Prognosis in myeloma. [Review]. Mayo Clin Proc 1994;69:895–902.

See Also

- Hyperglobulinemia

Neutropenia

Indications and Timing for Referral

- Absolute neutrophil count less than 1,000 and patient afebrile

Timing: Expedited (less than 1 week)

- Diagnostic uncertainty

Timing: Routine (less than 4 weeks)

Advice for referral

- Absolute neutrophil count less than 1,000 and febrile patient require immediate medical attention.
- If associated with viral syndrome, monitor for 4 weeks before referring
- Before referral, consider stopping all possible medications.
- Records of previous blood counts, medication history and any autoimmune disorder are vital.

Tests to Prepare for Consult

- CBC

Tests Not Useful Before Consult

- None

Tests Consultant May Need to Do

- CBC with blood smear
- ANA
- Antineutrophil antibody
- RF
- Immunophenotyping
- Bone marrow aspirate and biopsy
- Cytogenetics on marrow aspirate
- HIV antibody testing
- CMV antibody
- EBV antibody
- Hepatitis A antibody
- HB_sAb
- Hepatitis C antibody

Follow-up Visits Generally Required

- One

Suggested Readings

Shastri KA, Logue GL. Autoimmune neutropenia [see comments]. [Review]. Blood 1993;81:1984–1995.

Dall DC. Neutropenia. In: Beutler E, Lichtman MA, Coller BS, eds. Williams Hematology. 5th ed. New York: McGraw Hill, 1995:815–824.

Hathorn JW, Lyke K. Empirical treatment of febrile neutropenia: evolution of current therapeutic approaches. [Review] [72 refs]. Clin Infect Dis 1997;24(Suppl 2): S256–S265.

HEMATOLOGY

Pancytopenia, Elevated Reticulocyte Count

Indications and Timing for Referral
- Absolute neutrophil count less than 1,000 without fever
- Platelet count less than 20,000

Timing: Urgent (less than 24 hours)

- Diagnostic uncertainty
- Assistance with management

Timing: Expedited (less than 1 week)

Advice for Referral
- Presence of fever or bleeding require immediate medical care.
- A complete medication history is vital.
- Serious consideration should be given to having such patients co-managed by a hematologist.
- Consideration should be given to HLA typing of patient and family members.

Tests to Prepare for Consult
- CBC
- Reticulocyte count
- ALT, AST, alkaline phosphatase
- Folate, red cell level
- Vitamin B_{12}, serum

Tests Not Useful Before Consult
- Bone marrow aspirate and biopsy

Tests Consultant May Need to Do
- CBC with blood smear
- Reticulocyte count
- Antineutrophil antibody
- Coombs', direct and indirect
- Sucrose hemolysis
- Urine hemosiderin
- Bone marrow aspirate and biopsy
- In vitro marrow culture
- Flow cytometry on marrow aspirate
- HIV antibody testing
- EBV antibody
- CMV antibody
- Hepatitis A antibody
- HB_sAb
- Hepatitis C antibody
- CT scan, liver and spleen

Follow-up Visits Generally Required
- Co-management, see *Advice for Referral*

Suggested Readings
Tabbara IA. Hemolytic anemias. Diagnosis and management. [Review]. Med Clin North Am 1992;76:649–668.

See Also
- Pancytopenia, normal or low reticulocyte count
- Anemia, normocytic, elevated corrected reticulocyte count

Pancytopenia, Normal or Low Reticulocyte Count

Indications and Timing for Referral

- Absolute neutrophil count less than 1,000 without fever
- Platelet count less than 20,000

Timing: Urgent (less than 24 hours)

- Diagnostic uncertainty
- Assistance with management

Timing: Expedited (less than 1 week)

Advice for Referral

- Presence of fever or bleeding requires immediate medical care.
- A complete medication history is vital.
- Consideration should be given to having such patients co-managed by a hematologist.
- Serious consideration should be given to HLA typing of patient and family members.

Tests to Prepare for Consult

- CBC
- Reticulocyte count
- ALT, AST, alkaline phosphatase
- Serum folate level
- Vitamin B$_{12}$, serum

Tests Not Useful Before Consult

- Bone marrow aspirate and biopsy

Tests Consultant May Need to Do

- CBC with blood smear
- Reticulocyte count
- Bone marrow aspirate and biopsy
- In vitro marrow culture
- Flow cytometry on marrow aspirate
- Cytogenetics on marrow aspirate
- Antiparvovirus antibody
- HIV antibody testing
- EBV antibody
- CMV antibody
- Hepatitis A antibody
- HB$_s$Ab
- Hepatitis C antibody

Follow-up Visits Generally Required

- Co-management, see *Advice for Referral*

Suggested Readings

Keisu M, Ost A. Diagnoses in patients with severe pancytopenia suspected of having aplastic anemia. Eur J Haematol 1990;45:11–14.

Nissen C, Gratwohl A, Speck B. Management of aplastic anemia. [Review]. Eur J Haematol 1991;46:193–197.

Selected Guidelines

Bacigalupo A. Guidelines for the treatment of severe aplastic anemia. Working Party on Severe Aplastic Anemia (WPSAA) of the European Group of Bone Marrow Transplantation (EBMT). Haematologica 1994;79:438–444.

See Also

- Anemia, normocytic, normal or low corrected reticulocyte count
- Thrombocytopenia
- Pancytopenia, elevated reticulocyte count

HEMATOLOGY

Paroxysmal Nocturnal Hemoglobinuria

Indications and Timing for Referral

- Assistance with management

Timing: Routine (less than 4 weeks)

Advice for Referral

- Medical records establishing diagnosis, hemolytic manifestations of disease, and past treatments are vital.
- Serious consideration should be given to having such patients co-managed by a hematologist.

Tests to Prepare for Consult

- CBC
- Reticulocyte count

Tests Not Useful Before Consult

- None

Tests Consultant May Need to Do

- HAM test
- Sucrose hemolysis
- Urine hemosiderin
- Bone marrow aspirate and biopsy
- Flow cytometry on marrow aspirate

Follow-up Visits Generally Required

- Co-management, see *Advice for Referral*

Suggested Readings

Rosse WF. Paroxysmal nocturnal hemoglobinuria: the biochemical defects and the clinical syndrome. [Review]. Blood Rev 1989;3:192–200.

Nakakuma H. Mechanism of intravascular hemolysis in paroxysmal nocturnal hemoglobinuria (PNH). [Review] [71 refs]. Am J Hematol 1996;53:22–29.

Socie G, Mary JY, de Gramont A, et al. Paroxysmal nocturnal haemoglobinuria: long-term Follow-up and prognostic factors. French Society of Haematology [see comments]. Lancet 1996;348:573–577.

See Also

- Anemia, hemolytic

THE CONSULTATION GUIDE

Polycythemia Vera

Indications and Timing for Referral

- Confirmation of diagnosis
- Assistance with management

Timing: Routine (less than 4 weeks)

Advice for Referral

- Records of red cell mass or other finding establishing diagnosis are vital.
- Records of past blood counts are helpful.
- Serious consideration should be given to having such patients co-managed by a hematologist.

Tests to Prepare for Consult

- CBC × 2
- Erythropoietin level
- Red cell mass

Tests Not Useful Before Consult

- Bone marrow aspirate and biopsy

Consultant May Need to Do

- CBC with blood smear
- Reticulocyte count
- Leukocyte alkaline phosphatase
- Uric acid
- Red cell mass
- Bone marrow aspirate and biopsy
- Cytogenetics on marrow aspirate
- In vitro marrow culture
- CT scan, abdomen

Follow-up Visits Generally Required

- Co-management, see *Advice for Referral*

Suggested Readings

Pearson TC, Messinezy M. The diagnostic criteria of polycythaemia rubra vera. [Review] [45 refs]. Leuk Lymphoma 1996;22(Suppl 1):87–93.

Landaw SA. Polycythemia vera and other polycythemic states. [Review]. Clin Lab Med 1990;10:857–871.

Consensus conference on the diagnosis, prognosis and treatment of polycythaemia vera supported by the French Society of Haematology. Paris, France, June 21, 1993. [Review]. Nouvelle Revue Francaise d Hematologie 1994;36:139–208.

HEMATOLOGY

Porphyria, Acute, Intermittent

Indications and Timing for Referral

- Assistance with management and/or counseling

Timing: Routine (less than 4 weeks)

Advice for Referral

- Medical records establishing diagnosis, history of manifestations of disease, and past treatments are vital.
- Serious consideration should be given to having such patients co-managed by a hematologist.

Tests to Prepare for Consult

- None

Tests Not Useful Before Consult

- None

Tests Consultant May Need to Do

- Red cell PBG deaminase
- Urine porphobilinogens
- Urine ALA

Follow-up Visits Generally Required

- Co-management, see *Advice for Referral*

Suggested Readings

Tefferi A, Colgan JP, Solberg LA Jr. Acute porphyrias: diagnosis and management. [Review]. Mayo Clin Proc 1994;69:991–995.

Desnick RJ. The porphyrias. In: Fauci AS, Braunwald E, Isselbacher KJ, et al., eds. Harrison's Principles of Internal Medicine. 14th ed. New York: McGraw Hill, 1998:2152–2158.

Sassa S. Porphyrias. In: Beutler E, Lichtman MA, Coller BS, eds. Williams Hematology. 5th ed. New York: McGraw Hill, 1995:726–747.

Splenomegaly

Indications and Timing for Referral
- Persistent for more than 4 weeks
- Diagnostic uncertainty
- Assistance with management

Timing: Routine (less than 4 weeks)

Advice for Referral
- Monospot or heterophile helpful in patients younger than 40 years old.
- Liver-spleen scan helpful in patients older than 30 years.

Tests to Prepare for Consult
- CBC
- Reticulocyte count
- ALT, AST, alkaline phosphatase
- Bilirubin
- Globulin
- Heterophil or monospot test

Tests Not Useful Before Consult
- Bone marrow aspirate and biopsy

Tests Consultant May Need to Do
- CBC with blood smear
- IEP, serum
- EBV antibody
- RF
- CT scan, abdomen
- Bone marrow aspirate and biopsy
- Flow cytometry on marrow aspirate
- Cytogenetics on marrow aspirate
- Barium swallow

Follow-up Visits Generally Required
- One

Suggested Readings
Henry PH, Longo DL. Enlargement of the lymph nodes and spleen. In: Fauci AS, Braunwald E, Isselbacher KJ, et al., eds. Harrison's Principles of Internal Medicine. 14th ed. New York: McGraw Hill, 1998:345–351.

See Also
- Hypersplenism

HEMATOLOGY

Thalassemia

Indications and Timing for Referral

- Confirmation of specific diagnosis
- Assistance with management and/or counseling

Timing: Routine (less than 4 weeks)

Tests to Prepare for Consult

- CBC
- Reticulocyte count
- Hb electrophoresis
- Ferritin
- Iron/TIBC
- ALT, AST, alkaline phosphatase
- Bilirubin

Tests Not Useful Before Consult

- Bone marrow aspirate and biopsy

Tests Consultant May Need to Do

- CBC with blood smear
- Reticulocyte count
- Hb electrophoresis
- Hb F level
- Hb H level

Follow-up Visits Generally Required

- One

Suggested Readings

Rund D, Rachmilewitz E. Advances in the pathophysiology and treatment of thalassemia [review]. Crit Rev Oncol Hematol 1995;20:237–254.

Dumars KW, Boehm C, Eckman JR, et al. Practical guide to the diagnosis of thalassemia. Council of Regional Networks for Genetic Services (CORN). Am J Med Genet 1996;62:29–37.

Kan YW. Development of DNA analysis for human diseases. Sickle cell anemia and thalassemia as a paradigm. [Review]. JAMA 1992;267:1532–1536.

Piomelli S, Loew T. Management of thalassemia major (Cooley's anemia). [Review]. Hematol Oncol Clin North Am 1991;5:557–569.

Thrombocytopenia

Indications and Timing for Referral

- Platelet count less than 20,000
- Bruising and petechiae present

Timing: Urgent (less than 24 hours)

- Platelet count 20,000 to 50,000

Timing: Expedited (less than 1 week)

- Persistently less than 150,000 for 7 days without explanation
- Determine underlying cause

Timing: Routine (less than 4 weeks)

Advice for referral

- Patient requires immediate medical attention if mucosal bleeding, wet purpura, or headache is present with thrombocytopenia, or if trauma occurs in patient with known thrombocytopenia.
- Complete medication history is vital.
- Serious consideration should be given to having such patients co-managed by a hematologist.

Tests to Prepare for Consult

- CBC
- Reticulocyte count
- RDW
- Blood smear examination
- Platelet count

Tests Not Useful Before Consult

- Bone marrow aspirate and biopsy

Tests Consultant May Need to Do

- CBC with blood smear
- Reticulocyte count
- Prothrombin time
- PTT
- Fibrin split products
- Fibrinogen
- Creatinine
- Bilirubin
- ALT, AST, alkaline phosphatase
- Urinalysis with microscopic
- Antiplatelet antibody
- ANA
- ALT, AST, alkaline phosphatase
- HIV antibody testing
- Bone marrow aspirate and biopsy

Follow-up Visits Generally Required

- Co-management, see *Advice for Referral*

Thrombocytopenia (continued)

Suggested Readings

George JN, Woolf SH, Raskob GE, et al. Idiopathic thrombocytopenic purpura: a practice guideline developed by explicit methods for the American Society of Hematology [see comments]. [Review] [295 refs]. Blood 1996;88:3–40.

Chong BH. Diagnosis, treatment and pathophysiology of autoimmune thrombocytopenias [review]. Crit Rev Oncol Hematol 1995;20:271–296.

Rutherford CJ, Frenkel EP. Thrombocytopenia. Issues in diagnosis and therapy. [Review]. Med Clin North Am 1994;78:555–575.

Goldstein KH, Abramson N. Efficient diagnosis of thrombocytopenia. Am Fam Physician 1996;53:915–920.

Vadhan-Raj S, Murray LJ, Bueso-Ramos C, et al. Stimulation of megakaryocyte and platelet production by a single dose of recombinant human thrombopoietin in patients with cancer [see comments]. Ann Intern Med 1997;126:673–681.

George JN, el-Harake MA, Raskob GE. Chronic idiopathic thrombocytopenic purpura [see comments]. [Review]. N Engl J Med 1994;331:1207–1211.

See Also

- Pancytopenia, normal or low reticulocyte count

Thrombocytosis

Indications and Timing for Referral

- Diagnostic uncertainty
- Assistance with management

Timing: Routine (less than 4 weeks)

- Preoperative assessment

Timing: Expedited (less than 1 week)

Advice for Referral

- Records of old blood counts are vital.

Tests to Prepare for Consult

- CBC
- ESR
- Ferritin

Tests Not Useful Before Consult

- Bone marrow aspirate and biopsy

Tests Consultant May Need to Do

- CBC with blood smear
- CT scan, liver and spleen
- Bone marrow aspirate and biopsy
- Cytogenetics on marrow aspirate

Follow-up Visits Generally Required

- One

Suggested Readings

Kutti J, Wadenvik H. Diagnostic and differential criteria of essential thrombocythemia and reactive thrombocytosis. [Review] [42 refs]. Leuk Lymphoma 1996;22(Suppl 1):41–45.

Kutti J. The management of thrombocytosis. [Review]. Eur J Haematol 1990;44:81–88.

Williams WJ. Thrombocytosis. In: Beutler E, Lichtman MA, Coller BS, eds. Williams Hematology. 5th ed. New York: McGraw Hill, 1995:1361–1364.

Vitamin B$_{12}$ Deficiency

Indications and Timing for Referral

- Unresponsive to conventional therapy
- Diagnostic uncertainty
- Assistance with management

Timing: Routine (less than 4 weeks)

Tests to Prepare for Consult

- CBC with differential
- Reticulocyte count
- Vitamin B$_{12}$, serum
- Red cell folate level
- RDW
- LDH

Tests Not Useful Before Consult

- Serum folate level
- Bone marrow aspirate and biopsy

Tests Consultant May Need to Do

- CBC with blood smear
- Reticulocyte count
- Vitamin B$_{12}$, serum
- Schilling test ± intrinsic factor
- TSH (assay sensitivity <0.1 mU/L)
- Anti-intrinsic factor antibody
- Antiparietal cell antibody
- Bone marrow aspirate and biopsy

Follow-up Visits Generally Required

- One

Suggested Readings

Green R. Screening for vitamin B$_{12}$ deficiency—caveat emptor. Ann Intern Med 1996;124:509–511.

Hoffbrand V, Provan D. ABC of clinical haematology. Macrocytic anaemias. [Review] [0 refs]. Br Med J 1997;314:430–433.

Savage DG, Lindenbaum J, Stabler SP, Allen RH. Sensitivity of serum methylmalonic acid and total homocysteine determinations for diagnosing cobalamin and folate deficiencies. Am J Med 1994;96:239–246.

Beck WS. Diagnosis of megaloblastic anemia. [Review]. Annu Rev Med 1991;42:311–322.

Sumner AE, Chin MM, Abrahm JL, et al. Elevated methylmalonic acid and total homocysteine levels show high prevalence of vitamin B$_{12}$ deficiency after gastric surgery. Ann Intern Med 1996;124(5):469.

Clementz GL, Schade SG. The spectrum of vitamin B$_{12}$ deficiency [see comments]. [Review]. Am Fam Physician 1990;41:150–162.

Selected Guidelines

Guidelines on the investigation and diagnosis of cobalamin and folate deficiencies. A publication of the British Committee for Standards in Haematology. BCSH General Haematology Test Force. Clin Lab Haematol 1994;16:101–115.

CHAPTER 6

Infectious Diseases

Adenopathy
   Cervical 295
   Generalized 296
Carbuncles or Boils, Recurrent 297
Cough, in HIV-Positive Patient 298
Dementia, in HIV-Positive Patient 299
Diarrhea
   in HIV-Positive Patient 300
   History of Recent Foreign Travel 302
Dysphagia or Odynophagia in HIV-Positive Patient 303
Dysuria, Nonpyuric 304
Fatigue
   Chronic, Afebrile 305
   Chronic, Febrile 306
Fever
   of Unknown Origin (FUO) 308
   with Rash 310
Headache, in HIV-Positive Patient 311
Hepatitis Serology, Positive, Rejected by Blood Bank 312
Herpes Zoster, Chicken Pox, Shingles Exposure 313
Human Immunodeficiency Virus (HIV)
   Indeterminate Western Blot 314
   Positive Western Blot 315
Lower Leg Ulcers, Poorly Resolving 316
Lyme Titer
   Positive 317
   Positive, Typical Clinical Syndrome 318
Needlestick 319
Partner
   Is HIV-Positive 320
   with Gonorrhea, Asymptomatic 321
   with Herpes Simplex 322
   with Syphilis 323
Pneumonia, Recurrent 324
Pyuria 325

(continued)

Infectious Diseases (continued)

Rapid Plasma Reagin (RPR) Test, Venereal Disease Research Laboratories
  (VDRL) Test, Positive 326
Rubella Exposure 327
Sinusitis
  Persistent 328
  Recurrent 330
Soft Tissue Infection
  Poorly Resolving 332
  Recurrent 333
Sore Throat
  Recurrent 334
  Severe, *Streptococcus*-Negative 336
Tick Bite 337
Tuberculosis (TB) Skin Test
  Positive, Uncertain Duration 338
  Recent Conversion (Less Than 2 Years) 339
Urethral Discharge 340
Urinary Candidiasis 341
Urinary Tract Infections
  Recurrent 342
  with Indwelling Catheter 343

INFECTIOUS DISEASES

Adenopathy, Cervical

Indications and Timing for Referral
- Rapidly enlarging
- Clinical findings suggesting significant tracheal, esophageal or vascular compression
- Local signs of inflammation

Timing: Urgent (less than 24 hours)

- Unilateral or bilateral, unexplained for longer than 4 weeks

Timing: Expedited (less than 1 week)

Advice for Referral
- Nonspecific viral study panels are not recommended before seeing consultant.
- Should have lower threshold for referral in patient who is human immunodeficiency virus-positive (HIV+).
- If biopsy is anticipated, refer to M.D. capable of acquiring specimen for pathologic analysis.
- Dental consultation may be appropriate to identify occult site of infection.
- Factors favoring referral to infectious disease include:
    - Fever present
    - Local signs of inflammation
    - Elevated WBC or left shift
- Factors favoring referral to oncology/hematology or otorhinolaryngologist (ENT) include:
    - Adenopathy persists without inflammation

Tests To Prepare for Consult
- CBC with differential
- Glucose
- Creatinine
- ALT, AST, alkaline phosphatase

Tests Not Useful Before Consult
- None

Tests Consultant May Need to Do
- CBC with blood smear
- Heterophil or monospot test
- HIV antibody testing
- Anti-p24 antibody
- VDRL or RPR
- ANA
- Viral serology for suspected agents
- Anti-*Bartonella* antibody
- PPD
- Radiograph, chest
- CT scan, neck
- Indirect laryngoscopy
- Fine needle biopsy
- Surgical biopsy

Follow-up Visits Generally Required
- One

Suggested Readings
Swartz MN. Lymphadenitis and lymphangitis. In: Mandell GL, Bennett JE, Dolin R, eds. Principles and Practice of Infectious Diseases. 4th ed. NY: Churchill Livingstone, 1995:936–944.

Bailey RE. Diagnosis and treatment of infectious mononucleosis. [Review]. Am Fam Physician 1994;49:879–888.

Haynes BF. Enlargement of lymph nodes and spleen. In: Isselbacher KJ, Braunwald E, Wilson JD, et al., eds. Harrison's Principles of Internal Medicine. 13th ed. NY: McGraw-Hill Inc., 1994:323–329.

THE CONSULTATION GUIDE

Adenopathy, Generalized

Indications and Timing for Referral
- Rapidly enlarging
- Local compressive problem
- Clinically suspicious nodes

Timing: Urgent (less than 24 hours)

- Unilateral or bilateral, unexplained for longer than 4 weeks

Timing: Expedited (less than 1 week)

Advice for Referral
- Clinically suspicious nodes should be referred to M.D. capable of acquiring specimen for pathologic analysis.
- Factors favoring referral to infectious disease include:
  - Fever present
  - Elevated WBC or left shift
- Factors favoring referral to oncology/hematology or general surgeon include:
  - Biopsy anticipated
  - Adenopathy persists without inflammation

Tests To Prepare for Consult
- CBC with differential
- Creatinine
- ALT, AST, alkaline phosphatase
- VDRL or RPR
- Monospot test
- Radiograph, chest

Tests Not Useful Before Consult
- EBV antibody
- CT scan, abdomen

Tests Consultant May Need to Do
- CBC with differential
- ANA
- Heterophil or monospot test
- Bacterial serology for suspected agents
- Viral serology for suspected agents
- *Toxoplasma* serology
- Parasitic serologies for suspected agents
- Lyme (*Borrelia burgdorferi*) serology
- Anti-p24 antibody
- HIV antibody testing
- HIV, by PCR
- TSH (assay sensitivity <0.1 mU/L)
- CT scan, abdomen
- Fine needle biopsy
- Surgical biopsy

Follow-up Visits Generally Required
- Two

Suggested Readings
Haynes BF. Enlargement of lymph nodes and spleen. In: Isselbacher KJ, Braunwald E, Wilson JD, et al., eds. Harrison's Principles of Internal Medicine. 13th ed. NY: McGraw-Hill Inc., 1994:323–329.

Swartz MN. Lymphadenitis and lymphangitis. In: Mandell GL, Bennett JE, Dolin R, eds. Principles and Practice of Infectious Diseases. 4th ed. NY: Churchill Livingstone, 1995:936–944.

Bailey RE. Diagnosis and treatment of infectious mononucleosis. [Review]. Am Fam Physician 1994;49:879–888.

See Also
- Adenopathy, cervical

INFECTIOUS DISEASES

Carbuncles or Boils, Recurrent

Indications and Timing for Referral

Assistance with management

Timing: Routine (less than 4 weeks)

Advice for Referral

- Records of culture and sensitivity and treatment response are vital.

Tests To Prepare for Consult

- CBC with differential
- Glucose
- Creatinine
- Staphylococcal culture, nasal swab

Tests Not Useful Before Consult

- None

Tests Consultant May Need to Do

- WBC function studies
- IgE, quantitative

Follow-up Visits Generally Required

- One

Suggested Readings

Carson SC, Prose NS, Berg D. Infectious disorders of the skin. [Review]. Clin Plastic Surg 1993;20:67–76.

Williams RE, MacKie RM. The staphylococci. Importance of their control in the management of skin disease. [Review]. Dermatol Clin 1993;11:201–206.

Klempner MS, Styrt B. Prevention of recurrent staphylococcal skin infections with low-dose oral clindamycin therapy [see comments]. JAMA 1988;260:2682–2685.

See Also

- Soft tissue infection, recurrent
- Soft tissue infection, poorly resolving

THE CONSULTATION GUIDE

Cough, in HIV-Positive Patient

Indications and Timing for Referral

- Respiratory discomfort present

Timing: Urgent (less than 24 hours)

- Etiology unclear
- Assistance with management

Timing: Routine (less than 1 week)

Advice for Referral

- Oxygen saturation is helpful if available in physician's office.

Tests To Prepare for Consult

- CBC with differential
- Glucose
- Albumin, total protein
- Creatinine
- ALT, AST, alkaline phosphatase
- Radiograph, chest
- Sputum
  - Gram stain
  - Routine culture
  - AFB stain
- PPD
- T lymphocyte subsets

Tests Not Useful Before Consult

- None

Tests Consultant May Need to Do

- Arterial blood gas
- CD4 count
- HIV antigen load
- Blood cultures × 2
- Radiograph, chest
- Sputum Gram stain
- Sputum, routine culture
- AFB, induced sputum
- PCP, induced sputum

- Sputum, fungal stain
- Sputum, fungal culture
- Fungal serology for suspected agents
- PPD
- CT scan
  - Sinuses
  - Thorax
- Bronchoscopy

Follow-up Visits Generally Required

- Two

Suggested Readings

Freedberg KA, Tosteson AN, Cotton DJ, Goldman L. Optimal management strategies for HIV-infected patients who present with cough or dyspnea: a cost-effective analysis [see comments]. [Review]. J Gen Intern Med 1992;7:261–272.

Fever, cough, and dyspnea in a 38-year-old man with acquired immunodeficiency syndrome [clinical conference]. Am J Med 1995;98:85–94.

Murray JF, Mills J. Pulmonary infectious complications of human immunodeficiency virus infection. Part II. [Review]. Am Rev Respir Dis 1990;141:1582–1598.

Bernard EM, Sepkowitz KA, Telzak EE, Armstrong D. Pneumocystosis. [Review]. Med Clin North Am 1992;76:107–119.

Poulton TB. Chest manifestations of AIDS. [Review]. Am Fam Physician 1992;45:163–168.

Stansell JD. Pulmonary fungal infections in HIV-infected persons. [Review]. Semin Respir Infect 1993;8:116–123.

See Also

- Cough, chronic

INFECTIOUS DISEASES

Dementia, in HIV-Positive Patient

Indications and Timing for Referral

- Unexplained, new or change in baseline mental status

Timing: Expedited (less than 1 week)

Advice for Referral

- If outpatient monitoring is not assured and an acute problem is suspected, emergent evaluation is needed.
- When available, MR with enhancement is preferable test.

Tests To Prepare for Consult

- CBC with differential
- T lymphocyte subsets
- HIV antigen load
- *Toxoplasma* serology
- Cryptococcal antigen, serum
- CT or MR, cranial with contrast

Tests Not Useful Before Consult

- Skull films

Tests Consultant May Need to Do

- MR, cranial
- Lumbar puncture
- Albumin, CSF
- Protein, CSF
- Glucose, CSF
- Gram stain, CSF
- Culture and sensitivity, CSF
- VDRL or RPR, CSF
- Cryptococcal antigen, CSF
- HIV by PCR, CSF
- Fungal stain and culture, CSF
- Cytology, CSF
- Cell count, CSF
- CMV PCR, CSF
- Mycobacteria culture, CSF

Follow-up Visits Generally Required

- Two

Suggested Readings

Lipton SA, Gendelman HE. Seminars in medicine of the Beth Israel Hospital, Boston. Dementia associated with the acquired immunodeficiency syndrome. [Review]. N Engl J Med 1995;332:934–940.

Glass JD, Johnson RT. Human immunodeficiency virus and the brain. [Review] [149 refs]. Annu Rev Neurosci 1996;19:1–26.

Newton HB. Common neurologic complications of HIV-1 infection and AIDS. [Review]. Am Fam Physician 1995;51:387–398.

Atkinson JH, Grant I. Natural history of neuropsychiatric manifestations of HIV disease. [Review]. Psychiatr Clin North Am 1994;17:17–33.

Stern Y. Neuropsychological evaluation of the HIV patient. [Review]. Psychiatr Clin North Am 1994;17:125–134.

Melton ST, Kirkwood CK, Ghaemi SN. Pharmacotherapy of HIV dementia. [Review] [90 refs]. Ann Pharmacother 1997;31:457–473.

See Also

- Mental status change, acute or subacute
- Mental status change, chronic dementia

THE CONSULTATION GUIDE

Diarrhea, in HIV-Positive Patient

Indications and Timing for Referral

- Patient has marked systemic symptoms without control and/or diagnosis

Timing: Urgent (less than 24 hours)

- Patient has systemic symptoms without control and/or diagnosis

Timing: Expedited (less than 1 week)

- No systemic symptoms present
- Diagnostic uncertainty
- Assistance with management

Timing: Routine (less than 1 week)

Tests To Prepare for Consult

- CBC with differential
- Glucose
- Albumin, total protein
- Creatinine
- ALT, AST, alkaline phosphatase
- Electrolytes (Na, K, Cl, CO_2)
- T lymphocyte subsets
- Glucose
- Stool
  - C&S
  - O&P
  - WBC
- *Clostridium difficile* stool toxin

Tests Not Useful Before Consult

- Barium enema
- UGIS

Tests Consultant May Need to Do

- Blood culture
- CD4 count
- HIV antigen load
- *Giardia* antigen, stool
- Stool
  - C&S
  - O&P
  - WBC
- Stain for
  - *Cryptosporidium*, stool
  - Cyclospora, stool
  - Microsporidia, stool
- Stool culture for suspected agents
- Upper endoscopy
- Colonoscopy
- Sigmoidoscopy

Follow-up Visits Generally Required

- One

Diarrhea, in HIV-Positive Patient (continued)

Suggested Readings

Blanshard C, Francis N, Gazzard BG. Investigation of chronic diarrhoea in acquired immunodeficiency syndrome. A prospective study of 155 patients. Gut 1996;39:824–832.

Johanson JF. Diagnosis and management of AIDS-related diarrhea. [Review] [61 refs]. Can J Gastroenterol 1996;10:461–468.

Wilcox CM, Rabeneck L, Friedman S. AGA technical review: malnutrition and cachexia, chronic diarrhea, and hepatobiliary disease in patients with human immunodeficiency virus infection. [Review] [311 refs]. Gastroenterology 1996;111:1724–1752.

Grohmann GS, Glass RI, Pereira HG, et al. Enteric viruses and diarrhea in HIV-infected patients. Enteric Opportunistic Infections Working Group. [Review]. N Engl J Med 1993;329:14–20.

Smith PD. Infectious diarrheas in patients with AIDS. [Review]. Gastroenterol Clin North Am 1993;22:535–548.

Smith PD, Quinn TC, Strober W, et al. NIH conference. Gastrointestinal infections in AIDS [see comments]. [Review]. Ann Intern Med 1992;116:63–77.

Bartlett JG, Belitsos PC, Sears CL. AIDS enteropathy [see comments]. [Review]. Clin Infect Dis 1992;15:726–735.

See Also

- Diarrhea, chronic

Diarrhea, History of Recent Foreign Travel

Indications and Timing for Referral

- Diagnosis uncertain and persistent for longer than 10 days

Timing: Expedited (less than 1 week)

Advice for Referral

- *C. difficile* stool toxin required only in setting of prior antibiotic use.
- Fresh specimen needed to assess stool for C&S and O&P.

Tests To Prepare for Consult

- Stool
  - C&S
  - O&P
  - WBC
- *C. difficile* stool toxin

Tests Not Useful Before Consult

- Barium enema
- UGIS

Tests Consultant May Need to Do

- HIV antibody testing
- *Giardia*
  - Antigen, stool
  - Serology
- *Cryptosporidium* stain
- Cyclospora and *Isospora* stain
- Stool culture for suspected agents
- Stool O&P
- Sigmoidoscopy

Follow-up Visits Generally Required

- One

Suggested Readings

Larson SC. Traveler's diarrhea. [Review] [15 refs]. Emerg Med Clin North Am 1997;15:179–189.

Okhuysen PC, Ericsson CD. Travelers' diarrhea. Prevention and treatment. [Review]. Med Clin North Am 1992;76:1357–1373.

Heck JE, Cohen MB. Traveler's diarrhea. [Review]. Am Fam Physician 1993;48:793–800.

Kelsall BL, Guerrant RL. Evaluation of diarrhea in the returning traveler. [Review]. Infect Dis Clin North Am 1992;6:413–425.

Chak A, Banwell JG. Traveler's diarrhea. [Review]. Gastroenterol Clin North Am 1993;22:549–561.

Tellier R, Keystone JS. Prevention of traveler's diarrhea. [Review]. Infect Dis Clin North Am 1992;6:333–354.

INFECTIOUS DISEASES

Dysphagia or Odynophagia in HIV-Positive Patient

Indications and Timing for Referral

- Severe odynophagia, inability to swallow liquid, or evidence of dehydration

Timing: Urgent (less than 24 hours)

- Etiology unclear
- Assistance with management

Timing: Expedited (less than 1 week)

Tests To Prepare for Consult

- CBC with differential
- T lymphocyte subsets

Tests Not Useful Before Consult

- Barium swallow

Tests Consultant May Need to Do

- Orapharyngeal culture for specific viral agents
- Fungal culture, oropharyngeal
- CMV culture
- Herpes culture
- CD4 count
- Upper endoscopy

Follow-up Visits Generally Required

- One

Suggested Readings

Wilcox CM. Esophageal disease in the acquired immunodeficiency syndrome: etiology, diagnosis, and management [see comments]. [Review]. Am J Med 1992;92:412–421.

Raufman JP. Odynophagia/dysphagia in AIDS. [Review]. Gastroenterol Clin North Am 1988;17:599–614.

Rabeneck L, Laine L. Esophageal candidiasis in patients infected with the human immunodeficiency virus. A decision analysis to assess cost-effectiveness of alternative management strategies. Arch Intern Med 1994;154:2705–2710.

Selected Guidelines

Appropriate use of gastrointestinal endoscopy: a consensus statement from the American Society for Gastrointestinal Endoscopy. Manchester, MA: The Society. 1989;11:1995.

The role of endoscopy in the management of esophagitis. Guidelines for clinical application. Gastrointest Endosc 1988; 34(3 Suppl):9S.

THE CONSULTATION GUIDE

Dysuria, Nonpyuric

Indications and Timing for Referral

- Persistent for 6 weeks with no diagnostic urine analysis or culture

Timing: Routine (less than 4 weeks)

Advice for Referral

- Lab should identify all organisms.
- Gynecologic exam is necessary.
- In men, prostatitis should be considered before infectious disease referral.

Tests To Prepare for Consult

- Urinalysis with microscopic
- Urine, culture and sensitivity
- Pap smear

Tests Not Useful Before Consult

- None

Tests Consultant May Need to Do

- Urinalysis with microscopic
- Urine, culture and sensitivity
- KOH prep
- Wet prep
- Urethral swab for WBC
- *Chlamydia* culture, urethral swab
- Gonorrhea culture, urethral swab
- C&S, urethral swab
- Herpes simplex culture, urethral swab
- Ureaplasma culture, urethral swab

Follow-up Visits Generally Required

- One

Suggested Readings

Hamilton-Miller JM. The urethral syndrome and its management. [Review]. J Antimicrob Chemother 1994;33(Suppl A):63–73.

Neu HC. Urinary tract infections. [Review]. Am J Med 1992;92(Suppl 4A):63S–70S.

Pappas PG. Laboratory in the diagnosis and management of urinary tract infections. [Review]. Med Clin North Am 1991;75:313–325.

Osterberg E, Aspevall O, Grillner L, Persson E. Young women with symptoms of urinary tract infection—prevalence and diagnosis of chlamydial infection and evaluation of rapid screening of bacteriuria. Scan J Prim Health Care 1996;14:43–49.

See Also

- Urinary candidiasis
- Urinary tract infection, with indwelling catheter
- Urinary tract infections, recurrent
- Pyuria
- Urethral discharge

INFECTIOUS DISEASES

Fatigue, Chronic, Afebrile

Indications and Timing for Referral
- Diagnosis uncertain and persistent for 3 months
- Interferes with patient's ability to perform activities of daily living

Timing: Routine (less than 4 weeks)

Tests To Prepare for Consult
- CBC with differential
- ESR
- TSH (assay sensitivity <0.1 mU/L)
- ALT, AST, alkaline phosphatase
- Electrolytes (Na, K, Cl, CO_2)
- Glucose
- Albumin, total protein
- Creatinine
- Bilirubin
- LDH
- Urinalysis with microscopic
- Radiograph, chest

Tests Not Useful Before Consult
- EBV antibody
- T_3
- *Candida* serology
- Lyme (*B. burgdorferi*) serology
- HSV serology
- Environmental allergen serologies
- Skin testing

Tests Consultant May Need to Do
- Immunoglobulins, quantitative
- ANA
- Anti-double stranded DNA
- Rheumatoid factor
- Testosterone, in men
- T lymphocyte subsets
- HIV antibody testing
- Free T_4
- ACTH stimulation test, 1-hour
- CT scan, abdomen

Follow-up Visits Generally Required
- Two

Suggested Readings
Epstein KR. The chronically fatigued patient. [Review]. Med Clin North Am 1995;79:315–327.

Fukuda K, Straus SE, Hickie I, et al. The chronic fatigue syndrome: a comprehensive approach to its definition and study. International Chronic Fatigue Syndrome Study Group. Ann Intern Med 1994;121:953–959.

Bates DW, Buchwald D, Lee J, et al. Clinical laboratory test findings in patients with chronic fatigue syndrome. Arch Intern Med 1995;155:97–103.

Schluederberg A, Straus SE, Peterson P, et al. NIH conference. Chronic fatigue syndrome research. Definition and medical outcome assessment. Ann Intern Med 1992;117:325–331.

Buchwald D, Umali P, Umali J, et al. Chronic fatigue and the chronic fatigue syndrome: prevalence in a Pacific Northwest health care system. Ann Intern Med 1995;123:81–88.

Wilson A, Hickie I, Lloyd A, et al. Longitudinal study of outcome of chronic fatigue syndrome [see comments]. Br Med J 1994;308:756–759.

Straus SE. Chronic fatigue syndrome. In: Fauci AS, Braunwald E, Isselbacher KJ, et al., eds. Harrison's Principles of Internal Medicine. 14th ed. New York: McGraw Hill, 1998:2483–2485.

See Also
- Fatigue, chronic, febrile
- Fever of unknown origin

THE CONSULTATION GUIDE

Fatigue, Chronic, Febrile

Indications and Timing for Referral

- Diagnostic uncertainty and temperature higher than 101°F sustained for more than 5 days on 2 occasions

Timing: Routine (less than 4 weeks)

Tests To Prepare for Consult

- CBC with differential
- Glucose
- Albumin, total protein
- Bilirubin
- Creatinine
- ALT
- AST
- Alkaline phosphatase
- LDH
- Calcium
- TSH (assay sensitivity <0.1 mU/L)
- ANA
- ESR
- HIV antibody testing
- Blood cultures × 3
- VDRL or RPR
- Urinalysis with microscopic
- Radiograph, chest

Tests Not Useful Before Consult

- EBV antibody
- Lyme (*B. burgdorferi*) serology

Tests Consultant May Need to Do

- CBC with differential
- Glucose
- Albumin, total protein
- Bilirubin
- Creatinine
- ALT, AST, alkaline phosphatase
- Anti-double stranded DNA
- Rheumatoid factor
- Blood cultures × 3
- IEP, serum and urine
- FTA-ABS
- For suspected agents:
  - Bacterial cultures
  - Bacterial serology
  - Viral serology
  - Viral cultures
- ACTH stimulation test, 1-hour
- PPD
- Urine metanephrines
- Anergy intradermal skin test panel
- CT scan
  - Abdomen
  - Thorax
  - Pelvis
- Small bowel follow through
- Barium enema
- Colonoscopy
- Temporal artery biopsy

Follow-up Visits Generally Required

- Two

INFECTIOUS DISEASES

Fatigue, Chronic, Febrile (*continued*)

Suggested Readings

Buchwald D, Umali P, Umali J, et al. Chronic fatigue and the chronic fatigue syndrome: prevalence in a Pacific Northwest health care system. Ann Intern Med 1995;123:81–88.

Hirschmann JV. Fever of unknown origin in adults. [Review] [21 refs]. Clin Infect Dis 1997;24:291–300.

Fukuda K, Straus SE, Hickie I, et al. The chronic fatigue syndrome: a comprehensive approach to its definition and study. International Chronic Fatigue Syndrome Study Group. Ann Intern Med 1994;121:953–959.

Bates DW, Buchwald D, Lee J, et al. Clinical laboratory test findings in patients with chronic fatigue syndrome. Arch Intern Med 1995;155:97–103.

Straus SE. Chronic fatigue syndrome. In: Fauci AS, Braunwald E, Isselbacher KJ, et al., eds. Harrison's Principles of Internal Medicine. 14th ed. New York: McGraw Hill, 1998:2483–2485.

See Also

- Fatigue, chronic, afebrile
- Fever of unknown origin

THE CONSULTATION GUIDE

Fever, of Unknown Origin (FUO)

Indications and Timing for Referral

- Temperature higher than 101°F for more than 3 weeks with unclear etiology after clinical and laboratory evaluation

Timing: Expedited (less than 1 week)

Tests To Prepare for Consult

- CBC with differential
- ESR
- Glucose
- Blood cultures × 3
- Albumin, total protein
- Creatinine
- Bilirubin
- ALT, AST, alkaline phosphatase
- LDH
- Calcium
- ANA
- HIV antibody testing
- VDRL or RPR
- Urinalysis with microscopic
- Radiograph, chest

Tests Not Useful Before Consult

- EBV antibody
- Lyme (*B. burgdorferi*) serology

Tests Consultant May Need to Do

- CBC with differential
- Glucose
- Albumin, total protein
- Bilirubin
- Creatinine
- ALT, AST, alkaline phosphatase
- TSH (assay sensitivity <0.1 mU/L)
- Anti-double stranded DNA
- Rheumatoid factor
- Blood cultures × 3
- Immunoelectrophoresis, serum and urine
- FTA-ABS
- For suspected agents:
  - Bacterial cultures
  - Bacterial serology
  - Viral serology
  - Viral cultures
- Metanephrines, 24-hour urine
- ACTH stimulation test, 1-hour
- PPD
- Anergy intradermal skin test panel
- Echocardiogram with Doppler studies
- CT scan
  - Abdomen
  - Thorax
  - Pelvis
- Small bowel follow through
- Barium enema
- Colonoscopy
- Temporal artery biopsy

Fever, of Unknown Origin (FUO) (continued)

Follow-up Visits Generally Required
- Two

Suggested Readings
Hirschmann JV. Fever of unknown origin in adults. [Review] [21 refs]. Clin Infect Dis 1997;24:291–300.

Cunha BA. Fever of unknown origin. [Review] [64 refs]. Infect Dis Clin North Am 1996;10:111–127.

Knockaert DC, Dujardin KS, Bobbaers HJ. Long-term follow-up of patients with undiagnosed fever of unknown origin [review]. Arch Intern Med 1996;156:618–620.

Brusch JL, Weinstein L. Fever of unknown origin. [Review]. Med Clin North Am 1988;72:1247–1261.

Saxe SE, Gardner P. The returning traveler with fever. [Review]. Infect Dis Clin North Am 1992;6:427–439.

Gelfand JA, Dinarello CA. Fever of unknown origin. In: Fauci AS, Braunwald E, Isselbacher KJ, et al., eds. Harrison's Principles of Internal Medicine. 14th ed. New York: McGraw Hill, 1998:780–785.

See Also
- Fatigue, chronic, afebrile
- Fatigue, chronic, febrile

THE CONSULTATION GUIDE

Fever, with Rash

Indications and Timing for Referral

- Etiology unclear with systemic signs
- Patient immunosuppressed
- Rash with ulceration

Timing: Urgent (less than 24 hours)

Advice for Referral

- A purpuric rash requires emergent care.
- May require dermatology consultation for biopsy and culture.

Tests To Prepare for Consult

- CBC with differential
- Blood smear examination
- Glucose
- Albumin, total protein
- Creatinine
- ALT, AST, alkaline phosphatase
- VDRL or RPR
- Blood cultures × 2
- ESR
- Urinalysis with microscopic
- Radiograph, chest

Tests Not Useful Before Consult

- None

Tests Consultant May Need to Do

- Throat culture
- Monospot test
- ASLO titer
- HIV antibody testing
- Hepatitis A antibody
- HB_sAg
- Hepatitis C antibody
- Culture, lesions
- Smear for special stains
- Acute phase serology, hold serum for
- ANA
- Anti-double stranded DNA
- ECG
- Blood cultures × 2
- Lyme (*Borrelia burgdorferi*) serology
- FTA-ABS
- Biopsy, skin lesion

Follow-up Visits Generally Required

- Two

Suggested Readings

Schlossberg D. Fever and rash. [Review] [9 refs]. Infect Dis Clin North Am 1996;10:101–110.

Heymann WR. Noninfectious causes of fever and a rash. [Review]. Int J Dermatol 1989;28:145–156.

Kaye ET, Kaye KM. Fever and rash. In: Fauci AS, Braunwald E, Isselbacher KJ, et al., eds. Harrison's Principles of Internal Medicine. 14th ed. New York: McGraw Hill, 1998:90–97.

INFECTIOUS DISEASES

Headache, in HIV-Positive Patient

Indications and Timing for Referral

- Unexplained, new or change in pattern of chronic headache, and persistent for more than 48 hours

Timing: Expedited (less than 1 week)

Advice for Referral

- If fever and global or focal neurologic signs are present, emergent care is needed.
- If outpatient monitoring is not assured and an acute problem is suspected, emergent evaluation is needed.
- When available, MR with enhancement is the preferable test.
- Sinus CT, focused series (a limited series of appropriate regional cuts to include coronal images of the osteomeatal complex).

Tests To Prepare for Consult

- CBC
- T lymphocyte subsets
- *Toxoplasma* serology
- Cryptococcal antigen, serum
- CT or MR, cranial with contrast

Tests Not Useful Before Consult

- Skull films

Tests Consultant May Need to Do

- MR, cranial
- CT, sinuses, focused series (see *Advice for Referral*)
- Lumbar puncture
- Albumin, CSF
- Protein, CSF
- Glucose, CSF
- Gram stain, CSF
- Culture and sensitivity, CSF
- VDRL or RPR, CSF
- Cryptococcal antigen, CSF
- HIV by PCR, CSF
- Fungal stain and culture, CSF
- Cytology, CSF
- Cell count, CSF
- CMV PCR, CSF
- Mycobacteria culture, CSF

Follow-up Visits Generally Required

- Two

Suggested Readings

Singer EJ, Kim J, Fahy-Chandon B, et al. Headache in ambulatory HIV-1-infected men enrolled in a longitudinal study. Neurology 1996;47:487–494.

Brew BJ, Miller J. Human immunodeficiency virus-related headache. Neurology 1993;43:1098–1100.

Lipton RB, Feraru ER, Weiss G, et al. Headache in HIV-1-related disorders. Headache 1991;31:518–522.

Goldstein J. Headache and acquired immunodeficiency syndrome. [Review]. Neurol Clin 1990;8:947–960.

Selected Guidelines

Magnetic resonance imaging of the brain and spine: a revised statement. American College of Physicians [comment] [see comments]. Ann Intern Med 1994;120:872–875.

See Also

- Headache, chronic recurrent
- Headache, migraine
- Headache, acute

THE CONSULTATION GUIDE

Hepatitis Serology, Positive, Rejected by Blood Bank

Indications and Timing for Referral

- Assistance with management

Timing: Routine (less than 4 weeks)

Advice for Referral

- Record from blood bank is vital.

Tests To Prepare for Consult

- HB_sAb
- HB_sAg
- Hepatitis C antibody

Tests Not Useful Before Consult

- None

Tests Consultant May Need to Do

- HB_sAb
- HB_sAg
- Hepatitis C antibody
- Hepatitis C, PCR
- Hepatitis E antibody
- VDRL or RPR
- ALT, AST, alkaline phosphatase
- Bilirubin
- Anti-HTLV 1&2 antibodies
- HIV antibody testing

Follow-up Visits Generally Required

- One

Suggested Readings

Sjogren MH. Serologic diagnosis of viral hepatitis. [Review]. Gastroenterol Clin North Am 1994;23:457–477.

Rubin RA, Falestiny M, Malet PF. Chronic hepatitis C. Advances in diagnostic testing and therapy. [Review]. Arch Intern Med 1994;154:387–392.

See Also

- Hepatitis B
- Hepatitis C
- Hepatitis D
- Transaminase elevation

INFECTIOUS DISEASES

Herpes Zoster, Chicken Pox, Shingles Exposure

Indications and Timing for Referral

- Assist with management in pregnant, potentially pregnant, or immunocompromised patient who has no personal history of chicken pox or shingles

Timing: Urgent (less than 24 hours)

Tests To Prepare for Consult

- Varicella-zoster antibody
- Beta HCG, serum (quantitative)

Tests Not Useful Before Consult

- None

Tests Consultant May Need to Do

- None

Follow-up Visits Generally Required

- None

Suggested Readings

Holmes SJ. Review of recommendations of the Advisory Committee on Immunization Practices, Centers for Disease Control and Prevention, on varicella vaccine. J Infect Dis 1996;174(Suppl 3):S342–S344.

Whitley RJ, Weiss H, Gnann JW Jr, et al. Acyclovir with and without prednisone for the treatment of herpes zoster. A randomized, placebo-controlled trial. The National Institute of Allergy and Infectious Diseases Collaborative Antiviral Study Group. Ann Intern Med 1996;125:376–383.

Fox GN, Strangarity JW. Varicella-zoster virus infections in pregnancy [see comments]. [Review]. Am Fam Physician 1989;39:89–98.

Prevention of varicella: Recommendations of the Advisory Committee on Immunization Practices (ACIP). Centers for Disease Control and Prevention. MMWR Morb Mortal Wkly Rep 1996;45(RR-11):1–36.

THE CONSULTATION GUIDE

Human Immunodeficiency Virus (HIV), Indeterminate Western Blot

Indications and Timing for Referral

- Extreme patient concern

Timing: Expedited (less than 1 week)

- Diagnostic uncertainty
- Assistance with management

Timing: Routine (less than 4 weeks)

Tests To Prepare for Consult

- HIV antibody testing
- HIV antibody, by Western blot
- T lymphocyte subsets

Tests Not Useful Before Consult

- None

Tests Consultant May Need to Do

- HIV antibody testing
- HIV antibody, by Western blot
- T lymphocyte subsets
- HIV culture
- HIV, by PCR
- Anti-p24 antibody

Follow-up Visits Generally Required

- One

Suggested Readings

Proffitt MR, Yen-Lieberman B. Laboratory diagnosis of human immunodeficiency virus infection. [Review]. Infect Dis Clin North Am 1993;7:203–219.

Phair JP, Wolinsky S. Diagnosis of infection with the human immunodeficiency virus. [Review]. Clin Infect Dis 1992;15:13–16.

From the Centers for Disease Control and Prevention. Recommendations for HIV testing services for inpatients and outpatients in acute-care hospital settings. JAMA 1993;269:2071–2072.

Sloand EM, Pitt E, Chiarello RJ, Nemo GJ. HIV testing. State of the art. [Review]. JAMA 1991;266:2861–2866.

Bartlett JG. HIV serology and epidemiology. The Johns Hopkins Hospital 1997 Guide to Medical Care of Patients with HIV Infection. 7th ed. Baltimore: Williams & Wilkins, 1997;1–8.

See Also

- HIV, positive western blot
- Partner is HIV-positive

314

INFECTIOUS DISEASES

Human Immunodeficiency Virus (HIV), Positive Western Blot

Indications and Timing for Referral

- Assistance with management and assessment

Timing: Expedited (less than 1 week)

Advice for Referral

- Co-management with an infectious disease consultant is often required.

Tests To Prepare for Consult

- HIV antibody testing
- HIV antibody, by Western blot
- T lymphocyte subsets

Tests Not Useful Before Consult

- None

Tests Consultant May Need to Do

- HIV antibody testing
- HIV antibody, by Western blot
- HIV culture
- HIV, by PCR
- HIV antigen load
- Anti-p24 antibody
- CBC
- VDRL or RPR
- PPD
- Glucose
- Albumin, total protein
- Creatinine
- ALT, AST, alkaline phosphatase
- Radiograph, chest
- *Toxoplasma* serology
- Cryptococcal antigen, serum
- HB_sAb

Follow-up Visits Generally Required

- See *Advice for Referral*

Suggested Readings

Proffitt MR, Yen-Lieberman B. Laboratory diagnosis of human immunodeficiency virus infection. [Review]. Infect Dis Clin North Am 1993;7:203–219.

From the Centers for Disease Control and Prevention. Recommendations for HIV testing services for inpatients and outpatients in acute-care hospital settings. JAMA 1993;269:2071–2072.

Phair JP, Wolinsky S. Diagnosis of infection with the human immunodeficiency virus. [Review]. Clin Infect Dis 1992;15:13–16.

Sloand EM, Pitt E, Chiarello RJ, Nemo GJ. HIV testing. State of the art. [Review]. JAMA 1991;266:2861–2866.

See Also

- HIV, indeterminate western blot
- Partner is HIV-positive

THE CONSULTATION GUIDE

Lower Leg Ulcers, Poorly Resolving

Indications and Timing for Referral

- Rapidly progressing infection or signs of systemic sepsis

Timing: Urgent (less than 24 hours)

- Peripheral vascular disease, diabetes mellitus, or hemoglobinopathy present

Timing: Expedited (less than 1 week)

Advice for Referral

- Refer for biopsy (dermatology, or general surgery, or vascular surgical evaluation) may be appropriate.

Tests To Prepare for Consult

- CBC with differential
- Blood smear examination
- Glucose
- Albumin, total protein
- Creatinine
- ALT, AST, alkaline phosphatase

Tests Not Useful Before Consult

- None

Tests Consultant May Need to Do

- Rheumatoid factor
- Bacterial smear and culture
- Fungal smear and culture
- Lower extremity venous doppler study

Follow-up Visits Generally Required

- One

Suggested Readings

Pion IA, Buchness MR, Lim HW. Nonhealing leg ulcer. Arch Dermatol 1996;132:1105.

Margolis DJ, Cohen JH. Management of chronic venous leg ulcers: a literature-guided approach. [Review]. Clin Dermatol 1994;12:19–26.

Caputo GM, Cavanagh PR, Ulbrecht JS, et al. Assessment and management of foot disease in patients with diabetes [see comments]. [Review]. N Engl J Med 1994;331:854–860.

Mulder GD, Reis TM. Venous ulcers: pathophysiology and medical therapy. [Review]. Am Fam Physician 1990;42:1323–1330.

Spence RJ, Jones CE. Leg ulcers and varicose veins. In: Barker R, Burton JR, Zieve PD, eds. Principles of Ambulatory Medicine. 6th ed. Baltimore: Williams & Wilkins, 1998:1311–1320.

INFECTIOUS DISEASES

Lyme Titer, Positive

Indications and Timing for Referral

- Assistance with management
- Determine clinical significance

Timing: Routine (less than 4 weeks)

Advice for Referral

- Serologic tests for Lyme disease are poorly standardized and can be unreliable. There is controversy about the significance of positive serology in the absence of clinical illness compatible with Lyme disease.

Tests To Prepare for Consult

- RPR or VDRL

Tests Not Useful Before Consult

- ECG
- MR, cranial

Tests Consultant May Need to Do

- IgG anti-Lyme antibodies
- IgM anti-Lyme antibodies

Follow-up Visits Generally Required

- One

Suggested Readings

Tugwell P, Dennis DT, Weinstein A, et al. Laboratory evaluation in the diagnosis of Lyme disease. Ann Intern Med 1997;127:1109–1123.

Ledue TB, Collins MF, Craig WY. New laboratory guidelines for serologic diagnosis of Lyme disease: evaluation of the two-test protocol. J Clin Microbiol 1996;34:2343–2350.

Sivak SL, Aguero-Rosenfeld ME, Nowakowski J, et al. Accuracy of IgM immunoblotting to confirm the clinical diagnosis of early Lyme disease. Arch Intern Med 1996;156:2105–2109.

Schoen RT. Identification of Lyme disease. [Review]. Rheum Dis Clin North Am 1994;20:361–369.

Sigal LH. The Lyme disease controversy. Social and financial costs of misdiagnosis and mismanagement [see comments]. [Review] [30 refs]. Arch Intern Med 1996;156:1493–1500.

Kalish R. Lyme disease. [Review]. Rheum Dis Clin North Am 1993;19:399–3426.

Sigal LH. Lyme disease: testing and treatment. Who should be tested and treated for Lyme disease and how?. [Review]. Rheum Dis Clin North Am 1993;19:79–93.

Selected Guidelines

Guidelines for laboratory evaluation in the diagnosis of Lyme disease. American College of Physicians. Ann Intern Med 1997;127:1106–1108.

See Also

- Lyme titer, positive, typical clinical syndrome
- Tick bite
- Pain in a few joints (≤ 4)

Lyme Titer, Positive, Typical Clinical Syndrome

Indications and Timing for Referral

- Assistance with management

Timing: Expedited (less than 1 week)

Tests To Prepare for Consult

- None

Tests Not Useful Before Consult

- None

Tests Consultant May Need to Do

- ECG
- Lumbar puncture
- Cell count, CSF
- Glucose, CSF
- Protein, CSF
- Lyme titer, CSF
- Joint tap
- Cell count with differential, aspirated fluid
- Culture and sensitivity, aspirated fluid

Follow-up Visits Generally Required

- Two

Suggested Readings

From the Centers for Disease Control and Prevention. Lyme disease—United States, 1996. JAMA 1997;278:112.

Steere AC. Lyme disease [see comments]. [Review]. N Engl J Med 1989;321:586–596.

Kalish R. Lyme disease. [Review]. Rheum Dis Clin North Am 1993;19:399–426.

Rahn DW, Malawista SE. Lyme disease: recommendations for diagnosis and treatment [see comments]. [Review]. Ann Intern Med 1991;114:472–481.

Tugwell P, Dennis DT, Weinstein A, et al. Laboratory evaluation in the diagnosis of Lyme disease. Ann Intern Med 1997;127:1109–1123.

Selected Guidelines

Practice parameter: Diagnosis of patients with nervous system Lyme borreliosis (Lyme disease)—Summary statement. Report of the Quality Standards Subcommittee of the American Academy of Neurology. Neurology 1996;46:881–882.

Halperin JJ, Logigian EL, Finkel MF, Pearl RA. Practice parameters for the diagnosis of patients with nervous system Lyme borreliosis (Lyme disease). Quality Standards Subcommittee of the American Academy of Neurology. [Review] [66 refs]. Neurology 1996;46:619–627:

Guidelines for laboratory evaluation in the diagnosis of Lyme disease. American College of Physicians. Ann Intern Med 1997;127:1106–1108.

See Also

- Lyme titer, positive
- Tick bite
- Lyme disease, cause of neurologic findings
- Pain in a few joints (≤ 4)

INFECTIOUS DISEASES

Needlestick

Indications and Timing for Referral

- Assistance with management

Timing: Urgent (less than 24 hours)

Advice for Referral

- If the exposer is or is likely to be HIV+, the patient should be seen emergently for consideration of azidothymidine (AZT) prophylaxis.
- Records of the exposer's HIV antibody test, Hb_sAg, and hepatitis C antibody should be obtained whenever possible.
- Patient's previous serologic status to hepatitis B, if known, should be provided.
- The patient should be informed to seek medical evaluation for any acute illness that occurs during the 6 month follow-up period.
- During the 6 months after potential exposure, the patient should follow recommendations for preventing transmission of HIV.

Tests To Prepare for Consult

- None

Tests Not Useful Before Consult

- None

Tests Consultant May Need to Do

- HIV antibody testing
- HIV, by PCR
- HB_sAb
- HB_cAb
- Hepatitis C antibody

Follow-up Visits Generally Required

- One

Suggested Readings

Kasting G, Rollin PE. Wound care following needlestick injuries. JAMA 1997;277:517.

Gerberding JL. Prophylaxis for occupational exposure to HIV. [Review] [31 refs]. Ann Intern Med 1996;125:497–501.

Rich JD, Ramratnam B, Flanigan TP. Triple combination antiretroviral prophylaxis for needlestick exposure to HIV [letter]. Infect Control Hosp Epidemiol 1997;18:161.

Gerberding JL, Littell C, Tarkington A, et al. Risk of exposure of surgical personnel to patients' blood during surgery at San Francisco General Hospital [see comments]. N Engl J Med 1990;322:1788–1793.

From the Centers for Disease Control and Prevention. Update: provisional public health service recommendations for chemoprophylaxis after occupational exposure to HIV. JAMA 1996;276:90–92.

Anderson DC, Blower AL, Packer JM, Ganguli LA. Preventing needlestick injuries [published erratum appears in Br Med J 1991;302:1063] [see comments]. Br Med J 1991;302:769–770.

Selected Guidelines

From the Centers for Disease Control and Prevention. Evaluation of safety devices for preventing percutaneous injuries among health-care workers during phlebotomy procedures—Minneapolis-St Paul, New York City, and San Francisco, 1993–1995. JAMA 1997;277:449–450.

Recommendations for preventing transmission of human immunodeficiency virus and hepatitis B virus to patients during exposure-prone invasive procedures. MMWR Morb Mortal Wkly Rep 1991;40(RR-8):1–9.

THE CONSULTATION GUIDE

Partner, Is HIV-Positive

Indications and Timing for Referral

- Assistance with management

Timing: Expedited (less than 1 week)

Tests To Prepare for Consult

- HIV antibody testing

Tests Not Useful Before Consult

- None

Tests Consultant May Need to Do

- Herpes culture (if lesions present)
- *Chlamydia* culture
- Gonorrhea culture
- Wet prep
- Pap smear
- RPR or VDRL
- HIV antibody testing
- HB_sAg

Follow-up Visits Generally Required

- One

Suggested Readings

Jason J, Ou CY, Moore JL, et al. Prevalence of human immunodeficiency virus type 1 DNA in hemophilic men and their sex partners. Hemophilia-AIDS Collaborative Study Group. J Infect Dis 1989;160:789–794.

Proffitt MR, Yen-Lieberman B. Laboratory diagnosis of human immunodeficiency virus infection. [Review]. Infect Dis Clin North Am 1993;7:203–219.

Toomey KE, Cates W Jr. Partner notification for the prevention of HIV infection. [Review]. AIDS 1989;3(Suppl 1):S57–S62.

See Also

- HIV, positive western blot
- HIV, indeterminate western blot

INFECTIOUS DISEASES

Partner, with Gonorrhea, Asymptomatic

Indications and Timing for Referral

- Assistance with management

Timing: Urgent (less than 24 hours)

Tests To Prepare for Consult

- RPR or VDRL

Tests Not Useful Before Consult

- None

Tests Consultant May Need to Do

- Herpes culture (if lesions present)
- *Chlamydia* culture
- Gonorrhea culture
- Wet prep
- Pap smear
- RPR or VDRL
- HIV antibody testing
- HB_sAg

Follow-up Visits Generally Required

- One

Suggested Readings

Moy JG, Clasen ME. The patient with gonococcal infection. [Review]. Prim Care 1990;17:59–83.

Cates W, Holmes KK. Condom efficacy against gonorrhea and nongonococcal urethritis. Am J Epidemiol 1996;143:843–844.

Partner, with Herpes Simplex

Indications and Timing for Referral

- Assistance with management

Timing: Routine (less than 4 weeks)

Tests To Prepare for Consult

- None

Tests Not Useful Before Consult

- HSV serology

Tests Consultant May Need to Do

- Herpes culture (if lesions present)
- *Chlamydia* culture
- Gonorrhea culture
- Wet prep
- Pap smear
- RPR or VDRL
- HIV antibody testing
- HB_sAg

Follow-up Visits Generally Required

- One

Suggested Readings

Bryson Y, Dillon M, Bernstein DI, et al. Risk of acquisition of genital herpes simplex virus type 2 in sex partners of persons with genital herpes: a prospective couple study. J Infect Dis 1993;167:942–946.

Pereira FA. Herpes simplex: evolving concepts. [Review] [182 refs]. J Am Acad Dermatol 1996;35:503–520.

Mertz GJ. Epidemiology of genital herpes infections. [Review]. Infect Dis Clin North Am 1993;7:825–839.

INFECTIOUS DISEASES

Partner, with Syphilis

Indications and Timing for Referral

- Assistance with management

Timing: Routine (less than 4 weeks)

Advice for Referral

- If RPR-positive, do an FTA-ABS

Tests To Prepare for Consult

- RPR or VDRL
- FTA-ABS

Tests Not Useful Before Consult

- None

Tests Consultant May Need to Do

- Herpes culture (if lesions present)
- *Chlamydia* culture
- Gonorrhea culture
- Wet prep
- Pap smear
- HIV antibody testing
- HB_sAg

Follow-up Visits Generally Required

- One

Suggested Readings

Johnson PC, Farnie MA. Testing for syphilis. [Review]. Dermatol Clin 1994;12:9–17.

Thomas DL, Quinn TC. Serologic testing for sexually transmitted diseases. [Review]. Infect Dis Clin North Am 1993;7:793–824.

Hutchinson CM, Hook EW 3rd, Shepherd M, et al. Altered clinical presentation of early syphilis in patients with human immunodeficiency virus infection. Ann Intern Med 1994;121:94–100.

See Also

- RPR or VDRL, positive

Pneumonia, Recurrent

Indications and Timing for Referral

- More than 2, radiologically confirmed, suspected, bacterial pneumonias within 5 years without obvious cause, e.g., recurrent aspiration

Timing: Routine (less than 4 weeks)

Tests To Prepare for Consult

- CBC with differential
- Glucose
- Albumin, total protein
- Creatinine
- ALT, AST, alkaline phosphatase
- Radiograph, chest
- Radiograph, chest, obtain old films

Tests Not Useful Before Consult

- None

Tests Consultant May Need to Do

- Eosinophil count, total
- HIV antibody testing
- Immunoglobulins, quantitative
- PPD
- Sputum culture
- Spirometry, before and after bronchodilator
- Flow volume loops
- Cine esophagogram
- CT scan, thorax
- ANA
- Anti-double stranded DNA
- Anti-neutrophil cytoplasmic antibody

Follow-up Visits Generally Required

- One

Suggested Readings

Geppert EF. Chronic and recurrent pneumonia. [Review]. Semin Respir Infect 1992;7:282–288.

Fein AM, Feinsilver SH, Niederman MS. Nonresolving and slowly resolving pneumonia. Diagnosis and management in the elderly patient. [Review]. Clin Chest Med 1993;14:555–569.

Kirtland SH, Winterbauer RH. Slowly resolving, chronic, and recurrent pneumonia. [Review]. Clin Chest Med 1991;12:303–318.

Coley CM, Li YH, Medsger AR, et al. Preferences for home vs hospital care among low-risk patients with community-acquired pneumonia. Arch Intern Med 1996;156:1565–1571.

INFECTIOUS DISEASES

Pyuria

Indications and Timing for Referral
- Unexplained and persistent for 6 weeks
- More than 10 WBCs per high powered field in spun urine with negative urine C&S

Timing: Routine (less than 4 weeks)

Advice for Referral
- Laboratory to identify all organisms even if WBC count is low.
- Urinary tract malignancy work-up should be considered.

Tests To Prepare for Consult
- Urinalysis with microscopic
- Urine, culture & sensitivity
- PPD

Tests Not Useful Before Consult
- None

Tests Consultant May Need to Do
- Urinalysis with microscopic
- Urine, culture & sensitivity
- Cytology, urine
- AFB culture, urine
- *Chlamydia* culture, urethral swab
- Gonorrhea culture, urethral swab
- C&S, urethral swab
- Ureaplasma culture, urethral swab
- Fungal culture, urine
- Smear for special stains
- IVP

Follow-up Visits Generally Required
- One

Suggested Readings

Hooton TM. A simplified approach to urinary tract infection. [Review]. Hosp Pract (Off Ed) 1995;30:23–30.

Stamm WE. Criteria for the diagnosis of urinary tract infection and for the assessment of therapeutic effectiveness [see comments]. Infection 1992;20(Suppl 3):S151–S154.

Pappas PG. Laboratory in the diagnosis and management of urinary tract infections. [Review]. Med Clin North Am 1991;75:313–325.

Boscia JA, Abrutyn E, Levison ME, et al. Pyuria and asymptomatic bacteriuria in elderly ambulatory women. Ann Intern Med 1989;110:404–405.

See Also
- Dysuria, nonpyuric
- Urinary tract infections, recurrent
- Urinary tract infection, with indwelling catheter
- Urinary candidiasis
- Urethral discharge

THE CONSULTATION GUIDE

Rapid Plasma Reagin (RPR) Test, Venereal Disease Research Laboratories (VDRL) Test, Positive

Indications and Timing for Referral

- Assistance with management

Timing: Routine (less than 4 weeks)

Advice for Referral

- Records of previous test results and treatment are vital.

Tests To Prepare for Consult

- FTA-ABS

Tests Not Useful Before Consult

- None

Tests Consultant May Need to Do

- HIV antibody testing
- Lumbar puncture
- Cell count, CSF
- Protein, CSF
- VDRL or RPR, CSF

Follow-up Visits Generally Required

- One

Suggested Readings

Johnson PC, Farnie MA. Testing for syphilis. [Review]. Dermatol Clin 1994;12:9–17.

Thomas DL, Quinn TC. Serologic testing for sexually transmitted diseases. [Review]. Infect Dis Clin North Am 1993;7:793–824.

See Also

- Partner, with syphilis

INFECTIOUS DISEASES

Rubella Exposure

Indications and Timing for Referral

- Assistance with management in pregnant, potentially pregnant, or immunocompromised patient

Timing: Urgent (less than 24 hours)

Advice for Referral

- Order beta HCG if appropriate

Tests To Prepare for Consult

- Rubella antibody
- Beta HCG, serum (quantitative)

Tests Not Useful Before Consult

- None

Tests Consultant May Need to Do

- None

Follow-up Visits Generally Required

- None

Suggested Readings

Rushworth RL, Bell SM, Morrell S, Robertson PW. Rubella in mothers. Lancet 1996;347:1262.

Lindegren ML, Fehrs LJ, Hadler SC, Hinman AR. Update: rubella and congenital rubella syndrome, 1980–1990. [Review]. Epidemiol Rev 1991;13:341–348.

Mumps and rubella consensus conference. [Review]. Can Commun Dis Rep 1994;20:165–176.

See Also

- Herpes zoster, chicken pox, shingles exposure

Sinusitis, Persistent

Indications and Timing for Referral

- Marked signs and symptoms of related soft tissue inflammation
- Regional neurologic changes, especially visual
- Signs of systemic toxicity
- Severe pain

Timing: Urgent (less than 24 hours)

- Persistent for more than 4 weeks and refractory to treatment
- Associated allergic diathesis, especially if other clinical features of respiratory allergy are present
- Evidence of other recurrent infections, e.g., bronchitis, pneumonia

Timing: Routine (less than 4 weeks)

Advice for Referral

- Lower threshold for referral in HIV+ patient.
- Imaging should not be obtained during or within 2 weeks of an acute episode of sinusitis or other respiratory tract infection.
- In most practice settings, a focused sinus CT series is more informative than sinus radiographs.
- Sinus CT, focused series (a limited series of appropriate regional cuts to include coronal images of the osteomeatal complex).
- Factors favoring referral to infectious diseases include:
  - Evidence of other recurrent infections, e.g., bronchitis, pneumonia
- Factors favoring referral to an allergist/immunologist include:
  - Personal history of asthma
  - Family history of allergies
  - Symptoms related to specific environmental exposures
  - Normal sinus exam
- Factors favoring referral to ENT include:
  - Acute and severe sinusitis
  - Persistent or recurrent involvement of one sinus region
  - Bloody discharge
  - Evidence of extrasinus extension of infection e.g., orbit
  - Acute frontal sinusitis
  - History of sinofacial trauma

Sinusitis, Persistent (continued)

Tests To Prepare for Consult

- CBC with differential
- CT, sinuses, focused series (see *Advice for Referral*)

Tests Not Useful Before Consult

- Nasopharyngeal culture

Tests Consultant May Need to Do

- Eosinophil count, total
- Immunoglobulins, quantitative
- Radiograph, chest
- CBC with differential
- ESR
- Creatinine
- Urinalysis with microscopic
- Functional antibody response to immunization
- Immediate hypersensitivity skin testing
- RAST
- Fiberoptic rhinolaryngoscopy

Follow-up Visits Generally Required

- One

Suggested Readings

Wagner W. Changing diagnostic and treatment strategies for chronic sinusitis. [Review] [34 refs]. Cleve Clin J Med 1996;63:396–405.

Evans KL. Diagnosis and management of sinusitis. [Review]. Br Med J 1994;309:1415–1422.

Guarderas JC. Rhinitis and sinusitis: office management. [Review] [8 refs]. Mayo Clin Proc 1996;71:882–888.

Druce HM. Diagnosis of sinusitis in adults: history, physical examination, nasal cytology, echo, and rhinoscope. [Review]. J Allergy Clin Immunol 1992;90:436–441.

Wagenmann M, Naclerio RM. Complications of sinusitis. [Review]. J Allergy Clin Immunol 1992;90:552–554.

Spector SL. The role of allergy in sinusitis in adults. [Review]. J Allergy Clin Immunol 1992;90:518–520.

Zinreich SJ. Imaging of chronic sinusitis in adults: Radiograph, computed tomography, and magnetic resonance imaging. [Review]. J Allergy Clin Immunol 1992;90:445–451.

Lanza DC, Kennedy DW. Current concepts in the surgical management of chronic and recurrent acute sinusitis. [Review]. J Allergy Clin Immunol 1992;90:505–511.

See Also

- Sinusitis, recurrent

Sinusitis, Recurrent

Indications and Timing for Referral

- More than 3 documented episodes per year with purulent nasal discharge requiring antibiotic therapy
- Associated allergic diathesis, especially if other clinical features of respiratory allergy are present
- Evidence of other recurrent infections, e.g., bronchitis, pneumonia

Timing: Routine (less than 4 weeks)

Advice for Referral

- Lower threshold for referral if patient uses inhaled nasal steroids.
- Imaging should not be obtained during or within 2 weeks of an acute episode of sinusitis or other respiratory tract infection.
- In most practice settings, a focused sinus CT series is more informative than sinus radiographs.
- Dental evaluation may be appropriate for patients with recurring maxillary sinusitis.
- Sinus CT, focused series (a limited series of appropriate regional cuts to include coronal images of the osteomeatal complex).
- Factors favoring referral to infectious diseases include:
    - Evidence of other recurrent infections, e.g., bronchitis, pneumonia
- Factors favoring referral to an allergist/immunologist include:
    - Personal history of asthma
    - Family history of allergies
    - Symptoms related to specific environmental exposures
    - Normal sinus exam
    - Recurrent infection with suspicion of immunodeficiency
- Factors favoring referral to ENT include:
    - Acute and severe sinusitis
    - Persistent or recurrent involvement of one sinus region
    - Bloody discharge
    - Evidence of extrasinus extension of infection e.g., orbit
    - Acute frontal sinusitis
    - History of sinofacial trauma

Tests To Prepare for Consult

- CBC with differential
- Eosinophil count, total
- Nasal swab for eosinophils
- Immunoglobulins, quantitative
- Radiograph, chest
- CT, sinuses, focused series (see *Advice for Referral*)

Sinusitis, Recurrent (continued)

Tests Not Useful Before Consult
- Nasopharyngeal culture

Tests Consultant May Need to Do
- Nasal cytology
- Immunoglobulins, quantitative
- CBC
- ESR
- IgG subclasses
- HIV antibody testing
- Radiograph, chest
- RAST
- Immediate hypersensitivity skin testing
- Functional antibody response to immunization
- Fiberoptic rhinolaryngoscopy
- Pulmonary function tests

Follow-up Visits Generally Required
- Two

Suggested Readings
Galen BA. Chronic recurrent sinusitis. Recognition and treatment. [Review] [34 refs]. Lippincotts Prim Care Pract 1997;1:183–198.

Guarderas JC. Rhinitis and sinusitis: office management. [Review] [8 refs]. Mayo Clin Proc 1996;71:882–888.

Evans KL. Diagnosis and management of sinusitis. [Review]. Br Med J 1994;309:1415–1422.

Druce HM. Diagnosis of sinusitis in adults: history, physical examination, nasal cytology, echo, and rhinoscope. [Review]. J Allergy Clin Immunol 1992;90:436–441.

Spector SL. The role of allergy in sinusitis in adults. [Review]. J Allergy Clin Immunol 1992;90:518–520.

Zinreich SJ. Imaging of chronic sinusitis in adults: Radiograph, computed tomography, and magnetic resonance imaging. [Review]. J Allergy Clin Immunol 1992;90:445–451.

Selected Guidelines
Allergy testing. American College of Physicians [see comments]. Ann Intern Med 1989;110:317–320.

See Also
- Sinusitis, persistent

THE CONSULTATION GUIDE

Soft Tissue Infection, Poorly Resolving

Indications and Timing for Referral

- Rapidly progressing or signs of systemic sepsis present

Timing: Urgent (less than 24 hours)

- Refractory to conventional treatment
- Patient immunosuppressed, diabetic, or has a known history of peripheral vascular disease

Timing: Expedited (less than 1 week)

Advice for Referral

- Records of C&S and treatment response are vital.

Tests To Prepare for Consult

- CBC with differential
- Glucose
- Creatinine

Tests Not Useful Before Consult

- None

Tests Consultant May Need to Do

- Blood culture
- HIV antibody testing
- Radiograph, CT, or MR of affected region
- Smear and stain, needle aspirate of lesion
- Culture, needle aspiration of lesion
- Biopsy, skin lesion

Follow-up Visits Generally Required

- Two

Suggested Readings

Lindsey D. Soft tissue infections. [Review]. Emerg Med Clin North Am 1992;10:737–751.

Canoso JJ, Barza M. Soft tissue infections. [Review]. Rheum Dis Clin North Am 1993;19:293–309.

Carson SC, Prose NS, Berg D. Infectious disorders of the skin. [Review]. Clin Plast Surg 1993;20:67–76.

Sentochnik DE. Deep soft-tissue infections in diabetic patients. [Review]. Infect Dis Clin North Am 1995;9:53–64.

Lewis RT. Necrotizing soft-tissue infections. [Review]. Infect Dis Clin North Am 1992;6:693–703.

Lipsky BA, Pecoraro RE, Wheat LJ. The diabetic foot. Soft tissue and bone infection. [Review]. Infect Dis Clin North Am 1990;4:409–432.

See Also

- Soft tissue infection, recurrent
- Carbuncles or boils, recurrent

INFECTIOUS DISEASES

Soft Tissue Infection, Recurrent

Indications and Timing for Referral
- Predisposition unclear
- Assistance with appropriate management to prevent recurrence

Timing: Routine (less than 4 weeks)

Advice for Referral
- Records of C&S and treatment response are vital.

Tests To Prepare for Consult
- CBC with differential
- Glucose
- Albumin, total protein
- Creatinine
- ALT, AST, alkaline phosphatase

Tests Not Useful Before Consult
- Immunoglobulins, quantitative

Tests Consultant May Need to Do
- Staphylococcal culture, nasal swab
- WBC phagocyte function studies
- Biopsy, skin lesion

Follow-up Visits Generally Required
- One

Suggested Readings
Canoso JJ, Barza M. Soft tissue infections. [Review]. Rheum Dis Clin North Am 1993;19:293–309.

Falagas ME, Barefoot L, Griffith J, et al. Risk factors leading to clinical failure in the treatment of intra-abdominal or skin/soft tissue infections. Eur J Clin Microbiol Infect Dis 1996;15:913–921.

Lewis RT. Necrotizing soft-tissue infections. [Review]. Infect Dis Clin North Am 1992;6:693–703.

Lipsky BA, Pecoraro RE, Wheat LJ. The diabetic foot. Soft tissue and bone infection. [Review]. Infect Dis Clin North Am 1990;4:409–432.

Smith AJ, Daniels T, Bohnen JM. Soft tissue infections and the diabetic foot. [Review] [26 refs]. Am J Surg 1996;172(Suppl 6A): 7S–12S.

See Also
- Soft tissue infection, poorly resolving
- Carbuncles or boils, recurrent

THE CONSULTATION GUIDE

Sore Throat, Recurrent

Indications and Timing for Referral

- Patient HIV+ with fever or systemic symptoms

Timing: Urgent (less than 24 hours)

- Diagnostic uncertainty
- Unexplained treatment failure
- Extreme patient concern
- Severe, disabling with short duration between episodes
- Incomplete recovery between episodes

Timing: Routine (less than 4 weeks)

Advice for Referral

- Throat culture recommended only if inflammation is noted.
- Throat culture done without inflammation noted may lead to unnecessary treatment.
- Rule out reflux before seeking infectious disease consultation.
- Not unusual in daycare worker or patient with frequent exposure to children.
- Consider allergic rhinitis as a contributing factor.
- Imaging should not be obtained during or within 2 weeks of an acute episode of sinusitis or other respiratory tract infection.
- Sinus CT, focused series (a limited series of appropriate regional cuts to include coronal images of the osteomeatal complex).

Tests To Prepare for Consult

- CBC with differential
- Throat culture

Tests Not Useful Before Consult

- Monospot test
- Heterophil antibody
- Viral cultures, throat

Tests Consultant May Need to Do

- Throat culture
- *Chlamydia* culture, throat
- Gonorrhea culture, throat
- Mycoplasma culture, throat
- CT, sinuses, focused series (see *Advice for Referral*)
- CBC with differential
- ESR
- Eosinophil count, total
- Glucose
- Creatinine
- Albumin, total protein
- ALT, AST, alkaline phosphatase
- Immunoglobulins, quantitative
- IgE, quantitative
- HIV antibody testing
- Urinalysis with microscopic

Sore Throat, Recurrent (continued)

Follow-up Visits Generally Required

- One

Suggested Readings

Pichichero ME. Sore throat after sore throat after sore throat. Are you asking the critical questions? [Review] [22 refs]. Postgrad Med 1997;101:205–206.

Middleton DB. Pharyngitis. [Review] [52 refs]. Prim Care 1996;23:719–739.

Perkins A. An approach to diagnosing the acute sore throat. [Review] [25 refs]. Am Fam Physician 1997;55:131–138.

Goldstein MN. Office evaluation and management of the sore throat. [Review]. Otolaryngol Clin North Am 1992;25:837–842.

Kiselica D. Group A beta-hemolytic streptococcal pharyngitis: current clinical concepts. [Review]. Am Fam Physician 1994;49(5):1147–54.

Mossad SB, Macknin ML, Medendorp SV, Mason P. Zinc gluconate lozenges for treating the common cold. A randomized, double-blind, placebo-controlled study [see comments]. Ann Intern Med 1996;125:81–88.

Ruoff GE. Recurrent streptococcal pharyngitis—using practical treatment options to interrupt the cycle. Postgrad Med J 1996;99:211.

THE CONSULTATION GUIDE

Sore Throat, Severe, *Streptococcus*-Negative

Indications and Timing for Referral

- Patient is HIV+

Timing: Urgent (less than 1 week)

Advice for Referral

- If airway obstruction is present, requires emergent care.
- If drooling, pain, whispering voice, or difficulty swallowing are present associated with a high fever, consider epiglottitis and need for emergent care.
- Referral to ENT surgeon may be appropriate.
- Do not attempt throat culture if epiglottitis is likely.

Tests To Prepare for Consult

- CBC with differential
- Throat culture
- Monospot test

Tests Not Useful Before Consult

- Viral cultures, throat

Tests Consultant May Need to Do

- CBC with differential
- Monospot test
- EBV antibody
- Throat culture for suspected agents
- CT or MR, neck

Follow-up Visits Generally Required

- One

Suggested Readings

Gwattney JM Jr. Pharyngitis. In: Mandell GL, Bennett JE, Dolin R, eds. Principles and Practice of Infectious Diseases. 4th ed. New York: Churchill Livingstone, 1995:566–572.

See Also

- Adenopathy, generalized
- Sore throat, recurrent

INFECTIOUS DISEASES

Tick Bite

Indications and Timing for Referral

- Assistance with management

Timing: Routine (less than 4 weeks)

Advice for Referral

- If the patient becomes ill 2 weeks after a tick bite, he or she needs to be medically evaluated.
- Avoid inappropriate prophylactic antibiotics before the patient becomes symptomatic or sees infectious disease consultant.

Tests To Prepare for Consult

- Acute phase serology, hold serum for

Tests Not Useful Before Consult

- None

Tests Consultant May Need to Do

- Lyme (*Borrelia burgdorferi*) serology

Follow-up Visits Generally Required

- None

Suggested Readings

Doan-Wiggins L. Tick-borne diseases. [Review]. Emerg Med Clin North Am 1991;9:303–325.

Petri WA Jr. Tick-borne diseases. [Review]. Am Fam Physician 1988;37:95–104.

Magid D, Schwartz B, Craft J, Schwartz JS. Prevention of Lyme disease after tick bites. A cost-effectiveness analysis [see comments]. N Engl J Med 1992;327:534–541.

Shapiro ED, Gerber MA, Holabird NB, et al. A controlled trial of antimicrobial prophylaxis for Lyme disease after deer-tick bites [see comments]. N Engl J Med 1992;327:1769–1773.

Sood SK, Salzman MB, Johnson BJ, et al. Duration of tick attachment as a predictor of the risk of Lyme disease in an area in which Lyme disease is endemic. J Infect Dis 1997;175:996–999.

Tugwell P, Dennis DT, Weinstein A, et al. Laboratory evaluation in the diagnosis of Lyme disease. Ann Intern Med 1997;127:1109–1123.

Selected Guidelines

Guidelines for laboratory evaluation in the diagnosis of Lyme disease. American College of Physicians. Ann Intern Med 1997;127:1106–1108.

See Also

- Lyme titer, positive, typical clinical syndrome
- Lyme titer, positive

THE CONSULTATION GUIDE

Tuberculosis (TB) Skin Test, Positive, Uncertain Duration

Indications and Timing for Referral

- Assistance with management
- Patient is HIV+, diabetic, immunosuppressed, or has renal failure
- Immunosuppression or significant health impairment is anticipated

Timing: Routine (less than 4 weeks)

Tests To Prepare for Consult

- Radiograph, chest
- Urinalysis with microscopic

Tests Not Useful Before Consult

- None

Tests Consultant May Need to Do

- PPD
- CBC
- Glucose
- Creatinine
- ALT, AST, alkaline phosphatase
- HIV antibody testing
- Urinalysis with microscopic

Follow-up Visits Generally Required

- None

Suggested Readings

Murthy NK, Dutt AK. Tuberculin skin testing: present status. [Review]. Semin Respir Infect 1994;9:78–83.

Dutt AK, Stead WW. Tuberculosis in the elderly. [Review]. Med Clin North Am 1993;77:1353–1368.

Havlir DV, van der Kuyp F, Duffy E, et al. A 19-year follow-up of tuberculin reactors. Assessment of skin test reactivity and in vitro lymphocyte responses. Chest 1991;99:1172–1176.

Ciesielski SD. BCG vaccination and the PPD test: what the clinician needs to know. [Review]. J Family Pract 1995;40:76–80.

See Also

- TB skin test, recent conversion (less than 2 years)
- Cavitary lung lesion

INFECTIOUS DISEASES

Tuberculosis (TB) Skin Test, Recent Conversion (Less Than 2 Years)

Indications and Timing for Referral

- Assistance with management

Timing: Routine (less than 4 weeks)

Tests To Prepare for Consult

- Radiograph, chest
- Urinalysis with microscopic
- CBC
- ALT, AST, alkaline phosphatase

Tests Not Useful Before Consult

- None

Tests Consultant May Need to Do

- PPD
- CBC
- Glucose
- Creatinine
- ALT, AST, alkaline phosphatase
- HIV antibody testing
- Urinalysis with microscopic

Follow-up Visits Generally Required

- None

Suggested Readings

Camins BC, Bock N, Watkins DL, Blumberg HM. Acceptance of isoniazid preventive therapy by health care workers after tuberculin skin test conversion. JAMA 1996;275:1013–1015.

Miller B. Tuberculin skin testing of hospital workers. JAMA 1996;276:855.

Murthy NK, Dutt AK. Tuberculin skin testing: present status. [Review]. Semin Respir Infect 1994;9:78–83.

Barnes PF, Barrows SA. Tuberculosis in the 1990s [see comments]. [Review]. Ann Intern Med 1993;119:400–410.

See Also

- TB skin test, positive, uncertain duration
- Cavitary lung lesion

THE CONSULTATION GUIDE

Urethral Discharge

Indications and Timing for Referral

- Unexplained
- Unresponsive to conventional treatment

Timing: Routine (less than 4 weeks)

Advice for Referral

- Records of C&S and treatment response are vital.
- Postprostatic massage cultures and cell count are valuable.
- Rule out trauma.

Tests To Prepare for Consult

- Urinalysis with microscopic
- Urine, culture and sensitivity
- *Chlamydia* culture, urethral swab
- Gonorrhea culture, urethral swab
- Herpes simplex culture, urethral swab

Tests Not Useful Before Consult

- None

Tests Consultant May Need to Do

- Urinalysis with microscopic
- Urine, culture and sensitivity
- *Chlamydia* culture, urethral swab
- Gonorrhea culture, urethral swab
- Herpes simplex culture, urethral swab
- Ureaplasma culture, postprostatic massage
- Wet prep
- HIV antibody testing
- VDRL or RPR

Follow-up Visits Generally Required

- One

Suggested Readings

Bowie WR. Approach to men with urethritis and urologic complications of sexually transmitted diseases. [Review]. Med Clin North Am 1990;74:1543–1557.

Stamm WE. Diagnosis of *Chlamydia trachomatis* genitourinary infections. [Review]. Ann Intern Med 1988;108:710–717.

Krieger JN. Urethritis: Etiology, diagnosis, treatment, and complications. In: Gillenwater JY, ed. Adult and Pediatric Urology. 3rd ed. Philadelphia: Mosby-Year Book, 1998:1879–1915.

See Also

- Dysuria, nonpyuric
- Pyuria
- Urinary tract infections, recurrent
- Urinary tract infection, with indwelling catheter
- Urinary candidiasis

Urinary Candidiasis

Indications and Timing for Referral

- Patient symptomatic
- Following solid organ transplant
- Patient is diabetic
- Abnormal collecting system present

Timing: Routine (less than 4 weeks)

Tests To Prepare for Consult

- Urinalysis with microscopic
- Urine, culture and sensitivity
- Glucose
- Albumin, total protein
- Creatinine
- ALT, AST, alkaline phosphatase

Tests Not Useful Before Consult

- None

Tests Consultant May Need to Do

- Urine, culture and sensitivity
- Fungal culture, urine
- Ultrasound, renal
- IVP

Follow-up Visits Generally Required

- One

Suggested Readings

Gubbins PO, Piscitelli SC, Danziger LH. Candidal urinary tract infections: a comprehensive review of their diagnosis and management. [Review]. Pharmacotherapy 1993;13:110–127.

Ang BS, Telenti A, King B, et al. Candidemia from a urinary tract source: microbiological aspects and clinical significance. Clin Infect Dis 1993;17:662–666.

THE CONSULTATION GUIDE

Urinary Tract Infections, Recurrent

Indications and Timing for Referral

- In females, unexplained and more than 3 occurrences in 6 months
- In males, second episode
- Unexplained and unresponsive to therapy

Timing: Routine (less than 4 weeks)

Advice for Referral

- Records of C&S and treatment response are vital.
- In females, gynecologic examination is important to rule out atrophic vaginitis and other causes.
- When appropriate, a trial of antibiotics postcoitus should be attempted.
- If cancer or other obstructive lesion is suspected, a urologic work-up is indicated; otherwise, routine urologic work-up is usually not helpful.
- Homosexual men may have urinary tract infections caused by fecal flora, in the absence of structural abnormalities of the urinary tract. Treat identified organisms.
- Patients should be encouraged to void immediately after intercourse if relationship is apparent.

Tests To Prepare for Consult

- Urinalysis with microscopic
- Urine, culture and sensitivity

Tests Not Useful Before Consult

- Plain film, abdomen

Tests Consultant May Need to Do

- Urinalysis with microscopic
- Urine, culture and sensitivity
- Cytology, urine

- Ultrasound, renal
- IVP

Follow-up Visits Generally Required

- Two

Suggested Readings

Hooton TM, Scholes D, Hughes JP, et al. A prospective study of risk factors for symptomatic urinary tract infection in young women [see comments]. N Engl J Med 1996;335:468–474.

Bacheller CD, Bernstein JM. Urinary tract infections. [Review] [46 refs]. Med Clin North Am 1997;81:719–730.

Hooton TM. A simplified approach to urinary tract infection. [Review]. Hosp Pract (Off Ed) 1995;30:23–30.

Wisinger DB. Urinary tract infection. Current management strategies. [Review] [25 refs]. Postgrad Med 1996;100:229–236.

Stamm WE, Hooton TM. Management of urinary tract infections in adults [see comments]. [Review]. N Engl J Med 1993;329:1328–1334.

Nicolle LE. Prophylaxis: recurrent urinary tract infection in women. Infection 1992;20(Suppl 3):S203–S205.

Selected Guidelines

Common uses of intravenous pyelography in adults. American College of Physicians. Ann Intern Med 1989;111:83–84.

See Also

- Urinary tract infection, with indwelling catheter
- Urinary candidiasis
- Pyuria
- Dysuria, nonpyuric
- Urethral discharge

INFECTIOUS DISEASES

Urinary Tract Infections, with Indwelling Catheter

Indications and Timing for Referral

- Associated with decreased renal function
- Refractory to conventional antibiotic therapy

Timing: Routine (less than 4 weeks)

Advice for Referral

- Records of C&S and treatment response are vital.
- In females, gynecologic examination is necessary.

Tests To Prepare for Consult

- Urinalysis with microscopic
- Urine, culture and sensitivity

Tests Not Useful Before Consult

- Plain film, abdomen

Tests Consultant May Need to Do

- Urinalysis with microscopic
- Urine, culture and sensitivity
- Ultrasound, renal

Follow-up Visits Generally Required

- Two

Suggested Readings

Cardenas DD, Hooton TM. Urinary tract infection in persons with spinal cord injury. Arch Phys Med Rehabil 1995;76:272–280.

The prevention and management of urinary tract infections among people with spinal cord injuries. National Institute on Disability and Rehabilitation Research Consensus Statement. January 27–29, 1992. J Am Paraplegia Soc 1992;15:194–204.

Warren JW. The catheter and urinary tract infection. [Review]. Med Clin North Am 1991;75:481–493.

See Also

- Dysuria, nonpyuric
- Pyuria
- Urinary tract infections, recurrent
- Urinary candidiasis
- Urethral discharge

CHAPTER 7

Nephrology

Acidosis, with Renal Insufficiency 347
Creatinine Elevation 348
Glomerulonephritis
   History of 349
   in Scleroderma 350
   in Systemic Lupus Erythematosus 351
Hematuria
   Gross 352
   Microscopic 354
Hyperkalemia 356
Hypertension
   in Diabetes Mellitus 357
   Labile/Paroxysmal 358
   Renovascular 359
   Rule Out Secondary Cause 360
Hypokalemia 361
Hyponatremia 362
Kidneys
   Enlarged, Bilateral 363
   Enlarged, by Ultrasound, Computed Tomography, or Magnetic
      Resonance 364
   Small, Unilateral 365
Medullary Cystic Disease 366
Nephritis
   Chronic Tubulointerstitial 367
   Chronic Tubulointerstitial, Drug-Induced 368
   Chronic Tubulointerstitial, Industrial Exposure 369
Oliguria 370
Polycystic Kidneys
   History of, Abnormal Renal Function 371
   History of, Normal Renal Function 372
   Incidentally Detected 373
Polyuria 374
Proteinuria
   Trace to 1+ Positive 375
   Nephrotic Range 377

(continued)

THE CONSULTATION GUIDE

Nephrology (continued)

Pyelonephritis, Chronic 379
Red Blood Cell Casts 380
Renal Parenchymal Calcification 381
Renal Stone
    Initial 382
    Recurrent 383
    Calcium Oxalate 384
    Struvite 385
    Uric Acid 386
Uremia 387
Urine, Red 388

NEPHROLOGY

Acidosis, with Renal Insufficiency

Indications and Timing for Referral
- HCO_3 less than 15 mEq/L
- pH less than 7.3

Timing: Urgent (less than 24 hours)

- All patients with this as a new finding should see a nephrologist

Timing: Expedited (less than 1 week)

Advice for Referral
- Careful medication history is vital.

Tests to Prepare for Consult
- Electrolytes (Na, K, Cl, CO_2)
- Albumin, total protein
- BUN, creatinine
- Urinalysis with microscopic

Tests Not Useful Before Consult
- IVP
- MR, renal
- CT scan, renal

Tests Consultant May Need to Do
- Arterial blood gas
- Toxicology screen
- Urine
  - Chloride
  - Potassium
  - Sodium
- Urinalysis with microscopic
- Urine amino acids
- Osmolality, serum
- 24-hour urine creatinine for clearance
- 24-hour urine protein
- Immunoelectrophoresis, serum and urine
- Ultrasound, renal

Follow-up Visits Generally Required
- One

Suggested Readings

Smulders YM, Frissen PH, Slaats EH, Silberbusch J. Renal tubular acidosis. Pathophysiology and diagnosis. [Review] [63 refs]. Arch Intern Med 1996;156:1629–1636.

Bastani B, Gluck SL. New insights into the pathogenesis of distal renal tubular acidosis. [Review] [133 refs]. Miner Electrolyte Metab 1996;22:396–409.

Eiam-ong S, Kurtzman NA. Metabolic acidosis and bone disease. [Review]. Miner Electrolyte Metab 1994;20:72–80.

Giovannetti S, Cupisti A, Barsotti G. The metabolic acidosis of chronic renal failure: pathophysiology and treatment. [Review]. Contrib Nephrol 1992;100:48–57.

THE CONSULTATION GUIDE

Creatinine Elevation

Indications and Timing for Referral

- Rapidly progressive
- Associated with oliguria

Timing: Urgent (less than 24 hours)

- Elevation is new and persistently abnormal for two readings
- Diagnostic uncertainty

Timing: Expedited (less than 1 week)

Tests to Prepare for Consult

- CBC
- Electrolytes (Na, K, Cl, CO_2)
- Albumin, total protein
- Calcium, phosphorus
- BUN, creatinine
- Urinalysis with microscopic
- Urine sodium
- Urine creatinine
- 24-hour urine protein
- 24-hour urine creatinine for clearance
- Ultrasound, renal

Tests Not Useful Before Consult

- IVP
- CT scan, renal
- MR, renal

Tests Consultant May Need to Do

- Electrolytes (Na, K, Cl, CO_2)
- Albumin, total protein
- Calcium, phosphorus
- BUN, creatinine
- Urinalysis with microscopic
- 24-hour urine protein
- 24-hour urine creatinine for clearance
- ANA
- Anti-double stranded DNA
- Complement factors (C3, C4)
- Anti-neutrophil cytoplasmic antibody
- Osmolality, urine
- Immunoelectrophoresis, serum and urine
- Eosinophil count, serum and urine
- HIV antibody testing
- Ultrasound, renal

Follow-up Visits Generally Required

- Two

Suggested Readings

Perrone RD, Madias NE, Levey AS. Serum creatinine as an index of renal function: new insights into old concepts [see comments]. [Review]. Clin Chem 1992;38:1933–1953.

Levey AS, Perrone RD, Madias NE. Serum creatinine and renal function. [Review]. Annu Rev Med 1988;39:465–490.

Lafayette RA, Perrone RD, Levey AS. Laboratory evaluation of renal function. In: Schrier RW, Gottschalk CW, eds. Diseases of the Kidney. 6th ed. Boston: Little Brown, 1996:307–354.

See Also

- Uremia

NEPHROLOGY

Glomerulonephritis, History of

Indications and Timing for Referral
- Renal insufficiency present
- Active urine sediment present (e.g., proteinuria, RBCs, casts)
- Patient also has severe or difficult to control hypertension

Timing: Urgent (less than 24 hours)

Advice for Referral
- The need for renal biopsy may be apparent at the initial consultative visit. Actual procedures for preliminary discussion with primary care physician, authorization, and scheduling will depend upon the practice setting. If renal biopsy is performed an additional follow-up visit is appropriate.

Tests to Prepare for Consult
- Electrolytes (Na, K, Cl, CO_2)
- Albumin, total protein
- Calcium, phosphorus
- BUN, creatinine
- CBC
- Urinalysis with microscopic
- 24-hour urine protein
- 24-hour urine creatinine for clearance

Tests Not Useful Before Consult
- IVP
- CT scan, renal
- MR, renal

Tests Consultant May Need to Do
- Urinalysis with microscopic
- 24-hour urine creatinine for clearance
- 24-hour urine protein
- IEP, serum and urine
- ANA
- Anti-double stranded DNA
- Complement factors (C3, C4)
- Anti-neutrophil cytoplasmic antibody
- Hepatitis B, PCR
- HB_cAb
- HB_sAb
- HB_sAg
- Hepatitis C antibody
- HIV antibody testing
- Ultrasound, renal
- Renal biopsy

Follow-up Visits Generally Required
- Two

Suggested Readings
Cameron JS. The long-term outcome of glomerular diseases. In: Schrier RW, Gottschalk CW, eds. Diseases of the Kidney. 5th ed. Boston: Little, Brown, 1993:1895–1958.

Tisher CC, Croker BP. Indications for and interpretation of the renal biopsy: Evaluation by light, electron, and immunofluorescence microscopy. In: Schrier RW, Gottschalk CW, eds. Diseases of the Kidney. 5th ed. Boston: Little, Brown, 1993:485–512.

See Also
- Red blood cell casts
- Glomerulonephritis, in scleroderma
- Creatinine elevation

Glomerulonephritis, in Scleroderma

Indications and Timing for Referral

- Renal insufficiency present
- Active sediment, e.g., RBCs, casts, proteinuria
- Patient also has uncontrolled or difficult to control hypertension

Timing: Urgent (less than 24 hours)

Advice for Referral

- This condition often requires co-management with a nephrologist.
- The need for renal biopsy may be apparent at the initial consultative visit. Actual procedures for preliminary discussion with primary care physician, authorization, and scheduling will depend upon the practice setting. If renal biopsy is performed an additional follow-up visit is appropriate.

Tests to Prepare for Consult

- Electrolytes (Na, K, Cl, CO_2)
- Albumin, total protein
- BUN, creatinine
- CBC with differential
- 24-hour urine protein
- 24-hour urine creatinine for clearance

Tests Not Useful Before Consult

- IVP
- CT or MR, renal
- MR angiography

Tests Consultant May Need to Do

- Renal biopsy

Follow-up Visits Generally Required

- Co-management, see *Advice for Referral*

Suggested Readings

Shapiro AP, Medsger TA, Steen VD. Renal involvement in systemic sclerosis. In: Schrier RW, Gottschalk CW, eds. Diseases of the Kidney. 5th ed. Boston: Little, Brown, 1993:2039–2048.

Spencer RT, Arend WP, Woodruff E. Systemic sclerosis, rheumatoid arthritis, Sjögren's syndrome, and polymyositis-dermatomyositis. In: Schrier RW, Gottschalk CW, eds. Diseases of the Kidney. 6th ed. Boston: Little Brown, 1996:1801–1821.

See Also

- Glomerulonephritis, in systemic lupus erythematosus
- Hypertension, in diabetes mellitus

NEPHROLOGY

Glomerulonephritis, in Systemic Lupus Erythematosus

Indications and Timing for Referral

- Renal insufficiency present
- Active sediment, e.g., RBCs, casts, proteinuria
- Patient also has uncontrolled or difficult to control hypertension

Timing: Expedited (less than 1 week)

Advice for Referral

- This condition often requires co-management with a nephrologist.

Tests to Prepare for Consult

- Electrolytes (Na, K, Cl, CO_2)
- Albumin, total protein
- BUN, creatinine
- CBC with differential
- Urinalysis with microscopic
- 24-hour urine protein
- 24-hour urine creatinine for clearance
- ESR
- Complement factors (C3, C4)

Tests Not Useful Before Consult

- IVP
- CT scan, renal
- MR, renal
- MR angiography

Tests Consultant May Need to Do

- Complement factors (C3, C4)
- Anti-double stranded DNA
- Anti-ro (SS-A)
- Anti-la (SS-B)
- Ultrasound, renal
- Renal biopsy

Follow-up Visits Generally Required

- Co-management, see *Advice for Referral*

Suggested Readings

Gonzalez-Crespo MR, Lopez-Fernandez JI, et al. Outcome of silent lupus nephritis. [Review] [73 refs]. Semin Arthritis Rheum 1996;26:468–476.

Golbus J, McCune WJ. Lupus nephritis. Classification, prognosis, immunopathogenesis, and treatment. [Review]. Rheum Dis Clin North Am 1994;20:213–242.

Derksen RH, Hene RJ, Kater L. The long-term clinical outcome of 56 patients with biopsy-proven lupus nephritis followed at a single center. Lupus 1992;1:97–103.

Balow JE, Austin HA 3d. Renal disease in systemic lupus erythematosus. [Review]. Rheum Dis Clin North Am 1988;14:117–133.

Levey AS, Lan SP, Corwin HL, et al. Progression and remission of renal disease in the Lupus Nephritis Collaborative Study. Results of treatment with prednisone and short-term oral cyclophosphamide. Ann Intern Med 1992;116:114–123.

See Also

- Hypertension, in diabetes mellitus
- Glomerulonephritis, in scleroderma

THE CONSULTATION GUIDE

Hematuria, Gross

Indications and Timing for Referral

- Red cell casts present
- Renal dysfunction present
- High-grade proteinuria present

Timing: Urgent (less than 24 hours)

Advice for Referral

- An IVP is the test of choice if renal function is normal; however, renal ultrasound is preferred if there is renal dysfunction.
- The possibility of urologic problems should be considered before seeking nephrology consultation, e.g., prostatic hypertrophy.
- The presence of infection should be ruled out in both women and men before seeking nephrology consultation.
- The presence of menses should be excluded.
- The need for renal biopsy may be apparent at the initial consultative visit. Actual procedures for preliminary discussion with primary care physician, authorization, and scheduling will depend upon the practice setting. If renal biopsy is performed an additional follow-up visit is appropriate.

Tests to Prepare for Consult

- CBC
- BUN, creatinine
- Urinalysis with microscopic
- Urine, culture and sensitivity

Tests Not Useful Before Consult

- None

Tests Consultant May Need to Do

- CBC with blood smear
- PTT
- Prothrombin time
- Platelet count
- Urinalysis with microscopic
- 24-hour urine creatinine for clearance
- 24-hour urine protein
- Urine, culture and sensitivity
- Urine cytology
- Immunoelectrophoresis, serum and urine
- ANA
- Anti-double stranded DNA
- Complement factors (C3, C4)
- Anti-neutrophil cytoplasmic antibody
- Anti-GBM
- Hemoglobin electrophoresis
- Ultrasound, renal
- IVP
- Renal biopsy

Hematuria, Gross (*continued*)

Follow-up Visits Generally Required

- None

Suggested reading

McCarthy JJ. Outpatient evaluation of hematuria: locating the source of bleeding. [Review] [7 refs]. Postgrad Med 1997;101:125–128.

Ahmed Z, Lee J. Asymptomatic urinary abnormalities. Hematuria and proteinuria. [Review] [42 refs]. Med Clin North Am 1997;81:641–652.

Sutton JM. Evaluation of hematuria in adults [see comments]. [Review]. JAMA 1990;263:2475–2480.

Woolhandler S, Pels RJ, Bor DH, et al. Dipstick urinalysis screening of asymptomatic adults for urinary tract disorders. I. Hematuria and proteinuria [see comments]. JAMA 1989;262:1214–1219.

Selected Guidelines

Screening for asymptomatic bacteriuria, hematuria, and proteinuria. In: U. S. Preventive Services Task Force Guide to Clinical Preventive Services: an Assessment of the Effectiveness of 169 Interventions: Report of the U. S. Preventive Services Task Force. Baltimore: Williams & Wilkins, 1989: 155–161. 1995;U.S. Preventive Serv-61.

See Also

- Urine, red
- Hematuria, microscopic
- Red blood cell casts

Hematuria, Microscopic

Indications and Timing for Referral
- Red cell casts present
- Renal dysfunction present
- High-grade proteinuria present

Timing: Expedited (less than 1 week)

Advice for Referral
- An IVP is the test of choice if renal function is normal; however, renal ultrasound is preferred if there is renal dysfunction.
- The possibility of urologic problems should be considered before seeking nephrology consultation, e.g., prostatic hypertrophy, prostatitis.
- The presence of infection should be ruled out in both women and men before seeking nephrology consultation.
- Presence of menses should be excluded.
- Factors favoring nephrology consultation include:
  - Proteinuria present
  - Red cell casts present
  - Renal insufficiency

Tests to Prepare for Consult
- CBC
- BUN, creatinine
- Urinalysis with microscopic
- Urine, culture and sensitivity

Tests Not Useful Before Consult
- DSA, intra-arterial
- CT scan, renal
- MR angiography

Tests Consultant May Need to Do
- CBC
- Platelet count
- PTT
- Prothrombin time
- BUN, creatinine
- Urinalysis with microscopic
- 24-hour urine creatinine for clearance
- 24-hour urine protein
- Urine culture for TB
- Immunoglobulins, quantitative
- ANA
- Anti-double stranded DNA
- Complement factors (C3, C4)
- Anti-neutrophil cytoplasmic antibody
- HB_cAb
- Anti-GBM
- HB_sAb
- Cryoglobulins
- HB_sAg
- Hemoglobin electrophoresis
- Hepatitis C antibody
- PPD
- Ultrasound, renal

Hematuria, Microscopic (continued)

Follow-up Visits Generally Required
- One

Suggested Reading
Ahmed Z, Lee J. Asymptomatic urinary abnormalities. Hematuria and proteinuria. [Review] [42 refs]. Med Clin North Am 1997;81:641–652.

Fogazzi GB, Ponticelli C. Microscopic hematuria diagnosis and management [editorial]. [Review] [81 refs]. Nephron 1996;72:125–134.

McCarthy JJ. Outpatient evaluation of hematuria: locating the source of bleeding. [Review] [7 refs]. Postgrad Med 1997;101:125–128.

Yasumasu T, Koikawa Y, Uozumi J, et al. Clinical study of asymptomatic microscopic haematuria. Int Urol Nephrol 1994;26:1–6.

Sparwasser C, Cimniak HU, Treiber U, Pust RA. Significance of the evaluation of asymptomatic microscopic haematuria in young men. Br J Urol 1994;74:723–729.

Sutton JM. Evaluation of hematuria in adults [see comments]. [Review]. JAMA 1990;263:2475–2480.

Selected Guidelines
Screening for asymptomatic bacteriuria, hematuria, and proteinuria. In: U. S. Preventive Services Task Force Guide to Cinical Preventive Services: an Assessment of the Effectiveness of 169 Interventions: Report of the U. S. Preventive Services Task Force. Baltimore: Williams & Wilkins, 1989: 155–161. 1995;U.S. Preventive Serv-61.

See Also
- Urine, red
- Hematuria, gross
- Red blood cell casts

THE CONSULTATION GUIDE

Hyperkalemia

Indications and Timing for Referral

- Potassium level greater than 6.0 mEq/L or greater than 5.5 mEq/L with ECG changes warrants immediate evaluation
- Renal insufficiency present

Timing: Urgent (less than 24 hours)

- Confirmed potassium level 5.5 to 6.0 mEq/L without ECG changes

Timing: Expedited (less than 1 week)

Advice for Referral

- Stop all drugs that can elevate the potassium level, e.g., angiotensin-converting enzyme (ACE) inhibitors, potassium-sparing diuretics, trimethoprim, nonsteroidal anti-inflammatory drugs (NSAIDs), beta-blockers, potassium supplements, and angiotensin II receptor blockers.
- Spurious hyperkalemia (pseudohyperkalemia) may be caused by hemolysis, thrombocytosis, severe leukocytosis, prolonged tourniquet application, or intense fist clenching before sampling.

Tests to Prepare for Consult

- Electrolytes (Na, K, Cl, CO_2)
- Potassium, repeat
- Glucose
- Creatinine
- CBC with differential
- Platelet count
- Urinalysis with microscopic
- ECG

Tests Not Useful Before Consult

- None

Tests Consultant May Need to Do

- Electrolytes (Na, K, Cl, CO_2)
- Potassium, repeat
- Creatinine
- CBC with differential
- Platelet count
- Urinalysis with microscopic
- Urine potassium
- Urine sodium
- Osmolality
  - Urine
  - Serum
- ECG
- ACTH stimulation test, 1-hour
- Aldosterone suppression (salt load) test
- Renin stimulation (furosemide) test

Follow-up Visits Generally Required

- One

Suggested Readings

Mandal AK. Hypokalemia and hyperkalemia. [Review] [37 refs]. Med Clin North Am 1997;81:611–639.

Kamel KS, Quaggin S, Scheich A, Halperin ML. Disorders of potassium homeostasis: an approach based on pathophysiology. [Review]. Am J Kidney Dis 1994;24:597–613.

Latta K, Hisano S, Chan JC. Perturbations in potassium balance. [Review]. Clin Lab Med 1993;13:149–156.

Don BR, Sebastian A, Cheitlin M, et al. Pseudohyperkalemia caused by fist clenching during phlebotomy. N Engl J Med 1990;322:1290–1292.

Hypertension, in Diabetes Mellitus

Indications and Timing for Referral
- Renal insufficiency present
- Hypertension is uncontrolled
- High-grade proteinuria is present
- Patient has failed conventional therapy, e.g., ACE inhibitor, diuretic

Timing: Routine (less than 4 weeks)

Advice for Referral
- The goal of antihypertensive therapy in the patient with diabetes should be a blood pressure less than 130/85.
- See also recommendations for *Hypertension, Renovascular.*
- Co-management with a nephrologist may prove useful.

Tests to Prepare for Consult
- Electrolytes (Na, K, Cl, CO_2)
- Albumin, total protein
- BUN, creatinine
- Calcium, phosphorus
- CBC
- Glycohemoglobin
- Urinalysis with microscopic
- 24-hour urine protein
- 24-hour urine creatinine for clearance
- UA with microalbumin

Tests Not Useful Before Consult
- IVP

Tests Consultant May Need to Do
- Immunoelectrophoresis, serum and urine
- Ultrasound, renal

Follow-up Visits Generally Required
- Co-management, see *Advice for Referral*

Suggested Readings
Arauz-Pacheco C, Raskin P. Hypertension in diabetes mellitus. [Review] [173 refs]. Endocrinol Metab Clin North Am 1996;25:401–423.

Fatourechi V, Kennedy FP, Rizza RA, Hogan MJ. A practical guideline for management of hypertension in patients with diabetes. Mayo Clin Proc 1996;71:53–58.

Schrier RW, Estacio RO, Jeffers B. Appropriate blood pressure control in NIDDM (ABCD) Trial. Diabetologia 1996;39:1646–1654.

Hypertension in Diabetes Study IV. Therapeutic requirements to maintain tight blood pressure control. Diabetologia 1996;39:1554–1561.

Curb JD, Pressel SL, Cutler JA, et al. Effect of diuretic-based antihypertensive treatment on cardiovascular disease risk in older diabetic patients with isolated systolic hypertension. Systolic Hypertension in the Elderly Program Cooperative Research Group [published erratum appears in JAMA 1997;277:1356] [see comments]. JAMA 1996;276:1886–1892.

See Also
- Hypertension, labile/paroxysmal
- Hypertension, renovascular
- Hypertension, rule out secondary cause
- Glomerulonephritis, in systemic lupus erythematosus

THE CONSULTATION GUIDE

Hypertension, Labile/Paroxysmal

Indications and Timing for Referral
- Diagnostic uncertainty

Timing: Routine (less than 4 weeks)

Advice for Referral
- A complete medication history is vital.
- Ascertain presence of family history of endocrine tumors.

Tests to Prepare for Consult
- Calcium, phosphorus
- Electrolytes (Na, K, Cl, CO_2)
- Glucose
- Creatinine
- ALT, AST, alkaline phosphatase
- Urinalysis with microscopic
- 24-hour urine metanephrines

Tests Not Useful Before Consult
- IVP

Tests Consultant May Need to Do
- Captopril suppression test
- TSH (assay sensitivity <0.1 mU/L)
- Toxicology screen
- 24-hour urine catecholamines
- 24-hour urine metanephrines
- Ambulatory BP monitoring
- Ultrasound, renal
- Renal DTPA scan
- CT scan, abdomen

Follow-up Visits Generally Required
- Two

Suggested Readings
Reeves RA. Does this patient have hypertension? How to measure blood pressure. [Review]. JAMA 1995;273:1211–1218.

Littenberg B. A practice guideline revisited: screening for hypertension. [Review]. Ann Intern Med 1995;122:937–939.

Sheps SG, Canzanello VJ. Current role of automated ambulatory blood pressure and self-measured blood pressure determinations in clinical practice. Mayo Clin Proc 1994;69:1000–1005.

Haynes RB, Lacourciere Y, Rabkin SW, et al. Report of the Canadian Hypertension Society Consensus Conference: 2. Diagnosis of hypertension in adults. [Review]. Can Med Assoc J 1993;149:409–418.

Larson AW, Strong CG. Initial assessment of the patient with hypertension. [Review]. Mayo Clin Proc 1989;64:1533–1542.

See Also
- Hypertension, renovascular
- Hypertension, rule out secondary cause
- Hypertension, in diabetes mellitus

NEPHROLOGY

Hypertension, Renovascular

Indications and Timing for Referral

- Patient with known renovascular hypertension and poorly controlled symptoms
- Explore therapeutic options
- Renal dysfunction present

Timing: Routine (less than 4 weeks)

Tests to Prepare for Consult

- Electrolytes (Na, K, Cl, CO_2)
- Creatinine
- Urinalysis with microscopic
- CBC

Tests Not Useful Before Consult

- IVP

Tests Consultant May Need to Do

- Digital subtraction angiogram, intra-arterial
- Renal DTPA scan
- MR angiography
- Ultrasound
  - Renal
  - Abdomen
- Renal vein renins
- Arteriogram, renal

Follow-up Visits Generally Required

- Two

Suggested Readings

Romero JC, Feldstein AE, Rodriguez-Porcel MG, Cases-Amenos A. New insights into the pathophysiology of renovascular hypertension. [Review] [66 refs]. Mayo Clin Proc 1997;72:251–260.

Mitty HA, Shapiro RS, Parsons RB, Silberzweig JE. Renovascular hypertension. [Review] [49 refs]. Radiol Clin North Am 1996;34:1017–1036.

Mann SJ, Pickering TG. Detection of renovascular hypertension. State of the art: 1992 [see comments]. [Review]. Ann Intern Med 1992;117:845–853.

Pickering TG, Laragh JH, Sos TA. Renovascular hypertension. In: Schrier RW, Gottschalk CW, eds. Diseases of the Kidney. 5th ed. Boston: Little, Brown, 1993: 1451–1474.

Sheps SG, Blaufox MD, Nally JV Jr, Textor SC. Radionuclide scintrenography in the evaluation of patients with hypertension. American College of Cardiology position statement. J Am Coll Cardiol 1993;21:838–839.

Nally JV Jr, Chen C, Fine E, et al. Diagnostic criteria of renovascular hypertension with captopril renography. A consensus statement. Am J Hypertens 1991;4:749S–752S.

Selected Guidelines

1995 update of the working group reports on chronic renal failure and renovascular hypertension. National High Blood Pressure Education Program Working Group. [Review] [98 refs]. Arch Intern Med 1996;156:1938–1947.

See Also

- Hypertension, in diabetes mellitus
- Hypertension, labile/paroxysmal
- Hypertension, rule out secondary cause

Hypertension, Rule Out Secondary Cause

Indications and Timing for Referral

- Patient younger than 30 years old
- Patient over 60 years old with new onset of hypertension
- Diagnostic uncertainty with suspicion of secondary cause
- Hypertension uncontrolled

Timing: Routine (less than 4 weeks)

Advice for Referral

- If patient is female and under age 30, consider potential role of birth control pills.

Tests to Prepare for Consult

- CBC
- Electrolytes (Na, K, Cl, CO_2)
- Creatinine
- Urinalysis with microscopic

Tests Not Useful Before Consult

- None

Tests Consultant May Need to Do

- Catecholamines, plasma
- Electrolytes (Na, K, Cl, CO_2)
- Creatinine
- Urinalysis with microscopic
- 24-hour urine metanephrines
- 24-hour urinary aldosterone
- Renin stimulation (furosemide) test
- Aldosterone suppression (salt load) test
- Renal DTPA scan
- Toxicology screen
- Digital subtraction angiogram, intra-arterial
- Renal angiogram

Follow-up Visits Generally Required

- Two

Suggested Readings

Akpunonu BE, Mulrow PJ, Hoffman EA. Secondary hypertension: evaluation and treatment. [Review] [429 refs]. Dis Mon 1996;42:609–722.

Adcock BB, Ireland RB Jr. Secondary hypertension: a practical diagnostic approach. [Review] [23 refs]. Am Fam Physician 1997;55:1263–1270.

Setaro JF, Black HR. Refractory hypertension. [Review]. N Engl J Med 1992;327:543–547.

Mann SJ, Pickering TG. Detection of renovascular hypertension. State of the art: 1992 [see comments]. [Review]. Ann Intern Med 1992;117:845–853.

Larson AW, Strong CG. Initial assessment of the patient with hypertension. [Review]. Mayo Clin Proc 1989;64:1533–1542.

See Also

- Hypertension, in diabetes mellitus
- Hypertension, renovascular
- Hypertension, labile/paroxysmal

Hypokalemia

Indications and Timing for Referral

- Associated with hypertension
- Etiology unclear
- Potassium$_+$ less than 3.0 mEq/L off diuretic therapy
- Chronic and difficult to control

Timing: Expedited (less than 1 week)

Advice for Referral

- If patient on medical therapy known to cause hypokalemia, stop whenever possible and observe for 7 to 10 days before referring.

Tests to Prepare for Consult

- Electrolytes (Na, K, Cl, CO_2)
- Magnesium
- Phosphorus
- Creatinine
- Urinalysis with microscopic
- Urine potassium
- Urine chloride

Tests Not Useful Before Consult

- None

Tests Consultant May Need to Do

- Electrolytes (Na, K, Cl, CO_2)
- Magnesium
- Phosphorus
- BUN, creatinine
- Urinalysis with microscopic
- Urine potassium
- Urine sodium
- 24-hour urinary aldosterone
- Ultrasound, renal
- Aldosterone suppression (salt load) test
- Renin stimulation (furosemide) test
- Toxicology screen
- Diuretic screen
- Urine free cortisol, 24-hour
- Overnight dexamethasone suppression test, 1 mg
- Osmolality
  - Urine
  - Serum

Follow-up Visits Generally Required

- One

Suggested Readings

Mandal AK. Hypokalemia and hyperkalemia. [Review] [37 refs]. Med Clin North Am 1997;81:611–639.

Latta K, Hisano S, Chan JC. Perturbations in potassium balance. [Review]. Clin Lab Med 1993;13:149–156.

Coe FL. Fluids and electrolytes. In: Isselbacher KJ, Braunwald E, Wilson JD, et al., eds. Harrison's Principles of Internal Medicine. 13th ed. NY: McGraw-Hill Inc, 1994:242–252.

Hyponatremia

Indications and Timing for Referral

- Sodium level less than 120 mEq/L generally warrants immediate impatient evaluation and management
- Level less than 125 mEq/L and develops rapidly
- Patient moderately symptomatic

Timing: Urgent (less than 24 hours)

- Sodium level 125 to 133 mEq/L and patient not on diuretic therapy
- Sodium level less than 130 mEq/L and etiology unclear

Timing: Expedited (less than 1 week)

Advice for Referral

- Exclude hyperglycemia and hypertriglyceridemia.

Tests to Prepare for Consult

- Electrolytes (Na, K, Cl, CO_2)
- Total protein
- Glucose
- Creatinine
- Lipid profile, fasting (cholesterol, HDL, TG)
- Urinalysis with microscopic
- Osmolality, urine
- Urine sodium

Tests Not Useful Before Consult

- None

Tests Consultant May Need to Do

- Electrolytes (Na, K, Cl, CO_2)
- Creatinine
- ALT, AST, alkaline phosphatase
- Urinalysis with microscopic
- Urine potassium
- Urine sodium
- Osmolality
  - Urine
  - Serum
- Free T_4
- TSH
- Chest radiograph
- Diuretic screen
- ACTH stimulation test, 1-hour

Follow-up Visits Generally Required

- Two

Suggested Readings

Arieff AI. Management of hyponatraemia [see comments]. [Review]. BMJ 1993;307:305–308.

DeVita MV, Michelis MF. Perturbations in sodium balance. Hyponatremia and hypernatremia. [Review]. Clin Lab Med 1993;13:135–148.

Fried LF, Palevsky PM. Hyponatremia and hypernatremia. [Review] [120 refs]. Med Clin North Am 1997;81:585–609.

Laureno R, Karp BI. Myelinolysis after correction of hyponatremia. [Review] [49 refs]. Ann Intern Med 1997;126:57–62.

NEPHROLOGY

Kidneys, Enlarged, Bilateral

Indications and Timing for Referral
- Diagnostic uncertainty

Timing: Routine (less than 4 weeks)

Advice for Referral
- The need for renal biopsy may be apparent at the initial consultative visit. Actual procedures for preliminary discussion with primary care physician, authorization, and scheduling will depend upon the practice setting. If renal biopsy is performed an additional follow-up visit is appropriate.

Tests to Prepare for Consult
- Electrolytes (Na, K, Cl, CO_2)
- Albumin, total protein
- BUN, creatinine
- Calcium, phosphorus
- Glucose, fasting
- Glycohemoglobin
- CBC
- Urinalysis with microscopic
- 24-hour urine protein
- 24-hour urine creatinine for clearance
- Ultrasound, renal

Tests Not Useful Before Consult
- None

Tests Consultant May Need to Do
- Electrolytes (Na, K, Cl, CO_2)
- Albumin, total protein
- BUN, creatinine
- Calcium, phosphorus
- CBC with differential
- Urinalysis with microscopic
- 24-hour urine protein
- 24-hour urine creatinine
- Immunoelectrophoresis, serum and urine
- HIV antibody testing
- Renal biopsy
- Biopsy for amyloid, nonrenal

Follow-up Visits Generally Required
- None

Suggested Readings
Choyke PL. Inherited cystic diseases of the kidney. [Review] [57 refs]. Radiol Clin North Am 1996;34:925–946.

Gabow PA, Grantham JJ. Polycystic kidney disease. In: Schrier RW, Gottschalk CW, eds. Diseases of the Kidney. 5th ed. Boston: Little, Brown, 1993:535–570.

THE CONSULTATION GUIDE

Kidneys, Enlarged, by Ultrasound, Computed Tomography, or Magnetic Resonance

Indications and Timing for Referral
- Diagnostic uncertainty

Timing: Routine (less than 4 weeks)

Advice for Referral
- The need for renal biopsy may be apparent at the initial consultative visit. Actual procedures for preliminary discussion with primary care physician, authorization, and scheduling will depend upon the practice setting. If renal biopsy is performed an additional follow-up visit is appropriate.

Tests to Prepare for Consult
- Electrolytes (Na, K, Cl, CO_2)
- Albumin, total protein
- BUN, creatinine
- Calcium, phosphorus
- CBC with differential
- Glucose
- Urinalysis with microscopic
- 24-hour urine protein
- 24-hour urine creatinine for clearance
- Ultrasound, renal

Tests Not Useful Before Consult
- None

Tests Consultant May Need to Do
- Electrolytes (Na, K, Cl, CO_2)
- Albumin, total protein
- BUN, creatinine
- Calcium, phosphorus
- CBC with differential
- Glycohemoglobin
- Urinalysis with microscopic
- 24-hour urine protein
- 24-hour urine creatinine for clearance
- Immunoelectrophoresis, serum and urine
- HIV antibody testing
- Renal biopsy
- Biopsy for amyloid, nonrenal

Follow-up Visits Generally Required
- None

Suggested Readings

Gabow PA. Autosomal dominant polycystic kidney disease. [Review]. N Engl J Med 1993;329:332–342.

Gabow PA, Grantham JJ. Polycystic kidney disease. In: Schrier RW, Gottschalk CW, eds. Diseases of the Kidney. 5th ed. Boston: Little, Brown, 1993:535–570.

See Also
- Kidneys, enlarged, bilateral
- Polycystic kidneys, incidentally detected
- Polycystic kidneys, history of, normal renal function
- Polycystic kidneys, history of, abnormal renal function

NEPHROLOGY

Kidneys, Small, Unilateral

Indications and Timing for Referral

- Renal insufficiency present
- Associated hypertension
- Associated urinary tract infection

Timing: Routine (less than 4 weeks)

Tests to Prepare for Consult

- Electrolytes (Na, K, Cl, CO_2)
- BUN, creatinine
- CBC
- Urinalysis with microscopic
- Urine, culture and sensitivity
- 24-hour urine creatinine for clearance
- 24-hour urine protein
- Ultrasound, renal

Tests Not Useful Before Consult

- None

Tests Consultant May Need to Do

- Electrolytes (Na, K, Cl, CO_2)
- BUN, creatinine
- CBC
- Urinalysis with microscopic
- Urine, culture and sensitivity
- Ultrasound, renal
- Renal DTPA scan
- CT scan, abdomen
- MR, renal
- IVP

Follow-up Visits Generally Required

- None

Suggested Readings

Mitty HA, Shapiro RS, Parsons RB, Silberzweig JE. Renovascular hypertension. [Review] [49 refs]. Radiol Clin North Am 1996;34:1017–1036.

Mann SJ, Pickering TG. Detection of renovascular hypertension. State of the art: 1992 [see comments]. [Review]. Ann Intern Med 1992;117:845–853.

Selected Guidelines

1995 update of the working group reports on chronic renal failure and renovascular hypertension. National High Blood Pressure Education Program Working Group. [Review] [98 refs]. Arch Intern Med 1996;156(17):1938–1947.

Medullary Cystic Disease

Indications and Timing for Referral

- Renal insufficiency present
- Uncontrolled hypertension present
- Infection present
- Bleeding present
- Recurrent or persistent pain

Timing: Routine (less than 4 weeks)

Advice for Referral

- Co-management with a nephrologist is often useful.

Tests to Prepare for Consult

- Electrolytes (Na, K, Cl, CO_2)
- BUN, creatinine
- Calcium, phosphorus
- CBC
- Urinalysis with microscopic
- Urine, culture and sensitivity
- Ultrasound, renal

Tests Not Useful Before Consult

- 24-hour urine protein
- 24-hour urine creatinine for clearance

Tests Consultant May Need to Do

- None

Follow-up Visits Generally Required

- Co-management, see *Advice for Referral*

Suggested Readings

Gardner KD. Medullary and miscellaneous renal cystic disorders. In: Schrier RW, Gottschalk CW, eds. Diseases of the Kidney. 5th ed. Boston: Little, Brown, 1993:513–524.

Welling LW, Grantham JJ. Cystic and developmental diseases of the kidneys. In: Brenner BM, Rector FC, eds. Brenner and Rector's The Kidney. 5th ed. Philadelphia: WB Saunders, 1995:1828–1863.

NEPHROLOGY

Nephritis, Chronic Tubulointerstitial

Indications and Timing for Referral
- Renal insufficiency present
- Low-grade proteinuria present

Timing: Routine (less than 4 weeks)

Advice for Referral
- Complete drug history is vital, especially analgesics.
- The need for renal biopsy may be apparent at the initial consultative visit. Actual procedures for preliminary discussion with primary care physician, authorization, and scheduling will depend upon the practice setting. If renal biopsy is performed an additional follow-up visit is appropriate.

Tests to Prepare for Consult
- Electrolytes (Na, K, Cl, CO_2)
- BUN, creatinine
- Calcium, phosphorus
- CBC
- Urinalysis with microscopic
- Ultrasound, renal

Tests Not Useful Before Consult
- None

Tests Consultant May Need to Do
- Electrolytes (Na, K, Cl, CO_2)
- Albumin, total protein
- BUN, creatinine
- Calcium, phosphorus
- CBC
- Urinalysis with microscopic
- Urine, culture and sensitivity
- 24-hour urine creatinine for clearance
- 24-hour urine protein
- Osmolality, urine
- Urine culture for TB
- PPD
- Water deprivation test
- Arsenic, urine or hair
- Lead, serum
- Mercury, serum or urine
- Renal biopsy

Follow-up Visits Generally Required
- One

Suggested Readings
Eknoyan G. Chronic tubulointerstitial nephropathies. In: Schrier RW, Gottschalk CW, eds. Diseases of the Kidney. 5th ed. Boston: Little, Brown, 1993:1959–1992.

Kelly CJ, Neilson E. Chronic tubulointerstitial nephritis. In: Brenner, Rector FC, eds. Brenner and Rector's The Kidney. 5th ed. Philadelphia: WB Saunders, 1995:1655–1679.

See Also
- Nephritis, chronic tubulointerstitial, drug-induced
- Pyelonephritis, chronic
- Nephritis, chronic tubulointerstitial, industrial exposure

THE CONSULTATION GUIDE

Nephritis, Chronic Tubulointerstitial, Drug-Induced

Indications and Timing for Referral

- Renal insufficiency present
- Low-grade proteinuria present

Timing: Routine (less than 4 weeks)

Advice for Referral

- Complete medication history is vital.
- The need for renal biopsy may be apparent at the initial consultative visit. Actual procedures for preliminary discussion with primary care physician, authorization, and scheduling will depend upon the practice setting. If renal biopsy is performed an additional follow-up visit is appropriate.

Tests to Prepare for Consult

- Electrolytes (Na, K, Cl, CO_2)
- BUN, creatinine
- Calcium, phosphorus
- CBC
- Urinalysis with microscopic
- Ultrasound, renal

Tests Not Useful Before Consult

- None

Tests Consultant May Need to Do

- Electrolytes (Na, K, Cl, CO_2)
- Albumin, total protein
- BUN, creatinine
- Calcium, phosphorus
- Urinalysis with microscopic
- Urine, culture and sensitivity
- 24-hour urine creatinine for clearance
- 24-hour urine protein
- Osmolality, urine
- Urine culture for TB
- PPD
- Water deprivation test
- Arsenic, urine or hair
- Lead, serum
- Mercury, serum or urine
- Lithium level
- Eosinophil count, serum and urine
- Renal biopsy

Follow-up Visits Generally Required

- One

Suggested Readings

Cronin RE, Henrich WL. Toxic Nephropathy. In: Brenner, Rector FC, eds. Brenner and Rector's The Kidney. 5th ed. Philadelphia: WB Saunders, 1995:1680–1711.

See Also

- Nephritis, chronic tubulointerstitial
- Nephritis, chronic tubulointerstitial, industrial exposure

Nephritis, Chronic Tubulointerstitial, Industrial Exposure

Indications and Timing for Referral

- Renal insufficiency present
- Low-grade proteinuria present

Timing: Routine (less than 4 weeks)

Advice for Referral

- Complete occupational and medication history is vital.
- The need for renal biopsy may be apparent at the initial consultative visit. Actual procedures for preliminary discussion with primary care physician, authorization, and scheduling will depend upon the practice setting. If renal biopsy is performed an additional follow-up visit is appropriate.

Tests to Prepare for Consult

- Electrolytes (Na, K, Cl, CO_2)
- BUN, creatinine
- Calcium, phosphorus
- CBC
- Urinalysis with microscopic
- Ultrasound, renal

Tests Not Useful Before Consult

- None

Tests Consultant May Need to Do

- Electrolytes (Na, K, Cl, CO_2)
- Albumin, total protein
- BUN, creatinine
- Calcium, phosphorus
- CBC
- Urinalysis with microscopic
- Urine, culture and sensitivity
- 24-hour urine creatinine for clearance
- 24-hour urine protein
- Osmolality, urine
- Urine culture for TB
- PPD
- Water deprivation test
- Cadmium
- Arsenic, urine or hair
- Lead, serum
- Mercury, serum or urine
- Renal biopsy

Follow-up Visits Generally Required

- One

Suggested Readings

Eknoyan G. Chronic tubulointerstitial nephropathies. In: Schrier RW, Gottschalk CW, eds. Diseases of the Kidney. 5th ed. Boston: Little, Brown, 1993:1959–1992.

See Also

- Nephritis, chronic tubulointerstitial
- Nephritis, chronic tubulointerstitial, drug-induced

Oliguria

Indications and Timing for Referral

- Laboratory values indicative of renal failure

Timing: Urgent (less than 24 hours)

Advice for Referral

- A complete medication history is important.

Tests to Prepare for Consult

- Electrolytes (Na, K, Cl, CO_2)
- BUN, creatinine
- CBC
- Urinalysis with microscopic
- Urine sodium
- Urine creatinine

Tests Not Useful Before Consult

- IVP

Tests Consultant May Need to Do

- Electrolytes (Na, K, Cl, CO_2)
- BUN, creatinine
- CBC with blood smear
- Urinalysis with microscopic
- Osmolality, urine
- Urine sodium
- Urine creatinine
- ANA
- Anti-double stranded DNA
- Complement factors (C3, C4)
- Ultrasound, renal

Follow-up Visits Generally Required

- None

Suggested Readings

Wilson DR, Klahr S. Urinary tract obstruction. In: Schrier RW, Gottschalk CW, eds. Diseases of the Kidney. 5th ed. Boston: Little, Brown, 1993:657–688.

Polycystic Kidneys, History of, Abnormal Renal Function

Indications and Timing for Referral

- Uncontrolled hypertension present
- Infection present
- Bleeding present
- Recurrent or persistent pain

Timing: Routine (less than 4 weeks)

Advice for Referral

- Co-management with a nephrologist is often useful.

Tests to Prepare for Consult

- Electrolytes (Na, K, Cl, CO_2)
- BUN, creatinine
- Calcium, phosphorus
- CBC
- Urinalysis with microscopic
- 24-hour urine creatinine for clearance
- Ultrasound, renal

Tests Not Useful Before Consult

- None

Consultant May Need to Do

- Urine, culture and sensitivity
- 24-hour urine protein
- 24-hour urine creatinine for clearance
- MR, cranial

Follow-up Visits Generally Required

- Co-management, see *Advice for Referral*

Suggested Readings

Levine E. Acquired cystic kidney disease. [Review] [66 refs]. Radiol Clin North Am 1996;34:947–964.

Fick GM, Gabow PA. Natural history of autosomal dominant polycystic kidney disease. [Review]. Annu Rev Med 1994;45:23–29.

Choyke PL. Inherited cystic diseases of the kidney. [Review] [57 refs]. Radiol Clin North Am 1996;34:925–946.

Striker G. Report on a workshop to develop management recommendations for the prevention of progression in chronic renal disease. J Am Soc Nephrol 1995;5:1537–1540.

See Also

- Kidneys, enlarged, bilateral
- Kidneys, enlarged, by US, CT, or MR
- Polycystic kidneys, incidentally detected
- Polycystic kidneys, history of, normal renal function

THE CONSULTATION GUIDE

Polycystic Kidneys, History of, Normal Renal Function

Indications and Timing for Referral

- Uncontrolled hypertension present
- Infection present
- Bleeding present
- Recurrent or persistent pain

Timing: Routine (less than 4 weeks)

Advice for Referral

- Baseline renal consultation is often useful.

Tests to Prepare for Consult

- Electrolytes (Na, K, Cl, CO_2)
- BUN, creatinine
- Calcium, phosphorus
- CBC
- Urinalysis with microscopic
- Ultrasound, renal

Tests Not Useful Before Consult

- None

Tests Consultant May Need to Do

- Urine, culture and sensitivity
- 24-hour urine protein
- 24-hour urine creatinine for clearance
- MR, cranial

Follow-up Visits Generally Required

- See *Advice for Referral*

Suggested Readings

Fick GM, Gabow PA. Natural history of autosomal dominant polycystic kidney disease. [Review]. Annu Rev Med 1994;45:23–29.

Bennett WM, Elzinga LW. Clinical management of autosomal dominant polycystic kidney disease. [Review]. Kidney Int Suppl 1993;42:S74–S79.

Choyke PL. Inherited cystic diseases of the kidney. [Review] [57 refs]. Radiol Clin North Am 1996;34:925–946.

Chapman AB, Rubinstein D, Hughes R, et al. Intracranial aneurysms in autosomal dominant polycystic kidney disease [see comments]. N Engl J Med 1992;327:916–920.

Marple JT, MacDougall M, Chonko AM. Renal cancer complicating acquired cystic kidney disease [see comments]. [Review]. J Am Soc Nephrol 1994;4:1951–1956.

See Also

- Kidneys, enlarged, bilateral
- Polycystic kidneys, history of, abnormal renal function
- Kidneys, enlarged, by US, CT, or MR
- Polycystic kidneys, incidentally detected

NEPHROLOGY

Polycystic Kidneys, Incidentally Detected

Indications and Timing for Referral
- Renal insufficiency present
- Uncontrolled hypertension present
- Infection present
- Bleeding present
- Recurrent or persistent pain

Timing: Routine (less than 4 weeks)

Advice for Referral
- Genetics referral may be indicated.
- Baseline renal consultation is often useful.

Tests to Prepare for Consult
- Electrolytes (Na, K, Cl, CO_2)
- BUN, creatinine
- Calcium, phosphorus
- CBC
- Urinalysis with microscopic
- Ultrasound, renal

Tests Not Useful Before Consult
- IVP

Tests Consultant May Need to Do
- Urine, culture and sensitivity
- 24-hour urine protein
- 24-hour urine creatinine for clearance
- MR, cranial

Follow-up Visits Generally Required
- See *Advice for Referral*

Suggested Readings
Fick GM, Gabow PA. Natural history of autosomal dominant polycystic kidney disease. [Review]. Annu Rev Med 1994;45:23–29.

Choyke PL. Inherited cystic diseases of the kidney. [Review] [57 refs]. Radiol Clin North Am 1996;34:925–946.

Gabow PA. Autosomal dominant polycystic kidney disease. [Review]. N Engl J Med 1993;329:332–342.

Bennett WM, Elzinga LW. Clinical management of autosomal dominant polycystic kidney disease. [Review]. Kidney Int Suppl 1993;42:S74–S79.

Lieske JC, Toback FG. Autosomal dominant polycystic kidney disease. [Review]. J Am Soc Nephrol 1993;3:1442–14450.

See Also
- Kidneys, enlarged, bilateral
- Kidneys, enlarged, by US, CT, or MR
- Polycystic kidneys, history of, normal renal function
- Polycystic kidneys, history of, abnormal renal function

Polyuria

Indications and Timing for Referral
- Sudden onset
- Rapidly progressive
- Dehydration present

Timing: Urgent (less than 24 hours)

- Symptoms persist for 2 to 4 weeks without diagnosis after initial testing
- Volume is greater than 5 liters or twice baseline without diagnosis after initial testing
- Associated with renal dysfunction

Timing: Routine (less than 4 weeks)

Advice for Referral
- Differentiation of polyuria versus increased frequency with normal total volume is critical.
- Careful medication history is vital.
- Drug-induced polyuria is common in patients on lithium.
- Factors favoring referral to nephrology include:
    - Proteinuria present
    - Decreased renal function
- Factors favoring referral to endocrinology include:
    - Inappropriately dilute urine

Tests to Prepare for Consult
- Glucose
- Electrolytes (Na, K, Cl, CO_2)
- Calcium
- BUN, creatinine
- Albumin, total protein
- Urinalysis with microscopic
- Osmolality
    - Urine
    - Serum
- 24-hour urine volume

Tests Not Useful Before Consult
- Plain film, abdomen
- CT scan, renal
- IVP

Tests Consultant May Need to Do
- Glucose
- Electrolytes (Na, K, Cl, CO_2)
- Calcium
- BUN, creatinine
- Magnesium
- Urinalysis with microscopic
- Urine specific gravity
- Glucose, urine
- 24-hour urine
    - creatinine for clearance
    - Protein
    - Volume
- Osmolality
    - Urine
    - Serum
- Water deprivation test
- Ultrasound, renal
- MR or CT, cranial with contrast

Follow-up Visits Generally Required
- One

Suggested Readings
Robertson GL. Differential diagnosis of polyuria. [Review]. Annu Rev Med 1988;39:425–442.

Oster JR, Singer I, Thatte L, et al. The polyuria of solute diuresis. [Review] [42 refs]. Arch Intern Med 1997;157:721–729.

Corwyn HL. Urinalysis. In: Schrier RW, Gottschalk CW, eds. Diseases of the Kidney. 6th ed. Boston: Little Brown, 1996:295–306.

Proteinuria, Trace to 1+ Positive

Indications and Timing for Referral
- Proteinuria is present on 2 determinations more than 1 week apart in a patient with no systemic illness (e.g., diabetes mellitus, hypertension, or UTI)
- Abnormal renal function is present with active sediment (e.g., WBCs, RBCs, casts)
- Metabolic acidosis is present

Timing: Routine (less than 4 weeks)

Advice for Referral
- Trace levels of protein can be the result of fever or excessive exercise, and may be normal in concentrated urine.
- Complete medication history is vital.
- The need for renal biopsy may be apparent at the initial consultative visit. Actual procedures for preliminary discussion with primary care physician, authorization, and scheduling will depend upon the practice setting. If renal biopsy is performed an additional follow-up visit is appropriate.

Tests to Prepare for Consult
- CBC with differential
- Glucose, fasting
- Electrolytes (Na, K, Cl, CO_2)
- Albumin, total protein
- BUN, creatinine
- Calcium, phosphorus
- Urinalysis with microscopic
- 24-hour urine protein
- 24-hour urine creatinine for clearance
- Ultrasound, renal

Tests Not Useful Before Consult
- CT scan, renal
- MR, renal
- MR angiography

Tests Consultant May Need to Do
- CBC with differential
- Glucose, fasting
- Electrolytes (Na, K, Cl, CO_2)
- Albumin, total protein
- BUN, creatinine
- Calcium, phosphorus
- Urinalysis with microscopic
- 24-hour urine protein
- 24-hour urine creatinine for clearance
- Immunoelectrophoresis, serum and urine
- ANA
- Anti-double stranded DNA
- Complement factors (C3, C4)
- Hepatitis B, PCR
- Hepatitis C, PCR
- HB_sAg
- HB_sAb
- Hepatitis E antigen
- Hepatitis E antibody
- HIV antibody testing
- Renal biopsy

Follow-up Visits Generally Required
- None

Proteinuria, Trace to 1+ Positive (continued)

Suggested Readings

Ali H. Proteinuria. How much evaluation is appropriate?. [Review] [5 refs]. Postgrad Med 1997;101:173–175.

Moore J Jr, Carome MA. Proteinuria. [Review]. Clin Lab Med 1993;13:21–31.

Woolhandler S, Pels RJ, Bor DH, et al. Dipstick urinalysis screening of asymptomatic adults for urinary tract disorders. I. Hematuria and proteinuria [see comments]. JAMA 1989;262:1214–1219.

Tiu SC, Lee SS, Cheng MW. Comparison of six commercial techniques in the measurement of microalbuminuria in diabetic patients [see comments]. Diabetes Care 1993;16:616–620.

Winocour PH. Microalbuminuria [editorial]. Br Med J 1992;304:1196–1197.

Selected Guidelines

Screening for asymptomatic bacteriuria, hematuria, and proteinuria. In: U. S. Preventive Services Task Force Guide to Clinical Preventive Services: an Assessment of the Effectiveness of 169 Interventions: Report of the U. S. Preventive Services Task Force. Baltimore: Williams & Wilkins, 1989: 155–161. 1995;U.S. Preventive Serv-61.

See Also

- Proteinuria, nephrotic range

NEPHROLOGY

Proteinuria, Nephrotic Range

Indications and Timing for Referral

- Urine protein excretion greater than 3 grams/24 hours

Timing: Expedited (less than 1 week)

Advice for Referral

- The need for renal biopsy may be apparent at the initial consultative visit. Actual procedures for preliminary discussion with primary care physician, authorization, and scheduling will depend upon the practice setting. If renal biopsy is performed an additional follow-up visit is appropriate.

Tests to Prepare for Consult

- Glucose, fasting
- CBC with differential
- Electrolytes (Na, K, Cl, CO_2)
- Albumin, total protein
- BUN, creatinine
- Calcium, phosphorus
- Urinalysis with microscopic
- 24-hour urine protein
- 24-hour urine creatinine for clearance
- Lipid profile, fasting (cholesterol, HDL, TG)
- Ultrasound, renal

Tests Not Useful Before Consult

- IVP
- CT scan, renal
- MR, renal

Tests Consultant May Need to Do

- Glucose, fasting
- CBC with differential
- Electrolytes (Na, K, Cl, CO_2)
- Albumin, total protein
- BUN, creatinine
- Calcium, phosphorus
- Urinalysis with microscopic
- 24-hour urine protein
- 24-hour urine creatinine for clearance
- ANA
- Anti-double stranded DNA
- Complement factors (C3, C4)
- Anti-neutrophil cytoplasmic antibody
- Immunoelectrophoresis, serum and urine
- Anti-GBM
- Cryoglobulins
- HIV antibody testing
- HB_sAb
- HB_sAg
- Hepatitis E antibody
- Hepatitis E antigen
- Hepatitis C antibody
- Urine toxicology screen
- MR, renal
- Renal venography
- Renal biopsy

Follow-up Visits Generally Required

- Two

Proteinuria, Nephrotic Range (continued)

Suggested Readings

Moore J Jr, Carome MA. Proteinuria. [Review]. Clin Lab Med 1993;13:21–31.

Woolhandler S, Pels RJ, Bor DH, et al. Dipstick urinalysis screening of asymptomatic adults for urinary tract disorders. I. Hematuria and proteinuria [see comments]. JAMA 1989;262:1214–1219.

Selected Guidelines

Screening for asymptomatic bacteriuria, hematuria, and proteinuria. In: U. S. Preventive Services Task Force Guide to Clinical Preventive Services: an Assessment of the Effectiveness of 169 Interventions: Report of the U. S. Preventive Services Task Force. Baltimore: Williams & Wilkins, 1989:155–161. 1995;U.S. Preventive Serv-61.

See Also

- Proteinuria, trace to 1+ positive

NEPHROLOGY

Pyelonephritis, Chronic

Indications and Timing for Referral

- Renal insufficiency present

Timing: Routine (less than 4 weeks)

Advice for Referral

- Differentiate from chronic/recurrent UTIs.
- This is a common but indistinct term that can refer to recurrent acute pyelonephritis, chronic tubulointerstitial nephritis, or reflux nephropathy.
- The need for renal biopsy may be apparent at the initial consultative visit. Actual procedures for preliminary discussion with primary care physician, authorization, and scheduling will depend upon the practice setting. If renal biopsy is performed an additional follow-up visit is appropriate.

Tests to Prepare for Consult

- Electrolytes (Na, K, Cl, CO_2)
- BUN, creatinine
- Calcium, phosphorus
- CBC
- Urinalysis with microscopic
- Urine, culture and sensitivity
- Ultrasound, renal

Tests Not Useful Before Consult

- None

Tests Consultant May Need to Do

- Urine for eosinophils
- Renal biopsy

Follow-up Visits Generally Required

- One

Suggested Readings

Striker G. Report on a workshop to develop management recommendations for the prevention of progression in chronic renal disease. J Am Soc Nephrol 1995;5:1537–1540.

Hostetter TH, Nath KA, Hostetter MK. Infection-related chronic interstitial nephropathy. [Review]. Semin Nephrol 1988;8:11–16.

Kelly CJ, Neilson E. Chronic tubulointerstitial nephritis. In: Brenner, Rector FC, eds. Brenner and Rector's The Kidney. 5th ed. Philadelphia: WB Saunders, 1995:1655–1679.

See Also

- Nephritis, chronic tubulointerstitial

379

THE CONSULTATION GUIDE

Red Blood Cell Casts

Indications and Timing for Referral

- All patients presenting with this finding warrant renal evaluation

Timing: Urgent (less than 24 hours)

- Patients with a history of systemic lupus presenting with casts for the first time

Timing: Expedited (less than 1 week)

Advice for Referral

- The need for renal biopsy may be apparent at the initial consultative visit. Actual procedures for preliminary discussion with primary care physician, authorization, and scheduling will depend upon the practice setting. If renal biopsy is performed an additional follow-up visit is appropriate.

Tests to Prepare for Consult

- CBC
- Electrolytes (Na, K, Cl, CO_2)
- Calcium, phosphorus
- BUN, creatinine
- Urinalysis with microscopic
- Urine, culture and sensitivity
- ANA
- Antistreptolysin O assay (ASO)
- ESR

Tests Not Useful Before Consult

- None

Tests Consultant May Need to Do

- Urinalysis with microscopic
- 24-hour urine creatinine for clearance
- 24-hour urine protein
- Anti-neutrophil cytoplasmic antibody
- ANA
- Anti-double stranded DNA
- Complement factors (C3, C4)
- Anti-GBM
- Cryoglobulins
- HB_cAb
- HB_sAb
- HB_sAg
- Hepatitis C antibody
- HIV antibody testing
- Ultrasound, renal
- Renal biopsy

Follow-up Visits Generally Required

- Two

Suggested Readings

Fairley KF. Urinalysis. In: Schrier RW, Gottschalk CW, eds. Diseases of the Kidney. 5th ed. Boston: Little, Brown, 1993:355–360.

See Also

- Urine, red
- Glomerulonephritis, history of
- Hematuria, gross
- Hematuria, microscopic

NEPHROLOGY

Renal Parenchymal Calcification

Indications and Timing for Referral
- Renal insufficiency present
- Etiology unclear

Timing: Routine (less than 4 weeks)

Advice for Referral
- An IVP is the test of choice if renal function is normal; however, renal ultrasound is preferred if there is renal dysfunction.

Tests to Prepare for Consult
- Electrolytes (Na, K, Cl, CO_2)
- Albumin, total protein
- BUN, creatinine
- Calcium, phosphorus
- CBC
- Urinalysis with microscopic
- 24-hour urine creatinine
- 24-hour urine protein

Tests Not Useful Before Consult
- None

Tests Consultant May Need to Do
- Electrolytes (Na, K, Cl, CO_2)
- Albumin, total protein
- BUN, creatinine
- Calcium, phosphorus
- CBC
- Urine
  - pH
  - Culture and sensitivity
  - Culture for TB
- PTH
- 1,25-dihydroxyvitamin D
- Acid load test
- PPD
- Ultrasound, renal

Follow-up Visits Generally Required
- One

Suggested Readings
Kellete MK. Calculus disease and urothelial lesions: nephrocalcinosis. In: Grainger RG, Allison DY, eds. Diagnostic Radiology: An Anglo-American Textbook of Imaging. 3rd ed. New York: Churchill Livingstone, 1997:1391–1405.

Renal Stone, Initial

Indications and Timing for Referral

- Renal insufficiency present

Timing: Routine (less than 4 weeks)

Tests to Prepare for Consult

- Electrolytes (Na, K, Cl, CO_2)
- Calcium, phosphorus
- Creatinine
- Uric acid
- Urinalysis with microscopic
- Urine pH
- 24-hour urine
  - Calcium
  - Uric acid
  - Volume
  - Creatinine
- Plain film, abdomen
- IVP
- Stone analysis, when possible

Tests Not Useful Before Consult

- None

Tests Consultant May Need to Do

- Urine pH
- Urine, culture and sensitivity
- 24-hour urine
  - Calcium
  - Uric acid
  - Volume
  - Creatinine
  - Citrate
  - Oxalate
  - Sodium
- Acid load test
- PTH
- 25-hydroxyvitamin D
- Oral calcium deprivation and loading studies
- UGIS with small bowel follow through

Follow-up Visits Generally Required

- None

Suggested Readings

Saklayen MG. Medical management of nephrolithiasis. [Review] [56 refs]. Med Clin North Am 1997;81:785–799.

Pak CY. Southwestern Internal Medicine Conference: medical management of nephrolithiasis—a new, simplified approach for general practice. [Review] [29 refs]. Am J Med Sci 1997;313:215–219.

Levy FL, Adams-Huet B, Pak CY. Ambulatory evaluation of nephrolithiasis: an update of a 1980 protocol. Am J Med 1995;98:50–59.

Coe FL, Parks JH, Asplin JR. The pathogenesis and treatment of kidney stones [see comments]. [Review]. N Engl J Med 1992;327:1141–1152.

Uribarri J, Oh MS, Carroll HJ. The first kidney stone. [Review]. Ann Intern Med 1989;111:1006–1009.

Selected Guidelines

Segura JW, Preminger GM, Assimos DG, et al. Nephrolithiasis Clinical Guidelines Panel summary report on the management of staghorn calculi. The American Urological Association Nephrolithiasis Clinical Guidelines Panel. J Urol 1994;151:1648–1651.

See Also

- Renal stone, recurrent
- Renal stone, struvite
- Renal stone, uric acid
- Renal stone, calcium oxalate

NEPHROLOGY

Renal Stone, Recurrent

Indications and Timing for Referral
- Renal insufficiency present
- Etiology of stone diathesis unclear

Timing: Routine (less than 4 weeks)

Tests to Prepare for Consult
- Electrolytes (Na, K, Cl, CO_2)
- Calcium, phosphorus
- Creatinine
- Uric acid
- Urinalysis with microscopic
- Urine, culture and sensitivity
- 24-hour urine
  - Calcium
  - Uric acid
  - Creatinine
- Plain film, abdomen
- IVP
- Stone analysis, when possible

Tests Not Useful Before Consult
- None

Tests Consultant May Need to Do
- Urine pH
- 24-hour urine
  - Cystine
  - Calcium
  - Uric acid
  - Volume
  - Creatinine
  - Citrate
  - Oxalate
  - Sodium
- Acid load test
- Oral calcium deprivation and loading studies
- PTH
- Calcium
- 25-hydroxyvitamin D
- UGIS with small bowel follow through

Follow-up Visits Generally Required
- One

Suggested Readings
Levy FL, Adams-Huet B, Pak CY. Ambulatory evaluation of nephrolithiasis: an update of a 1980 protocol. Am J Med 1995;98:50–59.

Saklayen MG. Medical management of nephrolithiasis. [Review] [56 refs]. Med Clin North Am 1997;81:785–799.

Tiselius HG. Investigation of single and recurrent stone formers. [Review]. Miner Electrolyte Metab 1994;20:321–327.

Parks JH, Coe FL. An increasing number of calcium oxalate stone events worsens treatment outcome. Kidney Int 1994;45:1722–1730.

Selected Guidelines
Segura JW, Preminger GM, Assimos DG, et al. Nephrolithiasis Clinical Guidelines Panel summary report on the management of staghorn calculi. The American Urological Association Nephrolithiasis Clinical Guidelines Panel. J Urol 1994;151:1648–1651.

See Also
- Renal stone, initial
- Renal stone, calcium oxalate
- Renal stone, uric acid
- Renal stone, struvite

Renal Stone, Calcium Oxalate

Indications and Timing for Referral
- Renal insufficiency present
- Etiology of stone diathesis unclear

Timing: Routine (less than 4 weeks)

Tests to Prepare for Consult
- Electrolytes (Na, K, Cl, CO_2)
- Calcium, phosphorus
- Creatinine
- Uric acid
- Urinalysis with microscopic
- Urine, culture and sensitivity
- 24-hour urine
    - Calcium
    - Uric acid
    - Creatinine
- Plain film, abdomen
- IVP

Tests Not Useful Before Consult
- None

Tests Consultant May Need to Do
- Urine pH
- 24-hour urine
    - Calcium
    - Uric acid
    - Volume
    - Creatinine
    - Citrate
    - Oxalate
    - Sodium
- Acid load test
- PTH
- Calcium
- Oral calcium deprivation and loading studies
- 25-hydroxyvitamin D
- UGIS with small bowel follow through

Follow-up Visits Generally Required
- One

Suggested Readings
Parks JH, Coe FL. Pathogenesis and treatment of calcium stones. [Review] [89 refs]. Semin Nephrol 1996;16:398–411.

Ruml LA, Pearle MS, Pak CY. Medical therapy, calcium oxalate urolithiasis. [Review] [148 refs]. Urol Clin North Am 1997;24:117–133.

Breslau NA. Pathogenesis and management of hypercalciuric nephrolithiasis. [Review]. Miner Electrolyte Metab 1994;20:328–339.

Parks JH, Coe FL. An increasing number of calcium oxalate stone events worsens treatment outcome. Kidney Int 1994;45:1722–1730.

See Also
- Renal stone, uric acid
- Renal stone, struvite
- Renal stone, recurrent
- Renal stone, initial

Renal Stone, Struvite

Indications and Timing for Referral
- Renal insufficiency present

Timing: Routine (less than 4 weeks)

Tests to Prepare for Consult
- Electrolytes (Na, K, Cl, CO_2)
- BUN, creatinine
- Calcium, phosphorus
- CBC
- Urinalysis with microscopic
- Urine, culture and sensitivity
- 24-hour urine
  - Volume
  - Creatinine for clearance
  - Protein
- Ultrasound, renal
- IVP

Tests Not Useful Before Consult
- None

Tests Consultant May Need to Do
- Electrolytes (Na, K, Cl, CO_2)
- Albumin, total protein
- BUN, creatinine
- Calcium, phosphorus
- CBC
- Urinalysis with microscopic
- Urine, culture and sensitivity
- 24-hour urine
  - Volume
  - Creatinine for clearance
  - Protein

Follow-up Visits Generally Required
- One

Suggested Readings
Cohen TD, Preminger GM. Struvite calculi. [Review] [71 refs]. Semin Nephrol 1996;16:425–434.

Wang LP, Wong HY, Griffith DP. Treatment options in struvite stones. [Review] [149 refs]. Urol Clin North Am 1997;24:149–162.

Saklayen MG. Medical management of nephrolithiasis. [Review] [56 refs]. Med Clin North Am 1997;81:785–799.

See Also
- Renal stone, recurrent
- Renal stone, initial
- Renal stone, uric acid
- Renal stone, calcium oxalate

Renal Stone, Uric Acid

Indications and Timing for Referral

- Renal insufficiency present
- Etiology of stone diathesis unclear

Timing: Routine (less than 4 weeks)

Tests to Prepare for Consult

- Electrolytes (Na, K, Cl, CO_2)
- Creatinine
- Uric acid
- Urinalysis with microscopic
- Urine, culture and sensitivity
- 24-hour urine
  - Calcium
  - Uric acid
  - Creatinine
- IVP

Tests Not Useful Before Consult

- None

Tests Consultant May Need to Do

- Urine pH
- 24-hour urine
  - Uric acid
  - Volume
  - Calcium

Follow-up Visits Generally Required

- One

Suggested Readings

Asplin JR. Uric acid stones. [Review] [86 refs]. Semin Nephrol 1996;16:412–424.

Low RK, Stoller ML. Uric acid-related nephrolithiasis. [Review] [69 refs]. Urol Clin North Am 1997;24:135–148.

Halabe A, Sperling O. Uric acid nephrolithiasis. [Review]. Miner Electrolyte Metab 1994;20:424–431.

Saklayen MG. Medical management of nephrolithiasis. [Review] [56 refs]. Med Clin North Am 1997;81:785–799.

See Also

- Renal stone, recurrent
- Renal stone, calcium oxalate
- Renal stone, struvite
- Renal stone, initial

NEPHROLOGY

Uremia

Indications and Timing for Referral
- Rapidly progressive
- Associated with unexplained oliguria

Timing: Urgent (less than 24 hours)

- Persistently abnormal in absence of gastrointestinal bleeding, steroid or tetracycline use, excessive dietary protein, dehydration, or parenteral nutrition

Timing: Expedited (less than 1 week)

Tests to Prepare for Consult
- CBC
- Electrolytes (Na, K, Cl, CO_2)
- Albumin, total protein
- Calcium, phosphorus
- BUN, creatinine
- Urinalysis with microscopic
- Urine sodium
- Urine creatinine
- 24-hour urine protein
- 24-hour urine creatinine for clearance
- Ultrasound, renal

Tests Not Useful Before Consult
- IVP
- CT scan, renal
- MR, renal

Tests Consultant May Need to Do
- Electrolytes (Na, K, Cl, CO_2)
- Albumin, total protein
- Calcium, phosphorus
- BUN, creatinine
- Glucose
- Urinalysis with microscopic
- 24-hour urine protein
- 24-hour urine creatinine for clearance
- ANA
- Anti-double stranded DNA
- Complement factors (C3, C4)
- Anti-neutrophil cytoplasmic antibody
- Osmolality, urine
- Immunoelectrophoresis, serum and urine
- Eosinophil count, serum and urine
- HIV antibody testing

Follow-up Visits Generally Required
- Two

Suggested Readings
Luke RG. Uremia and the BUN. N Engl J Med 1981;305:1213–1215.

Lafayette RA, Perrone RD, Levey AS. Laboratory evaluation of renal function. In: Schrier RW, Gottschalk CW, eds. Diseases of the Kidney. 6th ed. Boston: Little, Brown, 1996:307–354.

See Also
- Creatinine elevation

Urine, Red

Indications and Timing for Referral
- Blood present in urine
- Urine negative for blood and diagnosis uncertain
- Dipstick positive without RBCs

Timing: Urgent (less than 24 hours)

Advice for Referral
- Careful medication history is vital e.g., rifampin, phenazopyridine.
- Careful dietary history is vital, e.g., red beets.

Tests to Prepare for Consult
- Electrolytes (Na, K, Cl, CO_2)
- CBC with differential
- BUN, creatinine
- Urinalysis, dipstick
- Urinalysis with microscopic
- CPK
- Myoglobin

Tests Not Useful Before Consult
- IVP

Tests Consultant May Need to Do
- Myoglobin
- Porphyrins

Follow-up Visits Generally Required
- None

Suggested Readings
Thompson WG. Things that go red in the urine—and others that don't. Lancet 1996;347:5–6.

McCarthy JJ. Outpatient evaluation of hematuria: locating the source of bleeding. [Review] [7 refs]. Postgrad Med 1997;101:125–128.

See Also
- Hematuria, microscopic
- Red blood cell casts
- Hematuria, gross

CHAPTER 8

Neurology

Alzheimer's Disease
    Diagnosis 391
    Management 393
Amyotrophic Lateral Sclerosis (ALS), Diagnosis 394
Brain Mass
    History of Primary Extracranial Malignancy 395
    No Known Extracranial Malignancy 396
Carotid Stenosis, Asymptomatic 397
Cervical Bruit, Asymptomatic 398
Cervical Spondylosis with Myelopathy 399
Cranial Neuropathy, Immunocompromised Patient 400
Diplopia 401
Dizziness, Nonvertiginous 402
Episodic Loss of Consciousness, Seizure Versus Syncope 403
Facial Weakness 405
Gait Disorders 406
Headache
    Acute 407
    Chronic Recurrent 408
    Migraine 409
    Post-traumatic 410
Imaging Abnormality
    Hydrocephalus 411
    Hygroma 412
    Subdural, Asymptomatic 413
    Unidentified Bright Objects (UBOs) 414
Lyme Disease, Possible Cause of Neurologic Findings 415
Memory Loss 416
Mental Status Change
    Acute or Subacute 417
    Chronic Dementia 419
    Immunocompromised Patient 421
Multiple Sclerosis
    Diagnosis 422
    Management 423
Myasthenia Gravis, Diagnosis 424

(continued)

THE CONSULTATION GUIDE

Neurology (continued)

Myopathic Weakness 425
Neuropathy, Peripheral 426
Paresthesias
    Feet 427
    Hands 428
Parkinsonian Syndrome, Atypical 429
Parkinson's Disease 430
Postconcussion Syndrome 431
Ptosis 432
Radiculopathy
    Cervical 433
    Thoracic 434
Seizures
    Generalized 435
    New Onset, in Adults 436
    Partial 438
Speech Disorder 439
Spells, Transient Ischemic Attack (TIA) Versus Seizure 440
Swallowing Disorder 441
Tics 442
Transient Ischemic Attacks (TIAs) 443
Tremor 445
Vertigo 446
Visual Loss, Monocular 447
Weakness, Generalized 448

Alzheimer's Disease, Diagnosis

Indications and Timing for Referral

- Diagnostic uncertainty

Timing: Routine (less than 4 weeks)

Advice for Referral

- A complete medication history is vital before consultation.

Tests to Prepare for Consult

- CBC
- Glucose
- Sodium
- Calcium
- Creatinine
- RPR or VDRL
- TSH (assay sensitivity <0.1 mU/L)
- Vitamin B_{12}, serum
- CT or MR, cranial, without contrast

Tests Not Useful Before Consult

- SPECT scan, cranial

Tests Consultant May Need to Do

- ESR
- ALT, AST
- Lyme (*Borrelia burgdorferi*) serology
- Toxicology screen
- EEG
- Neuropsychological testing
- Lumbar puncture
- Cell count, CSF
- Glucose, CSF
- Protein, CSF
- Culture and sensitivity, CSF
- Cytology, CSF
- Fungal stain and culture, CSF
- VDRL, CSF
- Lyme titer, CSF
- Cryptococcal antigen, CSF
- HIV antibody testing

Follow-up Visits Generally Required

- One

Suggested Readings

Geldmacher DS, Whitehouse PJ Jr. Differential diagnosis of Alzheimer's disease. [Review] [65 refs]. Neurology 1997;48(Suppl 6):S2–S9.

Morgan CD, Baade LE. Neuropsychological testing and assessment scales for dementia of the Alzheimer's type. [Review] [69 refs]. Psychiatr Clin North Am 1997;20:25–43.

Morris JC. Differential diagnosis of Alzheimer's disease. [Review]. Clin Geriatr Med 1994;10:257–276.

Reiman EM, Caselli RJ, Lang SY, et al. Preclinical evidence of Alzheimer's disease in persons homozygous for the E4 allele for apolipoprotein E. N Engl J Med 1996;334:752–758.

Post SG, Whitehouse PJ, Binstock RH, et al. The clinical introduction of genetic testing for Alzheimer disease. An ethical perspective. [Review] [75 refs]. JAMA 1997;277:832–836.

de Toledo-Morrell L, Morrell F. Alzheimer's disease: new developments for noninvasive detection of early cases. [Review]. Curr Opin Neurol Neurosurg 1993;6:113–118.

Alzheimer's Disease, Diagnosis (*continued*)

Selected Guidelines

Early identification of Alzheimer's disease and related dementias. Agency for Health Care Policy and Research. Clin Pract Guidel Quick Ref Guide Clin 1996;19:1–28.

Practice parameter for diagnosis and evaluation of dementia. (summary statement) Report of the Quality Standards Subcommittee of the American Academy of Neurology. Neurology 1994;44:2203–2206.

McKeith LG, Galasko D, Kosaka K, et al. Consensus guidelines for the clinical and pathologic diagnosis of dementia with Lewy bodies (DLB): report of the consortium on DLB international workshop. [Review] [49 refs]. Neurology 1996;47:1113–1124.

See Also

- Alzheimer's disease, management
- Memory loss
- Mental status change, immunocompromised patient
- Mental status change, chronic dementia
- Mental status change, acute or subacute

NEUROLOGY

Alzheimer's Disease, Management

Indications and Timing for Referral

- Assistance with management (e.g., Cognex use)
- Complete medication history is vital

Timing: Routine (less than 4 weeks)

Tests to Prepare for Consult

- CBC
- Glucose
- Sodium
- Calcium
- Creatinine

Tests Not Useful Before Consult

- None

Tests Consultant May Need to Do

- HIV antibody testing
- ALT, AST
- Magnesium

Follow-up Visits Generally Required

- None

Suggested Readings

Aisen PS, Davis KL. The search for disease-modifying treatment for Alzheimer's disease. [Review] [89 refs]. Neurology 1997;48:(Suppl 6):S35–S41.

Borson S, Raskind MA. Clinical features and pharmacologic treatment of behavioral symptoms of Alzheimer's disease. [Review] [71 refs]. Neurology 1997;48(Suppl 6):S17–S24.

Sano M, Ernesto C, Thomas RG, et al. A controlled trial of selegiline, alpha-tocopherol, or both as treatment for Alzheimer's disease. The Alzheimer's Disease Cooperative Study [see comments]. N Engl J Med 1997;336:1216–1222.

Selected Guidelines

Practice guideline for the treatment of patients with Alzheimer's disease and other dementias of late life. American Psychiatric Association. Am J Psychiatry 1997;154(Suppl):1–39.

Dementia: guidelines for diagnosis and treatment. 2nd ed. Washington, DC: Office of Geriatrics and Extended Care, Department of Veterans Affairs, Veterans Health Services and Research Administration, 1989; various pagings.

See Also

- Alzheimer's disease, diagnosis

THE CONSULTATION GUIDE

Amyotrophic Lateral Sclerosis (ALS), Diagnosis

Indications and Timing for Referral
- Diagnostic uncertainty

Timing: Routine (less than 4 weeks)

Advice for Referral
- Studies that differentiate ALS from multifocal motor neuropathy with conduction block are very operator-dependent and should be done by experts in electromyography.
- Co-management with a neurologist can be helpful in managing this disease.

Tests to Prepare for Consult
- None

Tests Not Useful Before Consult
- None

Test Consultant May Need to Do
- Anti-GM1 ganglioside antibody
- Lead, blood
- Mercury, serum or urine
- Electromyogram
- Nerve conduction study
- TSH (assay sensitivity <0.1 mU/L)

Follow-up Visits Generally Required
- Co-management, see *Advice for referral*

Suggested Readings
Rowland LP. Amyotrophic lateral sclerosis. [Review]. Curr Opin Neurol 1994;7:310–315.

Williams DB, Windebank AJ. Motor neuron disease (amyotrophic lateral sclerosis). [Review]. Mayo Clinic Proc 1991;66:54–82.

Belsh JM, Schiffman PL. Misdiagnosis in patients with amyotrophic lateral sclerosis. Arch Intern Med 1990;150:2301–2305.

Mitsumoto H, Olney RK. Drug combination treatment in patients with ALS: current status and future directions. [Review] [15 refs]. Neurology 1996;47(Suppl 2):S103–S107.

See Also
- Cervical spondylosis with myelopathy
- Myopathic weakness

Brain Mass, History of Primary Extracranial Malignancy

Indications and Timing for Referral
- Diagnostic uncertainty
- Assistance with management

Timing: Expedited (less than 1 week)

Advice for Referral
- MR with contrast can be valuable in distinguishing between primary brain tumor and metastatic disease.

Tests to Prepare for Consult
- MR, cranial with contrast

Tests Not Useful Before Consult
- None

Tests Consultant May Need to Do
- Urinalysis with microscopic
- Radiograph, chest
- EEG

Follow-up Visits Generally Required
- Two

Suggested Readings
O'Neill BP, Buckner JC, Coffey RJ, et al. Brain metastatic lesions. [Review]. Mayo Clin Proc 1994;69:1062–1068.

Das A, Hochberg FH. Clinical presentation of intracranial metastases. [Review] [65 refs]. Neurosurg Clin N Am 1996;7:377–391.

Cascino TL. Neurologic complications of systemic cancer. [Review]. Med Clin North Am 1993;77:265–278.

Merchut MP. Brain metastases from undiagnosed systemic neoplasms. Arch Intern Med 1989;149:1076–1080.

See Also
- Brain mass, no known extracranial malignancy

THE CONSULTATION GUIDE

Brain Mass, No Known Extracranial Malignancy

Indications and Timing for Referral
- Diagnostic uncertainty

Timing: Expedited (less than 1 week)

Advice for Referral
- MR with contrast can be valuable in distinguishing between primary brain tumor and metastatic disease.

Tests to Prepare for Consult
- Urinalysis with microscopic
- Bilirubin
- Calcium
- ALT, AST, alkaline phosphatase
- Radiograph, chest
- MR, cranial with contrast

Tests Not Useful Before Consult
- None

Tests Consultant May Need to Do
- HIV antibody testing
- EEG
- CT scan, thorax

Follow-up Visits Generally Required
- Two

Suggested Readings
Castillo M. Contrast enhancement in primary tumors of the brain and spinal cord. [Review]. Neuroimaging Clin North Am 1994;4:63–80.

Forsyth PA, Posner JB. Headaches in patients with brain tumors: a study of 111 patients. Neurology 1993;43:1678–1683.

Das A, Hochberg FH. Clinical presentation of intracranial metastases. [Review] [65 refs]. Neurosurg Clin N Am 1996;7:377–391.

See Also
- Brain mass, history of primary extracranial malignancy

Carotid Stenosis, Asymptomatic

Indications and Timing for Referral
- Assistance with decision-making regarding management

Timing: Routine (less than 4 weeks)

Tests to Prepare for Consult
- Carotid duplex study

Tests Not Useful Before Consult
- None

Tests Consultant May Need to Do
- MR angiography
- CT scan, cranial, spiral, with contrast
- Cerebral angiogram

Follow-up Visits Generally Required
- None

Suggested Readings

Rockman CB, Riles TS, Lamparello PJ, et al. Natural history and management of the asymptomatic, moderately stenotic internal carotid artery. J Vasc Surg 1997;25:423–431.

Goldstein LB, Bonito AJ, Matchar DB, et al. U. S. National Survey of Physician Practices for the secondary and tertiary prevention of ischemic stroke. Medical therapy in patients with carotid artery stenosis. Stroke 1996;27:1473–1478.

Rothwell PM, Slattery J, Warlow CP. A systematic comparison of the risks of stroke and death due to carotid endarterectomy for symptomatic and asymptomatic stenosis. [Review] [37 refs]. Stroke 1996;27:266–269.

Blakeley DD, Oddone EZ, Hasselblad V, et al. Noninvasive carotid artery testing. A meta-analytic review. Ann Intern Med 1995;122:360–367.

Endarterectomy for asymptomatic carotid artery stenosis. Executive Committee for the Asymptomatic Carotid Atherosclerosis Study [see comments]. JAMA 1995;273:1421–1428.

Selected Guidelines

Thiele BL, Jones AM, Hobson RW, et al. Standards in noninvasive cerebrovascular testing. Report from the Committee on Standards for Noninvasive Vascular Testing of the Joint Council of the Society for Vascular Surgery and the North American Chapter of the International Society for Cardiovascular Surgery. J Vasc Surg 1992;15:495–503.

American College of Physicians. Indications for carotid endarterectomy. Ann Intern Med 1989;111:675–677.

See Also
- Spells, TIA versus seizure
- Transient ischemic attacks (TIAs)
- Cervical bruit, asymptomatic

Cervical Bruit, Asymptomatic

Indications and Timing for Referral

- Assistance with decision-making regarding management

Timing: Routine (less than 4 weeks)

Advice for Referral

- See *Carotid Stenosis* if duplex is abnormal.
- Cerebral angiogram should be scheduled after preliminary review with neurology consultant.

Tests to Prepare for Consult

- Carotid duplex study

Tests Not Useful Before Consult

- None

Tests Consultant May Need to Do

- None

Follow-up Visits Generally Required

- None

Suggested Readings

Mackey AE, Abrahamowicz M, Langlois Y, et al. Outcome of asymptomatic patients with carotid disease. Asymptomatic Cervical Bruit Study Group. Neurology 1997;48:896–903.

Young B, Moore WS, Robertson JT, et al. An analysis of perioperative surgical mortality and morbidity in the asymptomatic carotid atherosclerosis study. ACAS Investigators. Asymptomatic Carotid Atherosclerosis Study. Stroke 1996;27:2216–2224.

Lord RS. Non-invasive testing for cerebrovascular disease. [Review] [96 refs]. Cardiovasc Surg 1996;4:424–437.

Bornstein NM, Norris JW. Management of patients with asymptomatic neck bruits and carotid stenosis. [Review]. Neurol Clin 1992;10:269–280.

Sauve JS, Thorpe KE, Sackett DL, et al. Can bruits distinguish high-grade from moderate symptomatic carotid stenosis? The North American Symptomatic Carotid Endarterectomy Trial. Ann Intern Med 1994;120:633–637.

Selected Guidelines

Thiele BL, Jones AM, Hobson RW, et al. Standards in noninvasive cerebrovascular testing. Report from the Committee on Standards for Noninvasive Vascular Testing of the Joint Council of the Society for Vascular Surgery and the North American Chapter of the International Society for Cardiovascular Surgery. J Vasc Surg 1992;15:495–503.

American College of Physicians. Indications for carotid endarterectomy. Ann Intern Med 1989;111:675–677.

See Also

- Transient ischemic attacks (TIAs)
- Carotid stenosis, asymptomatic
- Spells, TIA versus seizure

NEUROLOGY

Cervical Spondylosis with Myelopathy

Indications and Timing for Referral
- Diagnostic uncertainty
- Assistance with management

Timing: Routine (less than 4 weeks)

Advice for Referral
- Optimal timing of referral may be Urgent (less than 24 hours) or Expedited (less than 1 week) depending on the duration, severity, or progression of the syndrome.

Tests to Prepare for Consult
- None

Tests Not Useful Before Consult
- None

Tests Consultant May Need to Do
- Vitamin B_{12}, serum
- Glucose
- VDRL or RPR
- HIV antibody testing
- HTLV-I serology
- Radiograph, cervical spine
- MR, spine, without contrast
- MR, cranial, without contrast
- Electromyogram
- Nerve conduction study
- Cystometric study

Follow-up Visits Generally Required
- One

Suggested Readings
McCormack BM, Weinstein PR. Cervical spondylosis. An update. [Review] [116 refs]. West J Med 1996;165:43–51.

Krauss WE, McCormick PC. Cervical spondylotic myelopathy. [Review]. Semin Neurol 1993;13:343–348.

Long DM. Lumbar and cervical spondylosis and spondylotic myelopathy. [Review]. Curr Opin Neurol Neurosurg 1993;6:576–580.

Statham PF, Hadley DM, Macpherson P, et al. MRI in the management of suspected cervical spondylotic myelopathy. J Neurol Neurosurg Psychiatry 1991;54:484–489.

Selected Guidelines
Magnetic resonance imaging of the brain and spine: a revised statement. American College of Physicians [comment] [see comments]. Ann Intern Med 1994;120:872–875.

See Also
- Radiculopathy, cervical
- Radiculopathy, thoracic

Cranial Neuropathy, Immunocompromised Patient

Indications and Timing for Referral
- Assistance with management

Timing: Urgent (less than 24 hours)

Advice for Referral
- "Sinus CT, focused series" refers to a limited series of appropriate regional cuts to include coronal images of the osteo-meatal complex.

Tests to Prepare for Consult
- CBC
- VDRL
- CT or MR, cranial, with and without contrast
- Lumbar puncture
- Cell count, CSF
- Glucose, CSF
- Protein, CSF
- Culture and sensitivity, CSF
- Cytology, CSF
- Fungal stain and culture, CSF
- VDRL, CSF
- Cryptococcal antigen, CSF

Tests Not Useful Before Consult
- None

Tests Consultant May Need to Do
- CT, sinuses, focused series (see *Advice for Referral*)

Follow-up Visits Generally Required
- None

Suggested Readings
Cohen BA. Neurologic complications of HIV infection. Prim Care 1997;24(3):575–595.

Harindra V. Neurologic manifestations of HIV infection. Ann Intern Med 1995;122(11):883.

Simpson DM, Berger JR. Neurologic manifestations of HIV infection. Med Clin North Am 1996;80(6):1363–1394.

See Also
- Diplopia
- Ptosis
- Vertigo
- Headache, in HIV + Patient
- Dementia, in HIV + Patient
- Mental Status Change, Immunocompromised Patient

Diplopia

Indications and Timing for Referral

- Sudden onset or rapid progression

Timing: Immediate

- Unexplained

Timing: Routine (less than 4 weeks)

Advice for Referral

- Optimal timing of referral may be Urgent (less than 24 hours) or Expedited (less than 1 week) depending on the duration, frequency, severity, or progression of episodes.
- Preliminary ophthalmologic evaluation is necessary to exclude primary ophthalmologic disorders before consultation.

Tests to Prepare for Consult

- Glucose
- CBC
- ESR

Tests Not Useful Before Consult

- None

Tests Consultant May Need to Do

- Anti-acetylcholine receptor antibody
- Glycohemoglobin
- TSH (assay sensitivity <0.1 mU/L)
- Tensilon test
- MR or CT, cranial ± contrast
- Visual evoked response
- Brainstem-evoked responses
- Electromyogram
- Nerve conduction study
- Temporal artery biopsy
- Lumbar puncture
- Cell count, CSF
- Glucose, CSF
- Protein, CSF
- Culture and sensitivity, CSF
- Cytology, CSF

Follow-up Visits Generally Required

- One

Suggested Readings

Kutschke PJ. Taking a history of the patient with diplopia. Insight 1996;21:92–95.

Barton JJ, Corbett JJ. Neuro-ophthalmologic vascular emergencies in the elderly. [Review]. Clin Geriatr Med 1991;7:525–548.

Adams RA, Victor M, Ropper AH. Disorders of ocular movement and pupillary function. In: Adams RA, Victor M, Ropper AH, eds. Principles of Neurology. 6th ed. New York: McGraw Hill, 1997.

See Also

- Visual loss, monocular
- Ptosis

Dizziness, Nonvertiginous

Indications and Timing for Referral

- Persistent, unexplained symptoms

Timing: Routine (less than 4 weeks)

Advice for Referral

- Evaluation of orthostatic blood pressure is vital before consultation.
- A complete medication history is vital before consultation.

Tests to Prepare for Consult

- Glucose, fasting
- Electrolytes (Na, K, Cl, CO_2)
- Creatinine
- TSH (assay sensitivity <0.1 mU/L)
- ECG

Tests Not Useful Before Consult

- Tilt table test
- Posturography

Tests Consultant May Need to Do

- Carotid duplex study
- MR or CT, cranial ± contrast
- Ambulatory ECG (Holter)

Follow-up Visits Generally Required

- None

Suggested Readings

Linstrom CJ. Office management of the dizzy patient. [Review]. Otolaryngol Clin North Am 1992;25:745–780.

Kroenke K, Lucas CA, Rosenberg ML, et al. Causes of persistent dizziness. A prospective study of 100 patients in ambulatory care. Ann Intern Med 1992;117:898–904.

Brown JJ. A systematic approach to the dizzy patient. [Review]. Neurol Clin 1990;8:209–224.

Colledge NR, Barr-Hamilton RM, Lewis SJ, et al. Evaluation of investigations to diagnose the cause of dizziness in elderly people: a community based controlled study [see comments]. Br Med J 1996;313:788–792.

Sloane PD. Evaluation and management of dizziness in the older patient. [Review] [58 refs]. Clin Geriatr Med 1996;12:785–801.

Sullivan M, Clark MR, Katon WJ, et al. Psychiatric and otologic diagnoses in patients complaining of dizziness [see comments]. Arch Intern Med 1993;153:1479–1484.

See Also

- Vertigo

Episodic Loss of Consciousness, Seizure Versus Syncope

Indications and Timing for Referral
- Focal neurologic deficit present
- Prolonged loss of consciousness (longer than 5 minutes)

Timing: Expedited (less than 1 week)

Optimal timing of referral may be Urgent (less than 24 hours) or Routine (less than 4 weeks) depending on the duration, frequency, severity, or progression of episodes

Advice for Referral
- Because MRI is a more sensitive technique for identifying brain pathology that causes seizures, it is generally the procedure of choice when available and not contraindicated.
- Evaluation of orthostatic blood pressure is vital before consultation.

Tests to Prepare for Consult
- CBC
- Glucose
- Sodium
- Calcium
- Magnesium
- ALT, AST
- Creatinine
- ECG

Tests Not Useful Before Consult
- Tilt table test
- Carotid duplex study
- Cerebral angiogram
- Ocular plethysmography

Tests Consultant May Need to Do
- Toxicology screen
- EEG, wake and sleep study
- EEG, prolonged monitoring
- MR or CT, cranial ± contrast
- Ambulatory ECG (Holter)
- Echocardiogram

Follow-up Visits Generally Required
- One

Suggested Readings

Kapoor WN. Back to basics for the workup of syncope. J Gen Intern Med 1995;10:695–696.

Schmidt D. Syncopes and seizures. Curr Opin Neurol 1996;9:78–81.

Grubb BP, Kosinski D. Current trends in etiology, diagnosis, and management of neurocardiogenic syncope. Curr Opin Cardiol 1996;11:32–41.

Chabolla DR, Krahn LE, So EL, Rummans TA. Psychogenic nonepileptic seizures. Mayo Clin Proc 1996;71:493–500.

Morillo CA, Klein GJ, Gersh BJ. Can serial tilt testing be used to evaluate therapy in neurally mediated syncope. Am J Cardiol 1996;77:521.

Benditt DG, Remole S, Milstein S, Bailin S. Syncope: causes, clinical evaluation, and current therapy. [Review]. Annu Rev Med 1992;43:283–300.

Calkins H, Shyr Y, Frumin H, et al. The value of the clinical history in the differentiation of syncope due to ventricular tachycardia, atrioventricular block, and neurocardiogenic syncope. Am J Med 1995;98:365–373.

Episodic Loss of Consciousness, Seizure Versus Syncope (*continued*)

Selected Guidelines

Clinical policy for the initial approach to patients presenting with a chief complaint of seizure who are not in status epilepticus. American College of Emergency Physicians. Ann Emerg Med 1997;29:706–724.

See Also

- Seizure, new onset, in adults
- Spells, TIA versus seizure
- Seizures, generalized
- Seizures, partial
- Transient ischemic attacks (TIAs)

Facial Weakness

Indications and Timing for Referral

- Diagnostic uncertainty
- Assistance with management

Timing: Urgent (less than 24 hours)

Tests to Prepare for Consult

- Glucose, fasting

Tests Not Useful Before Consult

- None

Tests Consultant May Need to Do

- Radiograph, chest
- MR or CT, cranial ± contrast
- Lumbar puncture
- Cell count, CSF
- Glucose, CSF
- Protein, CSF
- Culture and sensitivity, CSF
- Cytology, CSF
- Lyme (*B. burgdorferi*) serology

Follow-up Visits Generally Required

- None

Suggested Readings

Brandle P, Satorettischefer S, Bohmer A, et al. Correlation of MRI, clinical, and electroneuronographic findings in acute facial nerve palsy. Am J Otology 1996;17:154–161.

May M, Klein SR. Differential diagnosis of facial nerve palsy. [Review]. Otolaryngol Clin North Am 1991;24:613–645.

Adour KK. Medical management of idiopathic (Bell's) palsy. [Review]. Otolaryngol Clin North Am 1991;24:663–673.

Adams RA, Victor M, Ropper AH. Diseases of the cranial nerves. In: Adams RA, Victor M, Ropper AH, eds. Principles Neurology. 6th ed. New York: McGraw Hill, 1997:1370–1385.

Gait Disorders

Indications and Timing for Referral

- Diagnostic uncertainty
- Assistance with management

Timing: Routine (less than 4 weeks)

Tests to Prepare for Consult

- CBC
- Glucose
- VDRL
- Vitamin B$_{12}$, serum

Tests Not Useful Before Consult

- None

Tests Consultant May Need to Do

- Electromyogram
- Nerve conduction study
- MR, spine
- MR, cranial, without contrast
- Lumbar puncture
- Cell count, CSF
- Glucose, CSF
- Protein, CSF
- Culture and sensitivity, CSF
- Cytology, CSF

Follow-up Visits Generally Required

- One

Suggested Readings

Alexander NB. Gait disorders in older adults [review]. J Am Geriatr Soc 1996;44:434–451.

Judge JO, Ounpuu S, Davis RB 3rd. Effects of age on the biomechanics and physiology of gait. [Review] [45 refs]. Clin Geriatr Med 1996;12:659–678.

Bloem BR, Haan J, Lagaay AM, et al. Investigation of gait in elderly subjects over 88 years of age. J Geriatr Psychiatry Neurol 1992;5:78–84.

NEUROLOGY

Headache, Acute

Indications and Timing for Referral

- Fever, change in mentation, stiff neck, or focal findings
- If described as "worst headache of my life"

Timing: Immediate

- Diagnostic uncertainty

Timing: Urgent (less than 24 hours)

Advice for Referral

- A complete medication history is vital before consultation.
- If subarachnoid hemorrhage is a clinical consideration, then a lumbar puncture with CSF studies is appropriate before consultation.

Tests to Prepare for Consult

- CT scan, cranial, without contrast

Tests Not Useful Before Consult

- None

Tests Consultant May Need to Do

- Toxicology screen
- MR, cranial, without contrast
- Lumbar puncture
- Cell count, CSF
- Glucose, CSF
- Protein, CSF
- Culture and sensitivity, CSF

Follow-up Visits Generally Required

- One

Suggested Readings

Dodick D. Headache as a symptom of ominous disease. What are the warning signals? [Review] [9 refs]. Postgrad Med 1997;101:46–50.

Evans RW. Diagnostic testing for the evaluation of headaches. [Review] [159 refs]. Neurol Clin 1996;14:1–26.

Silberstein SD, Lipton RB. Overview of diagnosis and treatment of migraine. [Review]. Neurology 1994;44(Suppl 7):S6–S16.

Alter M, Daube JR, Franklin G. Practice parameter: The utility of neuroimaging in the evaluation of headache in patients with normal neurological examinations. Neurology 1997;44:1353.

Selected Guidelines

Magnetic resonance imaging of the brain and spine: a revised statement. American College of Physicians [comment] [see comments]. Ann Intern Med 1994;120:872–875.

See Also

- Headache, chronic recurrent
- Headache, migraine
- Headache, post-traumatic

Headache, Chronic Recurrent

Indications and Timing for Referral

- Assistance with management

Timing: Routine (less than 4 weeks)

Advice for Referral

- A complete medication history (e.g., analgesics) is vital before consultation.
- Sleep studies should be requested only from centers with expertise in disordered breathing during sleep.
- The accuracy of home sleep studies remains to be established.

Tests to Prepare for Consult

- None

Tests Not Useful Before Consult

- None

Tests Consultant May Need to Do

- CBC
- ESR
- TSH (assay sensitivity <0.1 mU/L)
- MR or CT, cranial ± contrast
- Lumbar puncture
- Cell count, CSF
- Glucose, CSF
- Protein, CSF
- Culture and sensitivity, CSF
- Cytology, CSF
- Sleep study (see *Advice for Referral*)

Follow-up Visits Generally Required

- One

Suggested Readings

Ryan CW. Evaluation of patients with chronic headache. [Review] [14 refs]. Am Fam Physician 1996;54:1051–1057.

Mathew NT. Chronic refractory headache. [Review]. Neurology 1993;43(Suppl 3):S26–S33.

Sheftell FD. Chronic daily headache. [Review]. Neurology 1992;42(Suppl 2):32–36.

Silberstein SD. Tension-type and chronic daily headache. [Review]. Neurology 1993;43:1644–1649.

Dodick D. Headache as a symptom of ominous disease. What are the warning signals? [Review] [9 refs]. Postgrad Med 1997;101:46–50.

Olesen J, Rasmussen BK. The International Headache Society classification of chronic daily and near-daily headaches: a critique of the criticism. [Review] [33 refs]. Cephalalgia 1996;16:407–411.

Baumel B, Eisner LS. Diagnosis and treatment of headache in the elderly. [Review]. Med Clin North Am 1991;75:661–675.

Demaerel P, Boelaert I, Wilms G, Baert AL. The role of cranial computed tomography in the diagnostic work-up of headache. Headache 1996;36:347–348.

Selected Guidelines

Magnetic resonance imaging of the brain and spine: a revised statement. American College of Physicians [comment] [see comments]. Ann Intern Med 1994;120:872–875.

See Also

- Headache, post-traumatic
- Sinusitis, persistent
- Sinusitis, recurrent
- Headache, acute
- Headache, migraine

Headache, Migraine

Indications and Timing for Referral

- Assistance with management

Timing: Routine (less than 4 weeks)

Tests to Prepare for Consult

- None

Tests Not Useful Before Consult

- None

Tests Consultant May Need to Do

- CBC
- ESR
- TSH (assay sensitivity <0.1 mU/L)
- MR or CT, cranial ± contrast

Follow-up Visits Generally Required

- One

Suggested Readings

Capobianco DJ, Cheshire WP, Campbell JK. An overview of the diagnosis and pharmacologic treatment of migraine. [Review] [77 refs]. Mayo Clin Proc 1996;71:1055–1066.

Saper JR. Diagnosis and symptomatic treatment of migraine. [Review] [56 refs]. Headache 1997;37(Suppl 1):S1–S14.

Silberstein SD, Lipton RB. Overview of diagnosis and treatment of migraine. [Review]. Neurology 1994;44(Suppl 7):S6–S16.

Merikangas KR, Dartigues JF, Whitaker A, Angst J. Diagnostic criteria for migraine. A validity study. Neurology 1994;44(Suppl 4):S11–S16.

Diamond S. Migraine headaches. [Review]. Med Clin North Am 1991;75:545–566.

Welch KM. Drug therapy of migraine [see comments]. [Review]. N Engl J Med 1993;329:1476–1483.

Selected Guidelines

Pryse-Phillips WE, Dodick DW, et al. Guidelines for the diagnosis and management of migraine in clinical practice. Canadian Headache Society. [Review] [160 refs]. Can Med Assoc J 1997;156:1273–1287.

See Also

- Headache, acute
- Headache, chronic recurrent
- Headache, post-traumatic

THE CONSULTATION GUIDE

Headache, Post-traumatic

Indications and Timing for Referral

- Diagnostic uncertainty
- Assistance with management

Timing: Routine (less than 4 weeks)

Tests to Prepare for Consult

- None

Tests Not Useful Before Consult

- None

Tests Consultant May Need to Do

- Radiograph, cervical spine
- CT or MR, cranial, without contrast

Follow-up Visits Generally Required

- None

Suggested Readings

Haas DC. Chronic post-traumatic headaches classified and compared with natural headaches [see comments]. Cephalalgia 1996;16:486–493.

Evans RW. The postconcussion syndrome: 130 years of controversy. [Review]. Semin Neurol 1994;14:32–39.

Packard RC, Ham LP. Pathogenesis of posttraumatic headache and migraine: a common headache pathway?. [Review] [114 refs]. Headache 1997;37:142–152.

Goldstein J. Posttraumatic headache and the postconcussion syndrome. [Review]. Med Clin North Am 1991;75:641–651.

Weiss HD, Stern BJ, Goldberg J. Post-traumatic migraine: chronic migraine precipitated by minor head or neck trauma [see comments]. Headache 1991;31:451–456.

Warner JS, Fenichel GM. Chronic post-traumatic headache often a myth. Neurology 1996;46:915–916.

Macciocchi SN, Reid DB, Barth JT. Disability following head injury. [Review]. Curr Opin Neurol 1993;6:773–777.

Selected Guidelines

Magnetic resonance imaging of the brain and spine: a revised statement. American College of Physicians [comment] [see comments]. Ann Intern Med 1994;120:872–875.

See Also

- Headache, migraine
- Headache, acute
- Headache, chronic recurrent
- Postconcussion syndrome

Imaging Abnormality, Hydrocephalus

Indications and Timing for Referral

- Diagnostic uncertainty
- Assistance with management

Timing: Expedited (less than 1 week)

Tests to Prepare for Consult

- CT or MR, cranial with contrast

Tests Not Useful Before Consult

- None

Tests Consultant May Need to Do

- Lumbar puncture
- Cell count, CSF
- Glucose, CSF
- Protein, CSF
- Cytology, CSF
- Fungal stain and culture, CSF
- VDRL, CSF

Follow-up Visits Generally Required

- One

Suggested Readings

Vanneste J, Augustijn P, Tan WF, Dirven C. Shunting normal pressure hydrocephalus: the predictive value of combined clinical and CT data. J Neurol Neurosurg Psychiatry 1993;56:251–256.

Adams RA, Victor M, Ropper AH. Disturbances of cerebrospinal fluid: its circulation, including hydrocephalus and meningeal reactions. In: Adams RA, Victor M, Ropper AH, eds. Principles of Neurology. 6th ed. New York: McGraw Hill, 1997:123–141.

Selected Guidelines

Magnetic resonance imaging of the brain and spine: a revised statement. American College of Physicians [comment] [see comments]. Ann Intern Med 1994;120:872–875.

See Also

- Gait disorders

Imaging Abnormality, Hygroma

Indications and Timing for Referral
- Assessment of clinical significance

Timing: Routine (less than 4 weeks)

Advice for Referral
- Optimal timing of referral may be sooner if there are relevant clinical neurologic findings.

Tests to Prepare for Consult
- None

Tests Not Useful Before Consult
- None

Tests Consultant May Need to Do
- CT scan, cranial, without contrast

Follow-up Visits Generally Required
- One

Suggested Readings
Wippold FJ 2nd. Definition and pathophysiology of subdural hygroma. AJR 1996;167:1061.

Adams RA, Victor M, Ropper AH. Craniocerebral trauma. In: Adams RA, Victor M, Ropper AH, eds. Principles of Neurology. 6th ed. New York: McGraw Hill, 1997:1386–1401.

Imaging Abnormality, Subdural, Asymptomatic

Indications and Timing for Referral
- Assessment of clinical significance

Timing: Routine (less than 4 weeks)

Advice for Referral
- Optimal timing of referral may be sooner if there are relevant clinical neurologic findings.

Tests to Prepare for Consult
- None

Tests Not Useful Before Consult
- None

Tests Consultant May Need to Do
- CT scan, cranial, without contrast

Follow-up Visits Generally Required
- One

Suggested Readings
Merlicco G, Pierangeli E, Dipadova PL. Chronic subdural hematomas in adults—prognostic factors—analysis of 70 cases. Neurosurg Rev 1995;18:247–251.

Adams RA, Victor M, Ropper AH. Craniocerebral trauma. In: Adams RA, Victor M, Ropper AH, eds. Principles of Neurology. 6th ed. New York: McGraw Hill, 1997:874–901.

Selected Guidelines
Magnetic resonance imaging of the brain and spine: a revised statement. American College of Physicians [comment] [see comments]. Ann Intern Med 1994;120:872–875.

Imaging Abnormality, Unidentified Bright Objects (UBOs)

Indications and Timing for Referral
- Diagnostic uncertainty

Timing: Routine (less than 4 weeks)

Advice for Referral
- "UBOs" are not pathognomonic of multiple sclerosis. Their prevalence increases with age, and may accompany any cerebrovascular disorder.
- Evaluation and complete history regarding hypertension is important.

Tests to Prepare for Consult
- None

Tests Not Useful Before Consult
- None

Tests Consultant May Need to Do
- Visual evoked response
- Lumbar puncture
- Cell count, CSF
- Glucose, CSF
- Protein, CSF
- Oligoclonal bands, CSF
- IgG index/IgG synthesis rate, CSF

Follow-up Visits Generally Required
- None

Suggested Readings
Kertesz A, Black SE, Tokar G, et al. Periventricular and subcortical hyperintensities on magnetic resonance imaging. 'Rims, caps, and unidentified bright objects'. Arch Neurol 1988;45:404–408.

Kent DL, Haynor DR, Longstreth WT, Larson EB. The clinical efficacy of magnetic resonance imaging in neuroimaging. Ann Intern Med 1994;120:856–870.

Giang DW, Grow VM, Mooney C, et al. Clinical diagnosis of multiple sclerosis. The impact of magnetic resonance imaging and ancillary testing. Rochester-Toronto Magnetic Resonance Study Group. Arch Neurol 1994;51:61–66.

Selected Guidelines
Magnetic resonance imaging of the brain and spine: a revised statement. American College of Physicians [comment] [see comments]. Ann Intern Med 1994;120:872–875.

Lyme Disease, Possible Cause of Neurologic Findings

Indications and Timing for Referral

- Diagnostic uncertainty

Timing: Expedited (less than 1 week)

Advice for Referral

- Records of all previous Lyme titers.

Tests to Prepare for Consult

- Lyme (*B. burgdorferi*) serology

Tests Not Useful Before Consult

- None

Tests Consultant May Need to Do

- ECG
- Lumbar puncture
- Cell count, CSF
- Glucose, CSF
- Protein, CSF
- VDRL, CSF
- Lyme titer, CSF

Follow-up Visits Generally Required

- None

Suggested Readings

Coyle PK. Neurologic complications of Lyme disease. [Review]. Rheum Dis Clin North Am 1993;19:993–1009.

Coyle PK. Neurologic Lyme disease. [Review]. Semin Neurol 1992;12:200–208.

Pachner AR. Early disseminated Lyme disease: Lyme meningitis. [Review]. Am J Med 1995;98(Suppl 4A):30S–37S.

Magnarelli LA. Current status of laboratory diagnosis for Lyme disease. [Review]. Am J Med 1995;98(Suppl 4A):10S–12S.

Finkel MF, Halperin JJ. Nervous system Lyme borreliosis—revisited [see comments]. [Review]. Arch Neurol 1992;49:102–107.

See Also

- Needlestick
- Lyme titer, positive, typical clinical syndrome
- TB skin test, positive, uncertain duration

Memory Loss

Indications and Timing for Referral

- Diagnostic uncertainty

Timing: Routine (less than 4 weeks)

Tests to Prepare for Consult

- CBC
- Glucose
- Sodium
- Calcium
- Creatinine
- RPR or VDRL
- TSH
- Vitamin B_{12}, serum

Tests Not Useful Before Consult

- SPECT scan, cranial

Tests Consultant May Need to Do

- ESR
- ANA
- HIV antibody testing
- Lyme (*B. burgdorferi*) serology
- Toxicology screen
- ALT, AST
- Magnesium
- EEG
- Neuropsychological testing
- CT or MR, cranial, without contrast

Follow-up Visits Generally Required

- One

Suggested Readings

Crook TH 3d. Diagnosis and treatment of normal and pathologic memory impairment in later life. Semin Neurol 1989;9:20–30.

Gabrieli JD. Disorders of memory in humans. [Review]. Curr Opin Neurol Neurosurg 1993;6:93–97.

Loring DW, Lee GP, Meador KJ. Issues in memory assessment of the elderly. [Review]. Clin Geriatr Med 1989;5:565–581.

Vinson DC. Acute transient memory loss [see comments]. [Review]. Am Fam Physician 1989;39:249–254.

Korczyn AD. The clinical differential diagnosis of dementia: concept and methodology. [Review]. Psychiatr Clin North Am 1991;14:237–249.

Meharg SS, Pankratz L. The MILD interview: evaluating complaints of memory loss. [Review] [20 refs]. Am Fam Physician 1996;54:167–172.

Geldmacher DS, Whitehouse PJ Jr. Differential diagnosis of Alzheimer's disease. [Review] [65 refs]. Neurology 1997;48(Suppl 6):S2–S9.

Selected Guidelines

Early identification of Alzheimer's disease and related dementias. Agency for Health Care Policy and Research. Clin Pract Guidel Quick Ref Guide Clin 1996;19:1–28.

Practice parameter for diagnosis and evaluation of dementia. (summary statement) Report of the Quality Standards Subcommittee of the American Academy of Neurology. Neurology 1994;44:2203–2206.

See Also

- Alzheimer's disease, diagnosis
- Mental status change, acute or subacute
- Mental status change, chronic dementia
- Mental status change, immunocompromised patient

Mental Status Change, Acute or Subacute

Indications and Timing for Referral
- Diagnostic uncertainty

Timing: Expedited (less than 1 week)

Optimal timing of referral may be Urgent (less than 24 hours) depending on the duration, severity, or progression of syndrome

Advice for Referral
- A complete medication history is vital before consultation.

Tests to Prepare for Consult
- CBC
- Glucose
- Electrolytes (Na, K, Cl, CO_2)
- Magnesium
- ALT, AST, alkaline phosphatase
- Bilirubin
- BUN, creatinine
- Urinalysis with microscopic
- Toxicology screen

Tests Not Useful Before Consult
- None

Tests Consultant May Need to Do
- Arterial blood gas
- Ammonia
- TSH (assay sensitivity <0.1 mU/L)
- Blood culture
- HIV antibody testing
- PPD
- Radiograph, chest
- EEG
- Lumbar puncture
- Cell count, CSF
- Protein, CSF
- Glucose, CSF
- Culture and sensitivity, CSF
- Cytology, CSF
- Fungal stain and culture, CSF
- VDRL, CSF
- Cryptococcal antigen, CSF
- CT or MR, cranial, with and without contrast
- Calcium
- HIV antibody testing

Follow-up Visits Generally Required
- None

Mental Status Change, Acute or Subacute (continued)

Suggested Readings

Trzepacz PT. Delirium. Advances in diagnosis, pathophysiology, and treatment. [Review] [149 refs]. Psychiatr Clin North Am 1996;19:429–448.

Tangalos EG, Smith GE, Ivnik RJ, et al. The Mini-Mental State Examination in general medical practice: clinical utility and acceptance. Mayo Clin Proc 1996;71:829–837.

Stewart RB, Hale WE. Acute confusional states in older adults and the role of polypharmacy. [Review]. Ann Rev Public Health 1992;13:415–430.

O'Brien JG. Evaluation of acute confusion (delirium). [Review]. Prim Care 1989;16:349–360.

Selected Guidelines

U. S. Preventive Services Task Force. Screening for dementia. In: DiGuiseppi C, Atkins D, Woolf S, eds. Guide to Clinical Preventive Services. 2nd ed. Baltimore: Williams & Wilkins, 1996:531–540.

See Also

- Mental status change, chronic dementia
- Mental status change, immunocompromised patient
- Alzheimer's disease, diagnosis
- Alzheimer's disease, management
- Memory loss

NEUROLOGY

Mental Status Change, Chronic Dementia

Indications and Timing for Referral
- Diagnostic uncertainty

Timing: Routine (less than 4 weeks)

Advice for Referral
- A complete medication history is vital before consultation.

Tests to Prepare for Consult
- CBC
- Glucose
- Sodium
- Calcium
- Creatinine
- RPR or VDRL
- TSH (assay sensitivity <0.1 mU/L)
- Vitamin B_{12}, serum
- CT or MR, cranial, without contrast

Tests Not Useful Before Consult
- SPECT scan, cranial

Tests Consultant May Need to Do
- ESR
- ANA
- Magnesium
- ALT, AST
- Lyme (*B. burgdorferi*) serology
- Toxicology screen
- EEG
- Neuropsychological testing
- Lumbar puncture
- Cell count, CSF
- Glucose, CSF
- Protein, CSF
- Culture and sensitivity, CSF
- Cytology, CSF
- Fungal stain and culture, CSF
- VDRL, CSF
- Lyme titer, CSF
- Cryptococcal antigen, CSF

Follow-up Visits Generally Required
- One

Mental Status Change, Chronic Dementia (*continued*)

Suggested Readings

Geldmacher DS, Whitehouse PJ. Evaluation of dementia [see comments]. [Review] [39 refs]. N Engl J Med 1996;335:330–336.

Sandson TA, Price BH. Diagnostic testing and dementia [review]. Neurol Clin 1996;14:45.

Tangalos EG, Smith GE, Ivnik RJ, et al. The Mini-Mental State Examination in general medical practice: clinical utility and acceptance. Mayo Clin Proc 1996;71:829–837.

Korczyn AD. The clinical differential diagnosis of dementia: concept and methodology. [Review]. Psychiatr Clin North Am 1991;14:237–249.

Dalla Barba G, Boller F. Non-Alzheimer degenerative dementias. [Review]. Curr Opin Neurol 1994;7:305–309.

Morris JC. Differential diagnosis of Alzheimer's disease. [Review]. Clin Geriatr Med 1994;10:257–276.

Selected Guidelines

Early identification of Alzheimer's disease and related dementias. Agency for Health Care Policy and Research. Clin Pract Guidel Quick Ref Guide Clin 1996;19:1–28.

Practice parameter for diagnosis and evaluation of dementia. (summary statement) Report of the Quality Standards Subcommittee of the American Academy of Neurology. Neurology 1994;44:2203–2206.

McKeith LG, Galasko D, Kosaka K, et al. Consensus guidelines for the clinical and pathologic diagnosis of dementia with Lewy bodies (DLB): report of the consortium on DLB international workshop. [Review] [49 refs]. Neurology 1996;47:1113–1124.

Practice guideline for the treatment of patients with Alzheimer's disease and other dementias of late life. American Psychiatric Association. Am J Psychiatry 1997;154(Suppl):1–39.

U. S. Preventive Services Task Force. Screening for dementia. In: DiGuiseppi C, Atkins D, Woolf S, eds. Guide to Clinical Preventive Services. 2nd ed. Baltimore: Williams & Wilkins, 1996:531–540.

See Also

- Mental status change, immunocompromised patient
- Alzheimer's disease, diagnosis
- Memory loss
- Mental status change, acute or subacute

NEUROLOGY

Mental Status Change, Immunocompromised Patient

Indications and Timing for Referral

- Unexplained, new, or change in baseline mental status

Timing: Expedited (less than 1 week)

Optimal timing of referral may be Urgent (less than 24 hours) depending on the duration, severity, or progression of syndrome

Advice for Referral

- A complete medication history is vital before consultation.

Tests to Prepare for Consult

- CBC with differential
- Glucose
- Calcium
- Sodium
- ALT, AST
- Creatinine
- RPR or VDRL
- T lymphocyte subsets
- Cryptococcal antigen, serum
- *Toxoplasma* serology
- CT or MR, cranial with contrast

Tests Not Useful Before Consult

- None

Tests Consultant May Need to Do

- Toxicology screen
- Magnesium
- EEG
- MR, cranial
- Lumbar puncture
- Albumin, CSF
- Protein, CSF
- Glucose, CSF
- Gram stain, CSF
- Culture and sensitivity, CSF
- VDRL, CSF
- Cryptococcal antigen, CSF
- HIV by PCR, CSF
- Fungal stain and culture, CSF
- Cytology, CSF
- Cell count, CSF

Follow-up Visits Generally Required

- Two

Suggested Readings

Pajeau AK, Roman GC. HIV encephalopathy and dementia. [Review]. Psychiatr Clin North Am 1992;15:455–466.

Forstein M. The neuropsychiatric aspects of HIV infection. [Review]. Primary Care; Clin Off Pract 1992;19:97–117.

Trzepacz PT. Delirium. Advances in diagnosis, pathophysiology, and treatment. [Review] [149 refs]. Psychiatr Clin North Am 1996;19:429–48.

Selected Guidelines

Nomenclature and research case definitions for neurologic manifestations of human immunodeficiency virus-type 1 (HIV-1) infection. Report of a Working Group of the American Academy of Neurology AIDS Task Force [see comments]. [Review]. Neurology 1991;41:778–785.

See Also

- Mental status change, acute or subacute
- Mental status change, chronic dementia
- Alzheimer's disease, diagnosis
- Memory loss

Multiple Sclerosis, Diagnosis

Indications and Timing for Referral
- Diagnostic uncertainty

Timing: Routine (less than 4 weeks)

Tests to Prepare for Consult
- None

Tests Not Useful Before Consult
- None

Tests Consultant May Need to Do
- ESR
- ANA
- Lyme (*B. burgdorferi*) serology
- HIV antibody testing
- HTLV-I serology
- VLCFA
- MR, spine
- MR, cranial ± contrast
- Lumbar puncture
- Cell count, CSF
- Glucose, CSF
- Protein, CSF
- Lyme titer, CSF
- VDRL, CSF
- Oligoclonal bands, CSF
- IgG index/IgG synthesis rate, CSF
- Visual evoked response

Follow-up Visits Generally Required
- One

Suggested Readings
Swanson JW. Multiple sclerosis: update in diagnosis and review of prognostic factors. [Review]. Mayo Clinic Proc 1989;64(5):577–586.

Brod SA, Lindsey JW, Wolinsky JS. Multiple sclerosis: clinical presentation, diagnosis and treatment [published erratum appears in Am Fam Physician 1997;55(2):448]. [Review] [40 refs]. Am Fam Physician 1996;54(4):1301–1306.

Husted C. Contributions of neuroimaging to diagnosis and monitoring of multiple sclerosis. [Review]. Curr Opin Neurol 1994;7(3):234–241.

Weinshenker BG. Natural history of multiple sclerosis. [Review]. Ann Neurol 1994;36(Suppl):S6–S11.

Selected Guidelines
Magnetic resonance imaging of the brain and spine: a revised statement. American College of Physicians [comment] [see comments]. Ann Intern Med 1994;120(10):872–875.

See Also
- Gait disorders
- Multiple sclerosis, management

NEUROLOGY

Multiple Scleroisis, Management

Indications and Timing for Referral
- Assistance with management

Timing: Routine (less than 4 weeks)

Tests to Prepare for Consult
- None

Tests Not Useful Before Consult
- None

Tests Consultant May Need to Do
- CBC
- Glucose
- Urinalysis with microscopic
- Urine, culture and sensitivity
- Cystometric study

Follow-up Visits Generally Required
- None

Suggested Readings

Mitchell G. Update on multiple sclerosis therapy. [Review]. Med Clin North Am 1993;77:231–249.

Thompson AJ. Multiple sclerosis: symptomatic treatment. [Review] [62 refs]. J Neurol 1996;243:559–565.

Schapiro RT, Langer SL. Symptomatic therapy of multiple sclerosis. [Review]. Curr Opin Neurol 1994;7:229–233.

Lublin FD, Whitaker JN, Eidelman BH, et al. Management of patients receiving interferon beta-1b for multiple sclerosis: report of a consensus conference. [Review] [18 refs]. Neurology 1996;46:12–18.

Hunter SF, Weinshenker BG, Carter JL, Nosewortry JH. Rational clinical immunotherapy for multiple sclerosis. Mayo Clin Proc 1997;72:765–780.

Selected Guidelines

Miller DH, Albert PS, Barkhof F, et al. Guidelines for the use of magnetic resonance techniques in monitoring the treatment of multiple sclerosis. U. S. National MS Society Task Force. Ann Neurol 1996;39:6–16.

Whitaker JN. Expanded clinical trials of treatments for multiple sclerosis. The Advisory Committee on Clinical Trials of New Agents in Multiple Sclerosis of The National Multiple Sclerosis Society [see comments]. Ann Neurol 1993;34:755–756.

See Also
- Multiple sclerosis, diagnosis

Myasthenia Gravis, Diagnosis

Indications and Timing for Referral

- Compromised ventilation

Timing: Immediate

- Diagnostic uncertainty

Timing: Routine (less than 4 weeks)

Optimal timing of referral may be Urgent (less than 24 hours) or Expedited (less than 1 week) depending on the duration, severity, or progression of syndrome

Advice for Referral

- Co-management with a neurologist can be helpful when complications of the disease occur.

Tests to Prepare for Consult

- Anti-acetylcholine receptor antibody
- TSH (assay sensitivity <0.1 mU/L)
- ALT, AST
- Potassium
- Sodium
- Calcium
- Magnesium
- Glucose, fasting
- Radiograph, chest

Tests Not Useful Before Consult

- None

Tests Consultant May Need to Do

- ANA
- Vitamin B_{12}, serum
- Tensilon test
- Electromyogram, single fiber ± repetitive stimulation
- Nerve conduction study ± repetitive stimulation
- CT scan, thorax

Follow-up Visits Generally Required

- One

Suggested Readings

Beekman R, Kuks JB, Oosterhuis HJ. Myasthenia gravis: diagnosis and follow-up of 100 consecutive patients. J Neurol 1997;244:112–118.

Evoli A, Batocchi AP, Tonali P. A practical guide to the recognition and management of myasthenia gravis. [Review] [39 refs]. Drugs 1996;52:662–670.

Drachman DB. Myasthenia gravis. [Review]. N Engl J Med 1994;330:1797–1810.

Oosterhuis HJ, Kuks JB. Myasthenia gravis and myasthenic syndromes. [Review]. Curr Opin Neurol Neurosurg 1992;5:638–644.

Younger DS. Differential diagnosis of progressive flaccid weakness. [Review]. Semin Neurol 1993;13:241–246.

Sanders DB, Scoppetta C. The treatment of patients with myasthenia gravis. [Review]. Neurol Clin 1994;12:343–368.

See Also

- Weakness, generalized
- Myopathic weakness

Myopathic Weakness

Indications and Timing for Referral

- Diagnostic uncertainty

Timing: Routine (less than 4 weeks)

Optimal timing of referral may be Urgent (less than 24 hours) or Expedited (less than 1 week) depending on the duration, severity, or progression of syndrome

Advice for Referral

- A careful medical history regarding alcohol use, toxin exposure, familial incidence of diabetes mellitus, and possible cancer is vital before consultation.

Tests to Prepare for Consult

- CBC
- Glucose
- Electrolytes (Na, K, Cl, CO_2)
- Calcium, phosphorus
- ALT, AST
- Creatinine
- ESR
- CPK
- TSH (assay sensitivity <0.1 mU/L)

Tests Not Useful Before Consult

- None

Tests Consultant May Need to Do

- HIV antibody testing
- Magnesium
- Radiograph, chest
- Electromyogram
- Nerve conduction study
- Muscle biopsy

Follow-up Visits Generally Required

- One

Suggested Readings

Moxley RT 3rd. Evaluation of neuromuscular function in inflammatory myopathy. [Review]. Rheum Dis Clin North Am 1994;20:827–843.

Askanas V, Engel WK, Mirabella M. Idiopathic inflammatory myopathies: inclusion-body myositis, polymyositis, and dermatomyositis. [Review]. Curr Opin Neurol 1994;7:448–456.

Plotz PH, Dalakas M, Leff RL, et al. Current concepts in the idiopathic inflammatory myopathies: polymyositis, dermatomyositis, and related disorders. [Review]. Ann Intern Med 1989;111:143–157.

Drachman DB. Myasthenia gravis. [Review]. N Engl J Med 1994;330:1797–1810.

See Also

- Myasthenia gravis, diagnosis
- Cervical spondylosis with myelopathy
- Weakness, generalized
- Neuropathy, peripheral
- Amyotrophic lateral sclerosis

THE CONSULTATION GUIDE

Neuropathy, Peripheral

Indications and Timing for Referral
- Diagnostic uncertainty
- Assistance with management

Timing: Routine (less than 4 weeks)

Advice for Referral
- A careful medical history regarding alcohol use, toxin exposure, familial incidence of diabetes mellitus, and possible cancer is vital before consultation.
- Consider malignancy with proper targeted testing.

Tests to Prepare for Consult
- CBC
- Glucose, fasting
- Sodium
- Calcium
- Magnesium
- ALT, AST
- Creatinine
- VDRL
- Vitamin B_{12}, serum

Tests Not Useful Before Consult
- None

Tests Consultant May Need to Do
- Glycohemoglobin
- Porphobilinogen, plasma
- HIV antibody testing
- VLCFA
- Immunoelectrophoresis
  - Serum
  - Urine
- Radiograph, chest
- Skeletal survey
- Electromyogram
- Nerve conduction study
- Hair analysis for lead, mercury, argon, thorium
- Lumbar puncture
- Cell count, CSF
- Glucose, CSF
- Protein, CSF
- Cytology, CSF
- VDRL, CSF

Follow-up Visits Generally Required
- One

Suggested Readings
McLeod JG. Investigation of peripheral neuropathy. [Review]. J Neurol Neurosurg Psychiatry 1995;58:274–283.

Dyck PJ, Grant IA, Fealey RD. Ten steps in characterizing and diagnosing patients with peripheral neuropathy. Neurology 1996;47:10–17.

Richardson JK, Ashton-Miller JA. Peripheral neuropathy: an often-overlooked cause of falls in the elderly. [Review] [20 refs]. Postgrad Med 1996;99:161–172.

Partanen J. Natural history of peripheral neuropathy in patients with non–insulin-dependent diabetes mellitus. N Engl J Med 1995;333:89–94.

Simpson DM, Olney RK. Peripheral neuropathies associated with human immunodeficiency virus infection. [Review]. Neurol Clin 1992;10:685–711.

Smitt PS, Posner JB. Paraneoplastic peripheral neuropathy [review]. Baillieres Clinical Neurology 1995;4:443–468.

Quantitative sensory testing: a consensus report from the Peripheral Neuropathy Association. Neurology 1993;43:1050–1052.

See Also
- Weakness, generalized
- Myopathic weakness
- Paresthesias, hands
- Paresthesias, feet

NEUROLOGY

Paresthesias, Feet

Indications and Timing for Referral

- Extreme patient discomfort

Timing: Expedited (less than 1 week)

- Diagnostic uncertainty
- Complete history of alcohol intake important

Timing: Routine (less than 4 weeks)

Tests to Prepare for Consult

- CBC
- Glucose, fasting
- Creatinine
- Vitamin B_{12}, serum
- VDRL

Tests Not Useful Before Consult

- None

Tests Consultant May Need to Do

- Calcium
- HIV antibody testing
- Glycohemoglobin
- Electromyogram
- Nerve conduction study

Follow-up Visits Generally Required

- None

Suggested Readings

Dyck PJ, Grant IA, Fealey RD. Ten steps in characterizing and diagnosing patients with peripheral neuropathy. Neurology 1996;47:10–17.

McLeod JG. Investigation of peripheral neuropathy. [Review]. J Neurol Neurosurg Psychiatry 1995;58:274–283.

Quantitative sensory testing: a consensus report from the Peripheral Neuropathy Association. Neurology 1993;43:1050–1052.

See Also

- Paresthesias, hands
- Neuropathy, peripheral

THE CONSULTATION GUIDE

Paresthesias, Hands

Indications and Timing for Referral

- Extreme patient discomfort

Timing: Expedited (less than 1 week)

- Diagnostic uncertainty

Timing: Routine (less than 4 weeks)

Tests to Prepare for Consult

- CBC
- Glucose, fasting
- Calcium
- TSH

Tests Not Useful Before Consult

- None

Tests Consultant May Need to Do

- RPR or VDRL
- Vitamin B_{12}, serum
- Growth hormone
- Radiograph, cervical spine
- MR, cervical spine
- Electromyogram
- Nerve conduction study

Follow-up Visits Generally Required

- None

Suggested Readings

Asbury AK. Numbness, tingling, and sensory loss. In: Fauci AS, Braunwald E, Isselbacher KJ, et al., eds. Harrison's Principles of Internal Medicine. 14th ed. New York: McGraw Hill, 1998:122–125.

Selected Guidelines

Practice parameter for carpal tunnel syndrome (summary statement). Report of the Quality Standards Subcommittee of the American Academy of Neurology. Neurology 1993;43:2406–2409.

Practice parameter for electrodiagnostic studies in carpal tunnel syndrome: summary statement. American Association of Electrodiagnostic Medicine, American Academy of Neurology, American Academy of Physical Medicine and Rehabilitation [published erratum appears in Muscle Nerve 1994;17:262]. Muscle Nerve 1993;16:1390–1391.

See Also

- Paresthesias, feet
- Neuropathy, peripheral

NEUROLOGY

Parkinsonian Syndrome, Atypical

Indications and Timing for Referral

- Diagnostic uncertainty

Timing: Routine (less than 4 weeks)

Advice for Referral

- Co-management with a neurologist can be helpful when complications of the disease occur (e.g., hallucinations, worsening tremors).
- A complete medication history is vital before consultation.

Tests to Prepare for Consult

- None

Tests Not Useful Before Consult

- None

Tests Consultant May Need to Do

- Ceruloplasmin
- Trinucleotide repeats on CH4
- Slit lamp exam
- CT or MR, cranial, without contrast

Follow-up Visits Generally Required

- Co-management, see *Advice for Referral*

Suggested Readings

Koller WC. How accurately can Parkinson's disease be diagnosed? [Review]. Neurology 1992;42(Suppl 1):6–16.

Quinn N. Parkinsonism—recognition and differential diagnosis. [Review]. Br Med J 1995;310:447–452.

Stern MB. Parkinson's disease: early diagnosis and management. [Review]. J Fam Pract 1993;36:439–446.

Calne DB. Treatment of Parkinson's disease [see comments]. [Review]. N Engl J Med 1993;329:1021–1027.

Selected Guidelines

Practice parameters: initial therapy of Parkinson's disease (summary statement). Report of the Quality Standards Subcommittee of the American Academy of Neurology. Neurology 1993;43:1296–1297.

See Also

- Parkinson's disease
- Gait disorders
- Tremor

THE CONSULTATION GUIDE

Parkinson's Disease

Indications and Timing for Referral

- Diagnostic uncertainty
- Assistance with management

Timing: Routine (less than 4 weeks)

Advice for Referral

- Co-management with a neurologist can be helpful when complications of the disease occur (e.g., hallucinations, worsening tremors).

Tests to Prepare for Consult

- None

Tests Not Useful Before Consult

- None

Tests Consultant May Need to Do

- CT or MR, cranial, with and without contrast

Follow-up Visits Generally Required

- Co-management, see *Advice for Referral*

Suggested Readings

Quinn N. Parkinsonism—recognition and differential diagnosis. [Review]. Br Med J 1995;310:447–452.

Stern MB. Parkinson's disease: early diagnosis and management. [Review]. J Fam Pract 1993;36:439–446.

Hughes AJ, Daniel SE, Kilford L, Lees AJ. Accuracy of clinical diagnosis of idiopathic Parkinson's disease: a clinico-pathological study of 100 cases [see comments]. J Neurol Neurosurg Psychiatry 1992;55:181–184.

Poewe W. Clinical features, diagnosis, and imaging of parkinsonian syndromes. [Review]. Curr Opin Neurol Neurosurg 1993;6:333–338.

Bennett DA, Beckett LA, Murray AM, et al. Prevalence of parkinsonian signs and associated mortality in a community population of older people. N Engl J Med 1996;334:71–76.

Cleeves L, Findley LJ. Tremors. [Review]. Med Clin North Am 1989;73:1307–1319.

Hughes AJ. Drug treatment of Parkinson's disease in the 1990s. Achievements and future possibilities. [Review] [65 refs]. Drugs 1997;53:195–205.

Selected Guidelines

Practice parameters: initial therapy of Parkinson's disease (summary statement). Report of the Quality Standards Subcommittee of the American Academy of Neurology. Neurology 1993;43:1296–1297.

See Also

- Parkinsonian syndrome, atypical
- Gait disorders
- Tremor

NEUROLOGY

Postconcussion Syndrome

Indications and Timing for Referral

- Diagnostic uncertainty

Timing: Routine (less than 4 weeks)

Tests to Prepare for Consult

- None

Tests Not Useful Before Consult

- None

Tests Consultant May Need to Do

- EEG
- MR or CT, cranial ± contrast
- Neuropsychological testing
- Lumbar puncture
- Cell count, CSF
- Glucose, CSF
- Protein, CSF

Follow-up Visits Generally Required

- None

Suggested Readings

Goldstein J. Posttraumatic headache and the postconcussion syndrome. [Review]. Med Clin North Am 1991;75:641–651.

Haas DC, Lourie H. Trauma-triggered migraine: an explanation for common neurological attacks after mild head injury. Review of the literature. [Review]. J Neurosurg 1988;68:181–188.

Weiss HD, Stern BJ, Goldberg J. Post-traumatic migraine: chronic migraine precipitated by minor head or neck trauma [see comments]. Headache 1991;31:451–456.

Kelly JP, Rosenberg JH. Diagnosis and management of concussion in sports. [Review] [49 refs]. Neurology 1997;48:575–580.

Selected Guidelines

Practice parameter: the management of concussion in sports (summary statement). Report of the Quality Standards Subcommittee. Neurology 1997;48:581–585.

See Also

- Headache, post-traumatic

Ptosis

Indications and Timing for Referral
- Sudden onset or rapid progression

Timing: Urgent (less than 24 hours)

- Diagnostic uncertainty

Timing: Routine (less than 4 weeks)

Optimal timing of referral may be Urgent (less than 24 hours) or Expedited (less than 1 week) depending on the duration, frequency, severity, or progression of episodes

Tests to Prepare for Consult
- None

Tests Not Useful Before Consult
- None

Tests Consultant May Need to Do
- Glucose, fasting
- Anti-acetylcholine receptor antibody
- Nerve conduction study ± repetitive stimulation
- Electromyogram
- Tensilon test
- ECG
- MR or CT, cranial ± contrast
- Lumbar puncture
- Cell count, CSF
- Glucose, CSF
- Protein, CSF
- Culture and sensitivity, CSF
- Cytology, CSF
- RPR or VDRL

Follow-up Visits Generally Required
- One

Suggested Readings

Adams RA, Victor M, Ropper AH. Disorders of ocular movement and pupillary function. In: Adams RA, Victor M, Ropper AH, eds. Principles of Neurology. 6th ed. New York: McGraw Hill, 1997.

See Also
- Visual loss, monocular
- Diplopia

Radiculopathy, Cervical

Indications and Timing for Referral

- Diagnostic uncertainty
- Assistance with management

Timing: Routine (less than 4 weeks)

Advice for Referral

- Factors favoring referral to a neurologist or psychiatrist include:
  - Pain without other associated neurologic findings
- Factors favoring referral to a neurosurgeon include:
  - Associated weakness
  - Associated myelopathy
  - Intractable pain

Tests to Prepare for Consult

- None

Tests Not Useful Before Consult

- None

Tests Consultant May Need to Do

- MR, spine
- Electromyogram
- Nerve conduction study
- Radiograph, cervical spine

Follow-up Visits Generally Required

- One

Suggested Readings

Ahlgren BD, Garfin SR. Cervical radiculopathy. [Review] [30 refs]. Orthop Clin North Am 1996;27:253–263.

Connell MD, Wiesel SW. Natural history and pathogenesis of cervical disk disease. [Review]. Orthop Clin North Am 1992;23:369–380.

Selected Guidelines

Magnetic resonance imaging of the brain and spine: a revised statement. American College of Physicians [comment] [see comments]. Ann Intern Med 1994;120:872–875.

See Also

- Radiculopathy, thoracic
- Cervical spondylosis with myelopathy

Radiculopathy, Thoracic

Indications and Timing for Referral
- Diagnostic uncertainty
- Assistance with management

Timing: Routine (less than 4 weeks)

Tests to Prepare for Consult
- Radiograph, T-spine

Tests Not Useful Before Consult
- None

Tests Consultant May Need to Do
- MR, spine
- Radiograph, T-spine

Follow-up Visits Generally Required
- None

Suggested Readings
Long DM. Lumbar and cervical spondylosis and spondylotic myelopathy. [Review]. Curr Opin Neurol Neurosurg 1993;6:576–580.

Selected Guidelines
Magnetic resonance imaging of the brain and spine: a revised statement. American College of Physicians [comment] [see comments]. Ann Intern Med 1994;120:872–875.

See Also
- Radiculopathy, cervical
- Cervical spondylosis with myelopathy

NEUROLOGY

Seizures, Generalized

Indications and Timing for Referral

- Uncontrolled or change in pattern of seizures
- Assistance with optimization of treatment regimen
- Potential discontinuation of anti-seizure medication (e.g., pregnancy)

Timing: Routine (less than 4 weeks)

Advice for Referral

- Because MRI is a more sensitive technique for identifying brain pathology that causes seizures, it is generally the procedure of choice when available and not contraindicated.

Tests to Prepare for Consult

- Anti-epileptic drug levels

Tests Not Useful Before Consult

- None

Tests Consultant May Need to Do

- CBC
- Glucose
- Sodium
- Calcium
- Magnesium
- ALT, AST
- Creatinine
- CT or MR, cranial, with and without contrast
- EEG, wake and sleep study
- EEG, prolonged monitoring

Follow-up Visits Generally Required

- One

Suggested Readings

Gilliam F, Wyllie E. Diagnostic testing of seizure disorders [review]. Neurol Clin 1996;14:61.

Mosewich RK, So EL. A clinical approach to the classification of seizures and epileptic syndromes. Mayo Clin Proc 1996;71:405–414.

Pourmand R. Seizures and epilepsy in older patients—evaluation and management. Geriatrics 1996;51:39.

Consensus conference on driver licensing and epilepsy: American Academy of Neurology, American Epilepsy Society, and Epilepsy Foundation of America. Washington, DC, May 31–June 2, 1991. Proceedings. Epilepsia 1994;35:662–705.

Selected Guidelines

Guideline four: standards of practice in clinical electroencephalography. American Electroencephalographic Society. J Clin Neurophysiol 1994;11:14–15.

Clinical policy for the initial approach to patients presenting with a chief complaint of seizure who are not in status epilepticus. American College of Emergency Physicians. Ann Emerg Med 1997;29:706–724.

See Also

- Seizure, new onset, in adults
- Episodic loss of consciousness, seizure versus syncope
- Spells, TIA versus seizure
- Seizures, partial

Seizures, New Onset, in Adults

Indications and Timing for Referral

- Sustained seizure activity
- Residual neurological deficit

Timing: Immediate

- Diagnostic uncertainty without obvious cause (e. g., metabolic imbalance or alcohol withdrawal)

Timing: Expedited (less than 1 week)

Advice for Referral

- Because MRI is a more sensitive technique for identifying brain pathology that causes seizures, it is generally the procedure of choice when available and not contraindicated.
- If neurologic examination is normal, imaging (CT or MR) can generally be deferred until after preliminary consultation.
- Unless there is clinical suspicion of infection or subarachnoid hemorrhage, lumbar puncture with associated CSF studies is generally unnecessary.
- History of malignancy, even remote, should be sought and may justify early oncologic consultation.

Tests to Prepare for Consult

- CBC
- Glucose
- Sodium
- Calcium
- Magnesium
- ALT, AST
- Creatinine

Tests Not Useful Before Consult

- None

Tests Consultant May Need to Do

- EEG, wake and sleep study
- MR or CT, cranial ± contrast
- Lumbar puncture
- Cell count, CSF
- Glucose, CSF
- Protein, CSF
- Culture and sensitivity, CSF
- Cytology, CSF
- Fungal stain and culture, CSF
- VDRL, CSF
- Cryptococcal antigen, CSF
- Lyme (*B. burgdorferi*) serology

Follow-up Visits Generally Required

- One

Seizures, New Onset, in Adults (continued)

Suggested Readings

Mosewich RK, So EL. A clinical approach to the classification of seizures and epileptic syndromes. Mayo Clin Proc 1996;71: 405–414.

Gilliam F, Wyllie E. Diagnostic testing of seizure disorders [review]. Neurol Clin 1996;14:61.

Pourmand R. Seizures and epilepsy in older patients—evaluation and management. Geriatrics 1996;51:39.

Turnbull TL, Vanden Hoek TL, Howes DS, Eisner RF. Utility of laboratory studies in the emergency department patient with a new-onset seizure. Ann Emerg Med 1990;19:373–377.

Ng SK, Brust JC, Hauser WA, Susser M. Illicit drug use and the risk of new-onset seizures. Am J Epidemiol 1990;132:47–57.

Holtzman DM, Kaku DA, So YT. New-onset seizures associated with human immunodeficiency virus infection: causation and clinical features in 100 cases. Am J Med 1989;87:173–177.

Ng SK, Hauser WA, Brust JC, Susser M. Alcohol consumption and withdrawal in new-onset seizures. N Engl J Med 1988;319:666–673.

Henneman PL, DeRoos F, Lewis RJ. Determining the need for admission in patients with new-onset seizures. Ann Emerg Med 1994;24:1108–1114.

Selected Guidelines

Clinical policy for the initial approach to patients presenting with a chief complaint of seizure who are not in status epilepticus. American College of Emergency Physicians. Ann Emerg Med 1997;29:706–724.

Guideline four: standards of practice in clinical electroencephalography. American Electroencephalographic Society. J Clin Neurophysiol 1994;11:14–15.

See Also

- Seizures, partial
- Seizures, generalized
- Episodic loss of consciousness, seizure versus syncope
- Spells, TIA versus seizure

Seizures, Partial

Indications and Timing for Referral

- Assistance with management

Timing: Routine (less than 4 weeks)

Advice for Referral

- Because MRI is a more sensitive technique for identifying brain pathology that causes seizures, it is generally the procedure of choice when available and not contraindicated.
- Trough blood levels are often helpful in cases that are difficult to control.
- Co-management with a neurologist is often useful in cases that are difficult to control.

Tests to Prepare for Consult

- Anti-epileptic drug levels

Tests Not Useful Before Consult

- None

Tests Consultant May Need to Do

- CBC
- Glucose
- Sodium
- Calcium
- Magnesium
- ALT, AST
- Creatinine
- MR or CT, cranial ± contrast
- EEG, wake and sleep study
- EEG, prolonged monitoring

Follow-up Visits Generally Required

- Co-management, see *Advice for Referral*

Suggested Readings

Mosewich RK, So EL. A clinical approach to the classification of seizures and epileptic syndromes. Mayo Clin Proc 1996;71:405–414.

Cascino GD. Complex partial seizures. Clinical features and differential diagnosis. [Review]. Psychiatr Clin North Am 1992;15:373–382.

Gilliam F, Wyllie E. Diagnostic testing of seizure disorders [review]. Neurol Clin 1996;14:61.

So EL. Update on epilepsy. [Review]. Med Clin North Am 1993;77:203–214.

Luciano D. Partial seizures of frontal and temporal origin. [Review]. Neurol Clin 1993;11:805–822.

Consensus conference on driver licensing and epilepsy: American Academy of Neurology, American Epilepsy Society, and Epilepsy Foundation of America. Washington, DC, May 31–June 2, 1991. Proceedings. Epilepsia 1994;35:662–705.

Cascino GD. Intractable partial epilepsy: evaluation and treatment. [Review]. Mayo Clin Proc 1990;65:1578–1586.

Selected Guidelines

Guideline four: standards of practice in clinical electroencephalography. American Electroencephalographic Society. J Clin Neurophysiol 1994;11:14–15.

Guideline one: minimum technical requirements for performing clinical electroencephalography. American Electroencephalographic Society. J Clin Neurophysiol 1994;11:2–5.

See Also

- Episodic loss of consciousness, seizure versus syncope
- Spells, TIA versus seizure
- Seizures, new onset, in adults
- Seizures, generalized

NEUROLOGY

Speech Disorder

Indications and Timing for Referral

- Diagnostic uncertainty

Timing: Routine (less than 4 weeks)

Optimal timing of referral may be Urgent (less than 24 hours) or Expedited (less than 1 week) depending on the duration, frequency, severity, or progression of episodes

Advice for Referral

- Apopleptic onset requires immediate consultation.

Tests to Prepare for Consult

- None

Tests Not Useful Before Consult

- None

Tests Consultant May Need to Do

- CBC
- Glucose
- Sodium
- Calcium
- Magnesium
- ALT, AST
- Creatinine
- CPK
- TSH (assay sensitivity <0.1 mU/L)
- Anti-acetylcholine receptor antibody
- Tensilon test
- EEG, wake and sleep study
- Electromyogram
- Nerve conduction study ± repetitive stimulation
- MR or CT, cranial ± contrast
- Lumbar puncture
- Cell count, CSF
- Glucose, CSF
- Protein, CSF
- Culture and sensitivity, CSF
- Cytology, CSF

Follow-up Visits Generally Required

- One

Suggested Readings

Damasio AR. Aphasia [see comments]. [Review]. N Engl J Med 1992;326:531–539.

Albert ML, Helm-Estabrooks N. Diagnosis and treatment of aphasia. Part I. [Review]. JAMA 1988;259:1043–1047.

Albert ML, Helm-Estabrooks N. Diagnosis and treatment of aphasia. Part II. [Review]. JAMA 1988;259:1205–1210.

THE CONSULTATION GUIDE

Spells, Transient Ischemic Attack (TIA) Versus Seizure

Indications and Timing for Referral

- Diagnostic uncertainty

Timing: Routine (less than 4 weeks)

Optimal timing of referral may be Urgent (less than 24 hours) or Expedited (less than 1 week) depending on the duration, frequency, severity, or progression of episodes

Tests to Prepare for Consult

- CBC
- Glucose
- Sodium
- Calcium
- Magnesium
- ALT, AST
- Creatinine
- ECG

Tests Not Useful Before Consult

- None

Tests Consultant May Need to Do

- Carotid duplex study
- MR or CT, cranial ± contrast
- EEG, wake and sleep study
- EEG, prolonged monitoring
- Echocardiogram

Follow-up Visits Generally Required

- One

Suggested Readings

Gilliam F, Wyllie E. Diagnostic testing of seizure disorders [review]. Neurol Clin 1996;14:61.

Bots ML, van der Wilk EC, Koudstaal PJ, et al. Transient neurological attacks in the general population. Prevalence, risk factors, and clinical relevance. Stroke 1997;28:768–773.

Brown RD Jr, Evans BA, Wiebers DO, et al. Transient ischemic attack and minor ischemic stroke: an algorithm for evaluation and treatment. Mayo Clinic Division of Cerebrovascular Diseases [see comments]. [Review]. Mayo Clin Proc 1994;69:1027–1039.

Hankey GJ, Warlow CP. Symptomatic carotid ischaemic events: safest and most cost effective way of selecting patients for angiography, before carotid endarterectomy [see comments]. Br Med J 1990;300:1485–1491.

Selected Guidelines

Feinberg WM, Albers GW, Barnett HJ, et al. Guidelines for the management of transient ischemic attacks. From the Ad Hoc Committee on Guidelines for the Management of Transient Ischemic Attacks of the Stroke Council of the American Heart Association. Circulation 1994;89:2950–2965.

Guideline four: standards of practice in clinical electroencephalography. American Electroencephalographic Society. J Clin Neurophysiol 1994;11:14–15.

See Also

- Episodic loss of consciousness, seizure verus syncope
- Transient ischemic attacks (TIAs)
- Carotid stenosis, asymptomatic
- Cervical bruit, asymptomatic
- Seizures, new onset, in adults
- Syncope
- Seizures, partial
- Seizures, generalized

NEUROLOGY

Swallowing Disorder

Indications and Timing for Referral

- Diagnostic uncertainty
- Patients without obvious mechanical cause for dysphagia

Timing: Routine (less than 4 weeks)

Optimal timing of referral may be Urgent (less than 24 hours) or Expedited (less than 1 week) depending on the duration, frequency, severity, or progression of episodes

Advice for Referral

- Apopleptic onset requires immediate consultation.

Tests to Prepare for Consult

- None

Tests Not Useful Before Consult

- None

Tests Consultant May Need to Do

- CBC
- Glucose
- Sodium
- Calcium
- Magnesium
- ALT, AST
- Creatinine
- CPK
- TSH (assay sensitivity <0.1 mU/L)
- Anti-acetylcholine receptor antibody
- Tensilon test
- Swallowing study
- Electromyogram
- Nerve conduction study
- MR or CT, cranial ± contrast
- Lumbar puncture
- Cell count, CSF
- Glucose, CSF
- Protein, CSF
- Culture and sensitivity, CSF
- Cytology, CSF
- Esophageal manometry

Follow-up Visits Generally Required

- One

Suggested Readings

Buchholz DW. Neurogenic dysphagia: what is the cause when the cause is not obvious? [Review]. Dysphagia 1994;9:245–255.

Trate DM, Parkman HP, Fisher RS. Dysphagia. Evaluation, diagnosis, and treatment. [Review] [26 refs]. Prim Care 1996;23:417–432.

Kim CH, Weaver AL, Hsu JJ, et al. Discriminate value of esophageal symptoms: a study of the initial clinical findings in 499 patients with dysphagia of various causes [see comments]. Mayo Clin Proc 1993;68:948–954.

Koch WM. Swallowing disorders. Diagnosis and therapy. [Review]. Med Clin North Am 1993;77:571–582.

Mendez L, Friedman LS, Castell DO. Swallowing disorders in the elderly. [Review]. Clin Geriatr Med 1991;7:215–230.

Kelly JH. Use of manometry in the evaluation of dysphagia. Otolaryngol Head Neck Surg 1997;116:355–357.

Selected Guidelines

An American Gastroenterological Association medical position statement on the clinical use of esophageal manometry. American Gastroenterological Association. Gastroenterology 1994;107:1865.

THE CONSULTATION GUIDE

Tics

Indications and Timing for Referral

- Diagnostic uncertainty
- Assistance with management

Timing: Routine (less than 4 weeks)

Tests to Prepare for Consult

- None

Tests Not Useful Before Consult

- None

Tests Consultant May Need to Do

- Ceruloplasmin
- Slit lamp exam

Follow-up Visits Generally Required

- None

Suggested Readings

Jankovic J. Tourette syndrome. Phenomenology and classification of tics. [Review] [43 refs]. Neurol Clin 1997;15:267–275.

Kompoliti K, Goetz CG. Tourette syndrome. Clinical rating and quantitative assessment of tics. [Review] [49 refs]. Neurol Clin 1997;15:239–254.

Jankovic J. Diagnosis and classification of tics and Tourette syndrome. [Review]. Adv Neurol 1992;58:7–14.

Tolosa E, Berciano J. Choreas, hereditary and other ataxias, tics, myoclonus, and other movement disorders. [Review]. Curr Opin Neurol Neurosurg 1993;6:358–368.

NEUROLOGY

Transient Ischemic Attacks (TIAs)

Indications and Timing for Referral

- Assist with evaluation and management

Timing: Routine (less than 4 weeks)

Optimal timing of referral may be Immediate, Urgent (less than 24 hours), or Expedited (less than 1 week) depending on the duration, frequency, severity, or progression of episodes

Advice for Referral

- Carotid duplex study is only necessary if syndrome is consistent with hemispheric or retinal involvement.

Tests to Prepare for Consult

- CBC
- Platelet count
- Glucose
- Sodium
- ALT, AST
- Creatinine
- Prothrombin time
- PTT
- ECG
- Carotid duplex study

Tests Not Useful Before Consult

- Cerebral angiogram

Tests Consultant May Need to Do

- MR or CT, cranial ± contrast
- MR angiography
- Transcranial doppler study
- RPR or VDRL
- Echocardiogram
- Transesophageal echocardiography

Follow-up Visits Generally Required

- One

Suggested Readings

Bots ML, van der Wilk EC, Koudstaal PJ, et al. Transient neurological attacks in the general population. Prevalence, risk factors, and clinical relevance. Stroke 1997;28:768–773.

Brown RD Jr, Evans BA, Wiebers DO, et al. Transient ischemic attack and minor ischemic stroke: an algorithm for evaluation and treatment. Mayo Clinic Division of Cerebrovascular Diseases [see comments]. [Review]. Mayo Clin Proc 1994;69:1027–1039.

Hankey GJ, Warlow CP. Symptomatic carotid ischaemic events: safest and most cost effective way of selecting patients for angiography, before carotid endarterectomy [see comments]. Br Med J 1990;300:1485–1491.

Nadeau SE. Transient ischemic attacks: diagnosis, and medical and surgical management. [Review]. J Fam Pract 1994;38:495–504.

Transient Ischemic Attacks (TIAs) (continued)

Selected Guidelines

Feinberg WM, Albers GW, Barnett HJ, et al. Guidelines for the management of transient ischemic attacks. From the Ad Hoc Committee on Guidelines for the Management of Transient Ischemic Attacks of the Stroke Council of the American Heart Association. Circulation 1994;89:2950–2965.

See Also

- Episodic loss of consciousness, seizure versus syncope
- Vertigo
- Facial weakness
- Ptosis
- Diplopia
- Visual loss, monocular
- Swallowing disorder
- Speech disorder
- Carotid stenosis, asymptomatic
- Spells, TIA versus seizure
- Cervical bruit, asymptomatic

Tremor

Indications and Timing for Referral

- Diagnostic uncertainty
- Assistance with management

Timing: Routine (less than 4 weeks)

Advice for Referral

- A complete alcohol and medication history is vital (e.g., metoclopramide, theophylline, lithium).
- A careful dietary history is vital (e.g., caffeine intake).

Tests to Prepare for Consult

- None

Tests Not Useful Before Consult

- None

Tests Consultant May Need to Do

- TSH (assay sensitivity <0.1 mU/L)

Follow-up Visits Generally Required

- None

Suggested Readings

Findley LJ. Classification of tremors. [Review] [55 refs]. J Clin Neurophysiol 1996;13:122–132.

Cleeves L, Findley LJ. Tremors. [Review]. Med Clin North Am 1989;73:1307–1319.

Deuschl G, Krack P, Lauk M, Timmer J. Clinical neurophysiology of tremor. [Review] [79 refs]. J Clin Neurophysiol 1996;13:110–121.

Sandroni P, Young RR. Tremor: classification, diagnosis and management. [Review]. Am Fam Physician 1994;50:1505–1512.

Hopfensperger K, Koller WC. Non-parkinsonian tremor. [Review]. Curr Opin Neurol Neurosurg 1992;5:321–323.

Adams RA, Victor M, Ropper AH. Tremor, myoclonus, focal dystonias, and tics. In: Adams RA, Victor M, Ropper AH, eds. Principles of Neurology. 6th ed. New York: McGraw Hill, 1997:94–113.

See Also

- Parkinson's Disease
- Parkinsonian Syndrome, Atypical
- Thyrotoxicosis

THE CONSULTATION GUIDE

Vertigo

Indications and Timing for Referral

- Apopleptic onset with other brainstem signs

Timing: Immediate

- Suspicion of cerebellar or brainstem pathology

Timing: Urgent (less than 24 hours)

- Diagnostic uncertainty

Timing: Routine (less than 4 weeks)

Advice for Referral

- If MR is not available, CT with posterior fossae cuts is an alternative.
- A complete medication history is vital before consultation.
- Factors favoring referral to a neurologist include:
  - Accompanying signs or symptoms of cerebellar or brainstem lesion (e.g., diplopia, dysarthria, dysphagia, ataxia)
- Factors favoring referral to otorhinolaryngologist include:
  - Associated tinnitus
  - Diminished hearing

Tests to Prepare for Consult

- None

Tests Not Useful Before Consult

- Electronystamography
- Posturography

Tests Consultant May Need to Do

- MR angiography
- MR, cranial ± contrast
- Audiogram

Follow-up Visits Generally Required

- One

Suggested Readings

Froehling DA, Silverstein MD, Mohr DN, Beatty CW. Does this dizzy patient have a serious form of vertigo? [see comments]. JAMA 1994;271(5):385–388.

Kroenke K, Lucas CA, Rosenberg ML, et al. Causes of persistent dizziness. A prospective study of 100 patients in ambulatory care. Ann Intern Med 1992;117(11):898–904.

Luxon LM. Vertigo: new approaches to diagnosis and management. [Review] [22 refs]. Br J Hosp Med 1996;56(10):519–520.

Lewis RF. Vertigo: some uncommon causes of a common problem. [Review] [49 refs]. Semin Neurol 1996;16(1):55–62.

Colledge NR, Barr-Hamilton RM, Lewis SJ, Sellar RJ, Wilson JA. Evaluation of investigations to diagnose the cause of dizziness in elderly people: a community based controlled study [see comments]. BMJ 1996;313(7060):788–792.

NEUROLOGY

Visual Loss, Monocular

Indications and Timing for Referral

- Sudden onset or rapid progression

Timing: Immediate

- Diagnostic uncertainty

Timing: Expedited (less than 1 week)

Advice for Referral

- Preliminary ophthalmologic evaluation is necessary to exclude primary ophthalmologic disorders before consultation.

Tests to Prepare for Consult

- CBC
- ESR

Tests Not Useful Before Consult

- None

Tests Consultant May Need to Do

- Carotid duplex study
- MR or CT, cranial ± contrast
- Formal visual field testing
- Visual evoked response
- Temporal artery biopsy
- Lumbar puncture
- Cell count, CSF
- Glucose, CSF
- Protein, CSF
- Culture and sensitivity, CSF
- Cytology, CSF
- OPG
- Temporal artery biopsy

Follow-up Visits Generally Required

- One

Suggested Readings

Lueck CJ. Investigation of visual loss: neuro-ophthalmology from a neurologist's perspective. [Review] [48 refs]. J Neurol Neurosurg Psychiatry 1996;60:275–280.

Miller NR. The optic nerve. Curr Opin Neurol 1996;9:5–15.

Wray SH. The management of acute visual failure. [Review]. J Neurol Neurosurg Psychiatry 1993;56:234–240.

Barton JJ, Corbett JJ. Neuro-ophthalmologic vascular emergencies in the elderly. [Review]. Clin Geriatr Med 1991;7:525–48.

THE CONSULTATION GUIDE

Weakness, Generalized

Indications and Timing for Referral

- Diagnostic uncertainty

Timing: Routine (less than 4 weeks)

Optimal timing of referral may be Urgent (less than 24 hours) or Expedited (less than 1 week) depending on the duration, severity, or progression of syndrome

Tests to Prepare for Consult

- CBC
- Glucose
- Electrolytes (Na, K, Cl, CO_2)
- Calcium, phosphorus
- ALT, AST
- Creatinine
- ESR
- CPK
- TSH (assay sensitivity <0.1 mU/L)
- Phosphorus

Tests Not Useful Before Consult

- None

Tests Consultant May Need to Do

- ANA
- HIV antibody testing
- Electromyogram
- Nerve conduction study
- MR, spine with contrast
- MR, cranial with contrast

Follow-up Visits Generally Required

- None

Suggested Readings

Oosterhuis HJ, Kuks JB. Myasthenia gravis and myasthenic syndromes. [Review]. Curr Opin Neurol Neurosurg 1992;5:638–644.

Younger DS. Differential diagnosis of progressive flaccid weakness. [Review]. Semin Neurol 1993;13:241–246.

LoVecchio F, Jacobson S. Approach to generalized weakness and peripheral neuromuscular disease. Emerg Clin North Am 1997;15:605–623.

Olney RK, Aminoff MJ. Weakness, abnormal movements, and imbalance. In: Fauci AS, Braunwald E, Isselbacher KJ, et al., eds. Harrison's Principles of Internal Medicine. 14th ed. New York: McGraw Hill, 1998:107–118.

Adams RA, Victor M, Ropper AH. Principles of clinical myology: diagnosis and classification of muscle diseases–general considerations. In: Adams RA, Victor M, Ropper AH, eds. Principles of Neurology. 6th ed. New York: McGraw Hill, 1997:1386–1401.

McLeod JG. Investigation of peripheral neuropathy. [Review]. J Neurol Neurosurg Psychiatry 1995;58:274–283.

CHAPTER 9

Oncology

Adenopathy, Supraclavicular	451
Back Pain, History of Cancer	452
Bone Lesion, Lytic	453
Breast Mass	454
Breast Cancer	
Family History of	455
History of	456
Head and Neck Irradiation, Childhood	457
Lung Cancer	
Small Cell, History of	458
Squamous Cell, History of	459
Lymphoma, History of	460
Mammogram, Suspicious	461
Mass, Extremity	462
Melanoma, History of	463
Prostate Cancer, History of	464
Renal Cell Cancer, History of	465
Sarcoma, History of	466
Testicular Cancer, History of	467
Thyroid Cancer	
History of	468
Medullary, Family History of	469

ONCOLOGY

Adenopathy, Supraclavicular

Indications and Timing for Referral

- Patients with this finding should be promptly evaluated by biopsy.

Timing: Expedited (less than 1 week)

Tests to Prepare for Consult

- None

Tests Not Useful Before Consult

- CT or MR, affected region
- Upper endoscopy

Tests Consultant May Need to Do

- Radiograph, chest
- Fine needle biopsy
- Surgical biopsy

Follow-up Visits Generally Required

- One

Suggested Readings

Fijten GH, Blijham GH. Unexplained lymphadenopathy in family practice. An evaluation of the probability of malignant causes and the effectiveness of physicians' workup. J Fam Pract 1988;27:373–376.

Van Overhagen H, Lameris JS, Berger MY, et al. Supraclavicular lymph node metastases in carcinoma of the esophagus and gastroesophageal junction: assessment with CT, US, and US-guided fine-needle aspiration biopsy. Radiology 1991;179:155–158.

Van Overhagen H, Lameris JS, Berger MY, et al. Improved assessment of supraclavicular and abdominal metastases in oesophageal and gastro-oesophageal junction carcinoma with the combination of ultrasound and computed tomography. Br J Radiol 1993;66:203–208.

THE CONSULTATION GUIDE

Back Pain, History of Cancer

Indications and Timing for Referral

- Presence of progressive neurologic impairment
- Suspicion of infection

Timing: Immediate

- Associated with trauma
- History of medical condition known to compromise structural integrity of central nervous system (CNS) and cord

Timing: Urgent (less than 24 hours)

- Associated with severe pain
- Associated radiologic abnormalities present

Timing: Expedited (less than 1 week)

- Diagnosis uncertain with persistent symptoms for longer than 4 weeks
- Failure to follow expected course with conventional therapy

Timing: Routine (less than 4 weeks)

Tests to Prepare for Consult

- Radiograph, affected region

Tests Not Useful Before Consult

- None

Tests Consultant May Need to Do

- Bone scan
- MR, spine

Follow-up Visits Generally Required

- One

Suggested Readings

Ruckdeschel JC. Spinal cord compression: the cancer patient with back pain. In: Abeloff MD, ed. Clinical Oncology. New York: Churchill-Livingstone, 1998:619–628.

Selected Guidelines

Magnetic resonance imaging of the brain and spine: a revised statement. American College of Physicians [comment] [see comments]. Ann Intern Med 1994;120:872–875.

ONCOLOGY

Bone Lesion, Lytic

Indications and Timing for Referral

- Present in weight-bearing joint
- Suspicion of impending fracture

Timing: Urgent (less than 24 hours)

- Etiology unclear

Timing: Expedited (less than 1 week)

Tests to Prepare for Consult

- CBC
- ALT, AST, alkaline phosphatase
- Bilirubin
- Albumin, total protein
- Calcium
- Creatinine
- Urinalysis with microscopic
- Radiograph, chest
- Radiograph, affected region
- Bone scan

Tests Not Useful Before Consult

- None

Tests Consultant May Need to Do

- Immunoelectrophoresis
  - Serum
  - Urine
- Bone scan
- Surgical biopsy

Follow-up Visits Generally Required

- One

Suggested Readings

Merrick MV, Beales JS, Garvie N, Leonard RC. Evaluation and skeletal metastases. [Review]. Br J Radiol 1992;65:803–806.

Gold RI, Seeger LL, Bassett LW, Steckel RJ. An integrated approach to the evaluation of metastatic bone disease. [Review]. Radiol Clin North Am 1990;28:471–483.

THE CONSULTATION GUIDE

Breast Mass

Indications and Timing for Referral

- Diagnostic uncertainty

Timing: Expedited (less than 1 week)

Advice for Referral

- Refer to M.D. capable of biopsy

Tests to Prepare for Consult

- Mammograms, bilateral

Tests Not Useful Before Consult

- Bone scan
- Tumor markers

Tests Consultant May Need to Do

- Ultrasound, breast
- Fine needle biopsy
- Surgical biopsy

Follow-up Visits Generally Required

- One

Suggested Readings

Donegan WL. Evaluation of a palpable breast mass [see comments]. [Review]. N Engl J Med 1992;327:937–942.

Fajardo LL, DeAngelis GA. The role of stereotactic biopsy in abnormal mammograms. [Review] [24 refs]. Surg Oncol Clin N Am 1997;6:285–299.

Hall FM. Technologic advances in breast imaging. Current and future strategies, controversies, and opportunities. [Review] [31 refs]. Surg Oncol Clin N Am 1997;6:403–409.

Giard RW, Hermans J. The value of aspiration cytologic examination of the breast. A statistical review of the medical literature. [Review]. Cancer 1992;69:2104–2110.

Rosenblatt DS, Foulkes WD, Narod SA. Genetic screening for breast cancer. N Engl J Med 1996;334:1200–1201.

Selected Guidelines

Mettlin C, Dodd GD. The American Cancer Society Guidelines for the cancer-related checkup: an update. CA Cancer J Clin 1991;41:279–282.

Dodd GD. American Cancer Society guidelines on screening for breast cancer. An overview. Cancer 1992;69(7 Suppl): 1885–1887.

See Also

- Breast cancer, family history of
- Mammogram, suspicious
- Breast cancer, history of

ONCOLOGY

Breast Cancer, Family History of

Indications and Timing for Referral

- Patient with criteria for significant family history of breast cancer

Timing: Routine (less than 4 weeks)

Advice for Referral

- These patients should become proficient and faithful in performing regular breast self-examination, and undergo yearly mammography.
- Consideration should be given to having such patients referred to a specialist in genetic risk for breast cancer.
- Records of all old mammograms are vital.

Tests to Prepare for Consult

- None

Tests Not Useful Before Consult

- None

Tests Consultant May Need to Do

- Mammogram
- BRCA-1

Follow-up Visits Generally Required

- One

Suggested Readings

Hoskins KF, Stopfer JE, Calzone KA, et al. Assessment and counseling for women with a family history of breast cancer. A guide for clinicians. JAMA 1995;273:577–585.

Krainer M, Silva-Arrieta S, FitzGerald MG, et al. Differential contributions of BRCA1 and BRCA2 to early-onset breast cancer [see comments]. N Engl J Med 1997;336:1416–1421.

Schrag D, Kuntz KM, Garber JE, Weeks JC. Decision analysis—effects of prophylactic mastectomy and oophorectomy on life expectancy among women with BRCA1 or BRCA2 mutations [see comments]. N Engl J Med 1997;336:1465–1471.

Struewing JP, Hartge P, Wacholder S, et al. The risk of cancer associated with specific mutations of BRCA1 and BRCA2 among Ashkenazi Jews [see comments]. N Engl J Med 1997;336:1401–1408.

Couch FJ, DeShano ML, Blackwood MA, et al. BRCA1 mutations in women attending clinics that evaluate the risk of breast cancer [see comments]. N Engl J Med 1997;336:1409–1415.

Evans DG, Fentiman IS, McPherson K, et al. Familial breast cancer [see comments]. [Review]. Br Med J 1994;308:183–187.

Selected Guidelines

Dodd GD. American Cancer Society guidelines on screening for breast cancer. An overview. Cancer 1992;69(7 Suppl):1885–1887.

See Also

- Breast mass
- Mammogram, suspicious
- Breast cancer, history of

THE CONSULTATION GUIDE

Breast Cancer, History of

Indications and Timing for Referral

- Clinical or mammographic findings suggest recurrent or secondary malignancy

Timing: Expedited (less than 1 week)

- Assistance with decision making regarding hormonal replacement therapy
- Assistance with decision making regarding termination of tamoxifen therapy

Timing: Routine (less than 4 weeks)

Advice for Referral

- See specific finding (e.g., S*uspicious Mammogram, Breast Mass*) for additional testing that is potentially appropriate for consultant.
- Optimal plan for oncology follow-up is best defined by preliminary discussion with the consultant, considering the type and initial stage of disease, time since completion of anti-tumor treatment, and potential late complications of therapy.

Tests to Prepare for Consult

- None

Tests Not Useful Before Consult

- None

Tests Consultant May Need to Do

- None

Follow-up Visits Generally Required

- See *Advice for Referral*

Suggested Readings

Impact of follow-up testing on survival and health-related quality of life in breast cancer patients. A multicenter randomized controlled trial. The GIVIO Investigators [see comments]. JAMA 1994;271:1587–1592.

Rosselli Del Turco M, Palli D, Cariddi A, et al. Intensive diagnostic follow-up after treatment of primary breast cancer. A randomized trial. National Research Council Project on Breast Cancer follow-up [see comments]. JAMA 1994;271:1593–1597.

Wold LE, Ingle JN, Pisansky TM, et al. Prognostic factors for patients with carcinoma of the breast. [Review]. Mayo Clin Proc 1995;70:678–679.

Hall FM. Technologic advances in breast imaging. Current and future strategies, controversies, and opportunities. [Review] [31 refs]. Surg Oncol Clin N Am 1997;6:403–409.

See Also

- Breast cancer, family history of
- Breast mass
- Mammogram, suspicious

Head and Neck Irradiation, Childhood

Indications and Timing for Referral

- Clinical or laboratory evidence of thyroid dysfunction
- Uncertainty whether thyroid physical exam is normal

Timing: Routine (less than 4 weeks)

Tests to Prepare for Consult

- Calcium
- TSH

Tests Not Useful Before Consult

- None

Tests Consultant May Need to Do

- Calcium
- PTH
- Thyroglobulin
- Sonogram, thyroid
- Radionuclide thyroid scan
- Fine needle aspiration biopsy

Follow-up Visits Generally Required

- One

Suggested Readings

Sarne D, Schneider AB. External radiation and thyroid neoplasia. Endocrinol Metab Clin North Am 1996;25:181.

Schneider AB. Radiation-induced thyroid tumors. [Review]. Endocrinol Metab Clin North Am 1990;19:495–508.

See Also

- Thyroid cancer, medullary, family history of
- Thyroid cancer, history of

THE CONSULTATION GUIDE

Lung Cancer, Small Cell, History of

Indications and Timing for Referral

- Clinical or radiologic findings suggest recurrent malignancy

Timing: Expedited (less than 1 week)

- Serious consideration should be given to having such patients co-managed with an oncologist if less than 5 years since diagnosis

Timing: Routine (less than 4 weeks)

Advice for Referral

- Optimal plan for oncology follow-up is best defined by preliminary discussion with the consultant, considering the type and initial stage of disease, time since completion of anti-tumor treatment, and potential late complications of therapy.
- Careful neurologic exam important to detect late complications of therapy and/or CNS recurrence.

Tests to Prepare for Consult

- CBC
- Electrolytes (Na, K, Cl, CO_2)
- ALT, AST, alkaline phosphatase
- Calcium
- Creatinine
- Radiograph, chest

Tests Not Useful Before Consult

- CT or MR, chest

Tests Consultant May Need to Do

- CT or MR, affected region

Follow-up Visits Generally Required

- See *Advice for Referral*

Suggested Readings

Patel AM, Peters SG. Clinical manifestations of lung cancer. [Review]. Mayo Clin Proc 1993;68:273–277.

Feld R, Ginsberg RJ, Payne D, Shepherd FA. Lung. In: Abeloff MD, ed. Clinical Oncology. New York: Churchill-Livingstone, 1995:1083–1152.

Selected Guidelines

U. S. Preventive Services Task Force. Screening for lung cancer. In: DiGuiseppi C, Atkins D, Woolf S, eds. Guide to Clinical Preventive Services. 2nd ed. Baltimore: Williams & Wilkins, 1996:135–140.

See Also

- Lung cancer, squamous cell, history of

ONCOLOGY

Lung Cancer, Squamous Cell, History of

Indications and Timing for Referral

- Clinical or radiologic findings suggest recurrent malignancy

Timing: Expedited (less than 1 week)

- Serious consideration should be given to having such patients co-managed with an oncologist if less than 5 years since diagnosis

Timing: Routine (less than 4 weeks)

Advice for Referral

- Optimal plan for oncology follow-up is best defined by preliminary discussion with the consultant, considering the type and initial stage of disease, time since completion of anti-tumor treatment, and potential late complications of therapy.
- Careful evaluation for additional upper aerodigestive malignancies is vital (e.g., head and neck, esophageal).
- Concerted effort to encourage smoking cessation is essential.

Tests to Prepare for Consult

- CBC
- Electrolytes (Na, K, Cl, CO_2)
- Calcium
- Creatinine
- ALT, AST, alkaline phosphatase
- Radiograph, chest

Tests Not Useful Before Consult

- CT or MR, chest

Tests Consultant May Need to Do

- CT or MR, affected region

Follow-up Visits Generally Required

- See *Advice for Referral*

Selected Guidelines

U. S. Preventive Services Task Force. Screening for lung cancer. In: DiGuiseppi C, Atkins D, Woolf S, eds. Guide to Clinical Preventive Services. 2nd ed. Baltimore: Williams & Wilkins, 1996:135–140.

See Also

- Lung cancer, small cell, history of

Lymphoma, History of

Indications and Timing for Referral

- Clinical or radiologic findings suggest recurrent malignancy

Timing: Expedited (less than 1 week)

Advice for Referral

- Optimal plan for oncology follow-up is best defined by preliminary discussion with the consultant, considering the type and initial stage of disease, time since completion of anti-tumor treatment, and potential late complications of therapy.
- Old medical records are vital, including diagnostic studies and treatment regimens.

Tests to Prepare for Consult

- CBC with differential
- ALT, AST, alkaline phosphatase
- Creatinine
- TSH
- Radiograph, chest

Tests Not Useful Before Consult

- Radiocontrast studies

Tests Consultant May Need to Do

- CT or MR, affected region

Follow-up Visits Generally Required

- See *Advice for Referral*

Suggested Readings

Bhatia S, Robison LL, Oberlin O, et al. Breast cancer and other second neoplasms after childhood Hodgkin's disease. N Engl J Med 1996;334:745–752.

Hancock SL, Cox RS, McDougall R. Thyroid disease after treatment of Hodgkin's disease. N Engl J Med 1991;325:599–605.

Castellino RA. Diagnostic imaging evaluation of Hodgkin's disease and non-Hodgkin's lymphoma. [Review]. Cancer 1991;67(Suppl):1177–1180.

Cabanillas F, Fuller LM. The radiologic assessment of the lymphoma patient from the standpoint of the clinician. [Review]. Radiol Clin North Am 1990;28:683–695.

See Also

- Lymphoma, history of

ONCOLOGY

Mammogram, Suspicious

Indications and Timing for Referral

- Diagnostic uncertainty

Timing: Expedited (less than 1 week)

Advice for Referral

- Refer to M.D. capable of biopsy.

Tests to Prepare for Consult

- Mammogram

Tests Not Useful Before Consult

- Bone scan
- Tumor markers

Tests Consultant May Need to Do

- Ultrasound, breast
- Fine needle biopsy
- Surgical biopsy

Follow-up Visits Generally Required

- One

Suggested Readings

Fajardo LL, DeAngelis GA. The role of stereotactic biopsy in abnormal mammograms. [Review] [24 refs]. Surg Oncol Clin N Am 1997;6:285–299.

Hall FM. Technologic advances in breast imaging. Current and future strategies, controversies, and opportunities. [Review] [31 refs]. Surg Oncol Clin N Am 1997;6:403–409.

Schapira DV, Levine RB. Breast cancer screening and compliance and evaluation of lesions. Med Clin North Am 1996;80:15.

Lerman C, Trock B, Rimer BK, et al. Psychological and behavioral implications of abnormal mammograms. Ann Intern Med 1991;114:657–661.

Olson LK. Interpreting the mammogram report. [Review]. Am Fam Physician 1993;47:396–403.

Selected Guidelines

Quality determinants of mammography. [Anonymous] Washington, DC: Agency for Health Care Policy and Research. 1994; Report 95-0632. 1–70.

See Also

- Breast mass
- Breast cancer, history of
- Breast cancer, family history of

THE CONSULTATION GUIDE

Mass, Extremity

Indications and Timing for Referral

- Diagnostic uncertainty
- Assistance with management

Timing: Expedited (less than 1 week)

Advice for Referral

- Refer to M.D. capable of biopsy.

Tests to Prepare for Consult

- Radiograph, affected region

Tests Not Useful Before Consult

- None

Tests Consultant May Need to Do

- MR, relevant region
- Fine needle biopsy
- Surgical biopsy

Follow-up Visits Generally Required

- One

Suggested Readings

McClinton MA. Tumors and aneurysms of the upper extremity. [Review]. Hand Clinics 1993;9:15–1–69.

Panicek DM, Gatsonis C, Rosenthal DI, et al. CT and MR imaging in the local staging of primary malignant musculoskeletal neoplasms: Report of the Radiology Diagnostic Oncology Group. Radiology 1997;202:237–246.

Wolf RE, Enneking WF. The staging and surgery of musculoskeletal neoplasms. [Review] [21 refs]. Orthop Clin North Am 1996;27:473–481.

Murphy WA Jr. Imaging bone tumors in the 1990s. [Review]. Cancer 1991; 67(Suppl): 1169–1176.

See Also

- Sarcoma, history of
- Bone lesion, lytic

Melanoma, History of

Indications and Timing for Referral

- Locally recurrent disease
- Regional lymphadenopathy proximal to previously resected lesion

Timing: Expedited (less than 1 week)

Advice for Referral

- Family history is vital.
- Screen for additional primary lesions.
- Optimal plan for oncology follow-up is best defined by preliminary discussion with the consultant, considering the type and initial stage of disease, time since completion of anti-tumor treatment, and potential late complications of therapy.

Tests to Prepare for Consult

- None

Tests Not Useful Before Consult

- None

Tests Consultant May Need to Do

- Biopsy, skin lesion
- Fine needle biopsy, node
- Surgical biopsy, node

Follow-up Visits Generally Required

See *Advice for Referral*

Suggested Readings

Brobeil A, Rapaport D, Wells K, et al. Multiple primary melanomas: implications for screening and follow-up programs for melanoma. Ann Surg Oncol 1997;4:19–23.

Ahmed I. Malignant melanoma: prognostic indicators. [Review] [40 refs]. Mayo Clin Proc 1997;72:356–361.

NIH Consensus conference. Diagnosis and treatment of early melanoma [see comments]. [Review]. JAMA 1992;268:1314–1319.

Sober AJ. Diagnosis and management of early melanoma: a consensus view. [Review]. Semin Surg Oncol 1993;9:194–197.

Prostate Cancer, History of

Indications and Timing for Referral

- Clinical, laboratory, or radiologic finding suggests possible recurrence

Timing: Expedited (less than 1 week)

Advice for Referral

- Optimal plan for oncology follow-up is best defined by preliminary discussion with the consultant, considering the type and initial stage of disease, time since completion of anti-tumor treatment, and potential late complications of therapy.

Tests to Prepare for Consult

- PSA

Tests Not Useful Before Consult

- None

Tests Consultant May Need to Do

- Radiograph, affected region
- Bone scan
- CT scan
  - Abdomen
  - Pelvis

Follow-up Visits Generally Required

- See *Advice for Referral*

Suggested Readings

Coley CM, Barry MJ, Fleming C, Mulley AG. Early detection of prostate cancer. Part I: Prior probability and effectiveness of tests. The American College of Physicians. [Review] [181 refs]. Ann Intern Med 1997;126:394–406.

Coley CM, Barry MJ, Fleming C, et al. Early detection of prostate cancer. Part II: Estimating the risks, benefits, and costs. American College of Physicians [see comments]. Ann Intern Med 1997;126:468–479.

Freedman A, Hahn G, Love N. Follow-up after therapy for prostate cancer. Treating the problems and caring for the man. [Review] [18 refs]. Postgrad Med 1996;100:125–129.

Waxman S, Stevens AK, Walsh RA, et al. Management of asymptomatic rising PSA after prostatectomy or radiation therapy. [Review] [48 refs]. Oncology (Huntingt) 1997;11:457–460.

Garnick MB. Prostate cancer: screening, diagnosis, and management [see comments] [published erratum appears in Ann Intern Med 1994;120:698]. [Review]. Ann Intern Med 1993;118:804–818.

Smith JA Jr. Management of hot flushes due to endocrine therapy for prostate carcinoma. [Review] [22 refs]. Oncology (Huntingt) 1996;10:1319–1322.

Selected Guidelines

Screening for prostate cancer. American College of Physicians [comments]. [Review] [52 refs]. Ann Intern Med 1997;126:480–484.

American Urological Association releases guidelines for the management of localized prostate cancer. Am Fam Physician 1996;53:2751–2752.

ONCOLOGY

Renal Cell Cancer, History of

Indications and Timing for Referral

- Clinical, laboratory, or radiologic finding suggests possible recurrence

Timing: Expedited (less than 1 week)

Advice for Referral

- Optimal plan for oncology follow-up is best defined by preliminary discussion with the consultant, considering the type and initial stage of disease, time since completion of anti-tumor treatment, and potential late complications of therapy.

Tests to Prepare for Consult

- Creatinine
- Urinalysis with microscopic
- Calcium

Tests Not Useful Before Consult

- None

Tests Consultant May Need to Do

- Radiograph, chest
- CT scan
  - Abdomen
  - Pelvis

Follow-up Visits Generally Required

- See *Advice for Referral*

Suggested Readings

Motzer RJ, Bander NH, Nanus DM. Renal-cell carcinoma [see comments]. [Review] [150 refs]. N Engl J Med 1996;335:865–875.

Savage PD. Renal cell carcinoma. [Review]. Curr Opin Oncol 1994;6:301–307.

THE CONSULTATION GUIDE

Sarcoma, History of

Indications and Timing for Referral

- Clinical, laboratory, or radiologic finding suggests possible recurrence

Timing: Expedited (less than 1 week)

Advice for Referral

- Optimal plan for oncology follow-up is best defined by preliminary discussion with the consultant, considering the type and initial stage of disease, time since completion of antitumor treatment(s), and potential late complications of therapy.

Tests to Prepare for Consult

- CBC
- ALT, AST, alkaline phosphatase
- Radiograph, chest

Tests Not Useful Before Consult

- None

Tests Consultant May Need to Do

- Radiograph, affected region
- CT or MR, affected region

Follow-up Visits Generally Required

- See *Advice for Referral*

Suggested Readings

Elias AD. Advances in the diagnosis and management of sarcomas. [Review]. Curr Opin Oncol 1992;4:681–688.

Gascon P, Schwartz RA. Treatment of Kaposi's sarcoma. [Review]. Dermatol Clin 1994;12:451–456.

Pisters PWT, Brennan MF. Soft tissue sarcomas. In: Abeloff MD, ed. Clinical Oncology. New York: Churchill-Livingstone, 1998:1799–1832.

Bridge JA, Schwartz HS, Neff JR. Sarcomas of bone. In: Abeloff MD, ed. Clinical Oncology. New York: Churchill-Livingstone, 1998:1715–1797.

See Also

- Mass, extremity
- Bone lesion, lytic

Testicular Cancer, History of

Indications and Timing for Referral

- Clinical, laboratory, or radiologic finding suggests possible recurrence

Timing: Expedited (less than 1 week)

Advice for Referral

- Optimal plan for oncology follow-up is best defined by preliminary discussion with the consultant, considering the type and initial stage of disease, time since completion of anti-tumor treatment, and potential late complications of therapy.

Tests to Prepare for Consult

- None

Tests Not Useful Before Consult

- None

Tests Consultant May Need to Do

- Alpha-feto protein
- Beta HCG, serum
- Testosterone
- Radiograph, chest
- Sperm analysis
- Ultrasound, testicular
- CT scan
  - Abdomen
  - Pelvis

Follow-up Visits Generally Required

- See *Advice for Referral*

Suggested Readings

Beyer J, Kingreen D, Krause M, et al. Long-term survival of patients with recurrent or refractory germ cell tumors after high dose chemotherapy. Cancer 1997;79:161–168.

Bosl GJ, Motzer RJ. Testicular germ-cell cancer. [Review] [122 refs]. N Engl J Med 1997;337:242–253.

Sharir S, Foster RS, Donohue JP, Jewett MA. What is the appropriate follow-up after treatment?. [Review] [31 refs]. Semin Urol Oncol 1996;14:45–53.

Fossa SD, Kreuser ED, Roth GJ, Raghavan D. Long-term side effects after treatment of testicular cancer. Prog Clin Biol Res 1990;357:321–330.

Mead GM. Testicular cancer and related neoplasms [see comments]. [Review]. Br Med J 1992;304:1426–1429.

Rowland RG. Serum markers in testicular germ-cell neoplasms. [Review]. Hematol Oncol Clin North Am 1988;2:485–489.

Thyroid Cancer, History of

Indications and Timing for Referral

- Clinical, laboratory, or radiologic finding suggests possible recurrence

Timing: Expedited (less than 1 week)

Advice for Referral

- Optimal plan for oncology follow-up is best defined by preliminary discussion with the consultant, considering the type and initial stage of disease, time since completion of anti-tumor treatment, and potential late complications of therapy.
- Referral may be to an endocrinologist or oncologist depending on individual expertise.

Tests to Prepare for Consult

- TSH (sensitivity, < 0.1 mU/L)
- Thyroglobulin

Tests Not Useful Before Consult

- Bone scan

Tests Consultant May Need to Do

- Free T_4
- Radiograph, chest
- Ultrasound, neck
- ^{131}I total body scan

Follow-up Visits Generally Required

- See *Advice for Referral*

Suggested Readings

Hay ID, Klee GG. Thyroid cancer diagnosis and management. [Review]. Clin Lab Med 1993;13:725–734.

Ladenson PW, Braverman LE, Mazzaferri EL, et al. Comparison of administration of recombinant human thyrotropin with withdrawal of thyroid hormone for radioactive iodine scanning in patients with thyroid carcinoma. N Engl J Med 1997;337:888–896.

Brierley JD, Panzarella T, Tsang RW, et al. A comparison of different staging systems predictability of patient outcome. Thyroid carcinoma as an example. [Review] [30 refs]. Cancer 1997;79:2414–2423.

Robbins J, Merino MJ, Boice JD Jr, et al. Thyroid cancer: a lethal endocrine neoplasm. [Review]. Ann Intern Med 1991;115:133–147.

Mazzaferri EL, Jhiang SM. Long-term impact of initial surgical and medical therapy on papillary and follicular thyroid cancer. Am J Med 1994;97:418–428.

Maxon HR, Smith HS. Radioiodine-131 in the diagnosis and treatment of metastatic well differentiated thyroid cancer. Endocrinol Metab Clin N Amer 1990;19:685–718.

Ozata M, Suzuki S, Miyamoto T, et al. Serum thyroglobulin in the follow-up of patients with treated differentiated thyroid cancer. J Clin Endocrinol Metab 1994;74:98–105.

Selected Guidelines

Singer PA, Cooper DS, Daniels GH, et al. Treatment guidelines for patients with thyroid nodules and well-differentiated thyroid cancer. American Thyroid Association. Arch Intern Med 1996;156:2165–2172.

U. S. Preventive Services Task Force. Screening for thyroid cancer. In: DiGuiseppi C, Atkins D, Woolf S, eds. Guide to Clinical Preventive Services. 2nd ed. Baltimore: Williams & Wilkins, 1996:187–192.

See Also

- Head and neck irradiation, childhood
- Thyroid cancer, medullary, family history of

ONCOLOGY

Thyroid Cancer, Medullary, Family History of

Indications and Timing for Referral
- Patients with a positive family history should be referred for further evaluation

Timing: Routine (less than 4 weeks)

Advice for Referral
- Referral may be to an endocrinologist or oncologist depending on individual expertise.

Tests to Prepare for Consult
- Calcitonin

Tests Not Useful Before Consult
- None

Tests Consultant May Need to Do
- Calcium
- PTH
- 24-hour urine metanephrines
- Calcium/pentagastrin stimulation test
- RET proto-oncogene analysis
- Sonogram, thyroid
- Fine needle aspiration biopsy

Follow-up Visits Generally Required
- One

Suggested Readings
Nelkin BD, Ball DW, Baylin SB. Molecular abnormalities in tumors associated with multiple endocrine neoplasia type 2. [Review]. Endocrinol Metab Clin North Am 1994;23:187–213.

Dottorini ME, Assi A, Sironi M, et al. Multivariate analysis of patients with medullary thyroid carcinoma. Prognostic significance and impact on treatment of clinical and pathologic variables. Cancer 1996;77:1556–1565.

Heshmati HM, Gharib H, Khosla S, et al. Genetic testing in medullary thyroid carcinoma syndromes: mutation types and clinical significance. Mayo Clin Proc 1997;72:430–436.

Moley JF. The molecular genetics of multiple endocrine neoplasia type 2A and related syndromes. Annu Rev Med 1997;48:409–420.

Eng C, Clayton D, Schuffenecker I, et al. The relationship between specific RET proto-oncogene mutations and disease phenotype in multiple endocrine neoplasia type 2. International RET mutation consortium analysis. JAMA 1996;276:1575–1579.

See Also
- Thyroid cancer, history of
- Head and neck irradiation, childhood

CHAPTER 10

Pulmonary

Adenopathy, Hilar, Bilateral 473
Alpha-1-Antitrypsin (α_1-Antitrypsin) Deficiency 474
Asbestos Lung Disease 475
Asthma 476
    Cold- and Exercise-Induced 478
    During Pregnancy 479
    in the Elderly 480
    Occupational 481
Atelectasis 482
Cavitary Lung Lesion 483
Chronic Obstructive Pulmonary Disease (COPD) 484
Chronic Obstructive Pulmonary Disease (COPD), Premature 486
Cor Pulmonale 487
Cough, Chronic 488
Cystic Fibrosis 489
Disability Evaluation, Lung Disease 490
Dyspnea
    Chronic 491
    Episodic 492
    Nocturnal 493
Hemoptysis 494
Inhalation, Toxic 496
Lung Cancer, Non-Small Cell 497
Lung Disease
    Air Travel with 498
    Handicapped License Plates with 499
    Occupational 500
    Scuba Diving Clearance with 501
Pleural Effusion 502
Pneumonia
    Immunocompromised Host 503
    Lobar 504
    Poorly Resolving 505
Pneumothorax, Recurrent 506
Preoperative Pulmonary Assessment 507

(continued)

Pulmonary (continued)

Pulmonary Consolidation 508
Pulmonary Fibrosis, Interstitial 509
Pulmonary Hypertension, Primary 510
Pulmonary Infiltrate with Eosinophilia 511
Pulmonary Nodules
   Multiple 512
   Solitary, Central 513
   Solitary, Peripheral 514
Reactive Airway Dysfunction Syndrome 515
Sarcoidosis 516
Sleep Apnea/Snoring 517
Smoking Cessation 518

PULMONARY

Adenopathy, Hilar, Bilateral

Indications and Timing for Referral

- Symptomatic patient for whom treatment is indicated

Timing: Expedited (less than 1 week)

- Etiology unclear
- Tissue diagnosis needed
- Asymmetric bilateral involvement noted
- Significant physiologic impairment
- Possible fungus ball

Timing: Routine (less than 4 weeks)

Advice for Referral

- To confirm the diagnosis of sarcoidosis, additional referral may be required for biopsy of conjunctiva, lymph nodes or skin lesions.

Tests to Prepare for Consult

- Radiograph, chest, PA and lateral
- Electrolytes (Na, K, Cl, CO_2)
- Creatinine
- Calcium, phosphorus
- CBC
- Spirometry
- Lung CO diffusing capacity
- Anergy intradermal skin test panel
- PPD

Tests Not Useful Before Consult

- Mediastinoscopy

Tests Consultant May Need to Do

- Spirometry
- Lung volumes
- CT scan, thorax
- Bronchoscopy
- Transbronchial biopsy

Follow-up Visits Generally Required

- One

Suggested Readings

DeRemee RA. Sarcoidosis. [Review]. Mayo Clin Proc 1995;70:177–181.

Johns CJ, Scott PP, Schonfeld SA. Sarcoidosis. [Review]. Annu Rev Med 1989;40:353–371.

Alpha-1-Antitrypsin (α_1-Antitrypsin) Deficiency

Indications and Timing for Referral

- Any patient with a confirmed diagnosis of homozygous deficiency

Timing: Routine (less than 4 weeks)

Advice for Referral

- Patients with a confirmed diagnosis of α_1-antitrypsin deficiency should see a pulmonologist at least once for baseline evaluation.
- Patients on α_1-antitrypsin replacement therapy should be co-managed with a pulmonologist

Tests to Prepare for Consult

- Radiograph, chest, PA and lateral
- Spirometry
- α_1-antitrypsin level

Tests Not Useful Before Consult

- None

Tests Consultant May Need to Do

- Spirometry, before and after bronchodilator
- Lung volumes
- Flow volume loops
- Lung CO diffusing capacity
- Arterial blood gas
- ECG

Follow-up Visits Generally Required

- Co-management, see *Advice for Referral*

Suggested Readings

McElvaney NG, Stoller JK, Buist AS, et al. Baseline characteristics of enrollees in the National Heart, Lung and Blood Institute Registry of alpha 1 antitrypsin deficiency. Alpha 1-Antitrypsin Deficiency Registry Study Group. Chest 1997;111:394–403.

Perlmutter DH. Alpha-1-antitrypsin deficiency: biochemistry and clinical manifestations. [Review] [70 refs]. Ann Med 1996;28:385–394.

Snider GL. Pulmonary disease in alpha-1-antitrypsin deficiency. [Review]. Ann Intern Med 1989;111:957–959.

Hutchison DC. Natural history of alpha-1-protease inhibitor deficiency. [Review]. Am J Med 1988;84(6A):3–12.

Stockley RA. Alpha 1-antitrypsin and the pathogenesis of emphysema. Lung 1991;169:S205.

Crystal RG. Alpha-1 antitrypsin deficiency. In: Fishman AP, ed. Update: Pulmonary Diseases and Disorders. NY: McGraw-Hill, 1992:19–36.

See Also

- COPD, premature

PULMONARY

Asbestos Lung Disease

Indications and Timing for Referral

- Diagnosis uncertain after initial testing
- Symptoms poorly controlled

Timing: Routine (less than 4 weeks)

Tests to Prepare for Consult

- Radiograph, chest, PA and lateral
- Spirometry
- Lung volumes
- Lung CO diffusing capacity
- Radiograph, chest, obtain old films

Tests Not Useful Before Consult

- None

Tests Consultant May Need to Do

- Arterial blood gas
- CT scan, thorax
- Exercise test for oxygen titration

Follow-up Visits Generally Required

- One

Suggested Readings

Rudd RM. New developments in asbestos-related pleural disease [review]. Thorax 1996;51:210–216.

Yates DH, Browne K, Stidolph PN, Neville E. Asbestos-related bilateral diffuse pleural thickening—natural history of radiographic and lung function abnormalities. Am J Respir Crit Care Med 1996;153:301–306.

Lordi GM, Reichman LB. Pulmonary complications of asbestos exposure [see comments]. [Review]. Am Fam Physician 1993;48:1471–1477.

Muller NL. Imaging of the pleura. Radiology 1993;186:297.

Jones RN. The diagnosis of asbestosis [editorial; comment]. Am Rev Respir Dis 1991;144:477–478.

Asthma

Indications and Timing for Referral

- Multiple flares of asthma requiring unscheduled visits
- Pregnant patient with unstable asthma
- Excessive self-administration of β-adrenergic agonists

Timing: Expedited (less than 1 week)

- Persistent or recurrent symptoms interfering with daily activities or quality of life
- Management of disease requires continuous steroid therapy
- Side effects (i.e., tremors, palpitations) are present from medications needed to control the disease
- One or more episodes of respiratory failure requiring mechanical ventilation or with documented hypercapnia
- Uncontrolled nocturnal episodes of dyspnea, especially if worsening

Timing: Routine (less than 4 weeks)

Advice for Referral

- Factors favoring referral to an allergist/immunologist include:
  - Personal history of respiratory allergies
  - Allergy to aspirin
  - Family history of early-onset asthma
  - Adult onset of asthma
  - Presumed provocation by specific environmental exposure
  - Predictable seasonal exacerbation
- Factors favoring referral to pulmonologist include:
  - Incompletely reversible airway obstruction
  - History of smoking
  - History of respiratory failure
  - Abnormal chest radiograph
- Sinus CT, focused series (a limited series of appropriate regional cuts to include coronal images of the osteomeatal complex).

Tests to Prepare for Consult

- CBC with differential
- Radiograph, chest
- Spirometry, before and after bronchodilator
- Theophylline level (if on theophylline)
- Oxygen saturation level

Tests Not Useful Before Consult

- Immediate hypersensitivity skin testing
- RAST

Tests Consultant May Need to Do

- Spirometry, before and after bronchodilator
- Lung volumes
- Flow volume loops
- Lung CO diffusing capacity
- Arterial blood gas
- Theophylline level
- IgE, quantitative
- *Aspergillus* skin test
- Radiograph, chest
- Immediate hypersensitivity skin testing
- RAST
- CT, sinuses, focused series (see *Advice for Referral*)

Asthma (continued)

Follow-up Visits Generally Required

- Two

Suggested Readings

Goldstein RA, Paul WE, Metcalfe DD, et al. NIH conference. Asthma. Ann Intern Med 1994;121:698–708.

Grammer LC, Greenberger PA. Diagnosis and classification of asthma. [Review]. Chest 1992;101(Suppl):393S–395S.

Selected Guidelines

NHLBI issues updated guidelines for the diagnosis and management of asthma. Am Fam Physician 1997;56:621–623.

Practice parameters for the diagnosis and treatment of asthma. Joint Task Force on Practice Parameters, representing the American Academy of Allergy Asthma and Immunology, the American College of Allergy, Asthma and Immunology, and the Joint Council of Allergy, Asthma and Immunology. J Allergy Clin Immunol 1995;96:707–870.

Beveridge RC, Grunfeld AF, Hodder RV, Verbeek PR. Guidelines for the emergency management of asthma in adults. CAEP/CTS Asthma Advisory Committee. Canadian Association of Emergency Physicians and the Canadian Thoracic Society. [Review] [167 refs]. Can Med Assoc J 1996;155:25–37.

Sheffer AL, Taggart VS. The National Asthma Education Program. Expert panel report guidelines for the diagnosis and management of asthma. National Heart, Lung, and Blood Institute. Med Care 1993;31(3 Suppl):MS20–MS28.

Guidelines for the evaluation of impairment/disability in patients with asthma. American Thoracic Society. Medical Section of the American Lung Association [see comments]. Am Rev Respir Dis 1993;147:1056–1061.

North of England evidence based guidelines development project: summary version of evidence based guideline for the primary care management in adults. North of England Asthma Guideline Development Group. Br Med J 1996;312:762–766.

See Also

- Asthma, occupational
- Asthma, during pregnancy
- Asthma, cold- and exercise-induced
- Asthma, in the elderly

THE CONSULTATION GUIDE

Asthma, Cold- and Exercise-Induced

Indications and Timing for Referral

- Symptoms occurring with athletic activity

Timing: Routine (less than 4 weeks)

Advice for Referral

- Factors favoring referral to an allergist/immunologist include:
  - Personal history of respiratory allergies
  - Family history of early-onset asthma
  - Adult onset of asthma
  - Presumed provocation by specific environmental exposure
  - Predictable seasonal exacerbation
- Factors favoring referral to a pulmonologist include:
  - Incompletely reversible airway obstruction
  - History of smoking
  - History of respiratory failure
  - Abnormal chest radiograph

Tests to Prepare for Consult

- CBC with differential
- Spirometry

Tests Not Useful Before Consult

- Immediate hypersensitivity skin testing
- RAST

Tests Consultant May Need to Do

- Spirometry, before and after bronchodilator
- Lung volumes
- Flow volume loops
- Lung CO diffusing capacity
- Arterial blood gas
- Theophylline level
- Radiograph, chest
- Immediate hypersensitivity skin testing
- RAST
- Spirometry, before and after exercise

Follow-up Visits Generally Required

- One

Suggested Readings

McFadden ER Jr, Gilbert IA. Exercise-induced asthma. [Review]. N Engl J Med 1994;330:1362–1367.

Cypcar D, Lemanske RF, Jr. Asthma and exercise. [Review]. Clin Chest Med 1994;15:351–368.

Kyle JM. Exercise-induced pulmonary syndromes. [Review]. Med Clin North Am 1994;78:413–421.

Weiler JM. Exercise-induced asthma: a practical guide to definitions, diagnosis, prevalence, and treatment. [Review] [67 refs]. Allergy Asthma Proc 1996;17:315–325.

Hendrickson CD, Lynch JM, Gleeson K. Exercise induced asthma: a clinical perspective. [Review]. Lung 1994;172:1–14.

Mellion MB, Kobayashi RH. Exercise-induced asthma. [Review]. Am Fam Physician 1992;45:2671–2677.

NHLBI issues updated guidelines for the diagnosis and management of asthma. Am Fam Physician 1997;56:621–623.

See Also

- Asthma
- Asthma, in the elderly
- Asthma, during pregnancy
- Asthma, occupational

PULMONARY

Asthma, During Pregnancy

Indications and Timing for Referral

- Multiple flares of asthma requiring unscheduled visits

Timing: Expedited (less than 1 week)

- The duration, intensity, and/or frequency of the patient's symptoms are increasing

Timing: Routine (less than 4 weeks)

Advice for Referral

- Sinus CT, focused series (a limited series of appropriate regional cuts to include coronal images of the osteo-meatal complex).

Tests to Prepare for Consult

- Spirometry, before and after bronchodilator
- CBC with differential
- PPD

Tests Not Useful Before Consult

- None

Tests Consultant May Need to Do

- Spirometry, serial
- Lung volumes
- Flow volume loops
- Lung CO diffusing capacity
- Arterial blood gas
- Theophylline level
- CT, sinuses, focused series (see *Advice for Referral*)

Follow-up Visits Generally Required

- Two

Suggested Readings

Mabie WC. Asthma in pregnancy. [Review] [44 refs]. Clin Obstet Gynecol 1996;39:56–69.

Greenberger PA. Asthma in pregnancy. [Review]. Clin Chest Med 1992;13:597–605.

Huff RW. Asthma in pregnancy. [Review]. Med Clin North Am 1989;73:653–660.

Zeldis SM. Dyspnea during pregnancy. Distinguishing cardiac from pulmonary causes. [Review]. Clin Chest Med 1992;13:567–585.

Selected Guidelines

National Asthma Education Program Working Group. Management of asthma during pregnancy. [Anonymous] Bethesda, MD. The National Heart, Lung and Blood Institute. 1992; Report nr 93–3279A.

McDonald CF, Burdon JG. Asthma in pregnancy and lactation. A position paper for the Thoracic Society of Australia and New Zealand. Med J Aust 1996;165:485–488.

See Also

- Asthma, cold- and exercise-induced
- Asthma, occupational
- Asthma!

THE CONSULTATION GUIDE

Asthma, in the Elderly

Indications and Timing for Referral

- Multiple flares of asthma requiring unscheduled visits
- One or more episodes of respiratory failure requiring mechanical ventilation

Timing: Expedited (less than 1 week)

- Management of disease requires continuous steroid therapy
- Side effects (i.e., tremors, palpitations) are present from medications needed to control the disease

Timing: Routine (less than 4 weeks)

Advice for Referral

- In this setting, it is important to consider and exclude the possibility of heart failure and/or pulmonary embolism.
- Sinus CT, focused series (a limited series of appropriate regional cuts to include coronal images of the osteo-meatal complex).

Tests to Prepare for Consult

- CBC with differential
- Radiograph, chest
- Theophylline level (if on theophylline)
- Spirometry, before and after bronchodilator
- ECG

Tests Not Useful Before Consult

- None

Tests Consultant May Need to Do

- Spirometry, serial
- Lung volumes
- Flow volume loops
- Lung CO diffusing capacity
- Arterial blood gas
- Theophylline level
- Echocardiogram
- Cardiac exercise tolerance test
- CT, sinuses, focused series (see *Advice for Referral*)
- V/Q scan

Follow-up Visits Generally Required

- Two

Suggested Readings

Bauer BA, Reed CE, Yunginger JW, et al. Incidence and outcomes of asthma in the elderly. A population-based study in Rochester, Minnesota. Chest 1997;111:303–310.

Jack CIA, Lye M. Asthma in the elderly patient [review]. Gerontology 1996;42:61–68.

Braman SS. Asthma in the elderly patient. [Review]. Clin Chest Med 1993;14:413–422.

Braman SS. Drug treatment of asthma in the elderly. [Review] [41 refs]. Drugs 1996;51:415–423.

Selected Guidelines

National Asthma Education and Prevention Program Working Group. Considerations for diagnosing and managing asthma in the elderly. [Anonymous] Bethesda, MD. The National Heart, Lung and Blood Institute. 1996; Report nr 96–3662.

See Also

- Asthma, occupational
- Asthma, cold- and exercise-induced
- Asthma

Asthma, Occupational

Indications and Timing for Referral

- Diagnostic uncertainty
- Symptoms are poorly controlled

Timing: Routine (less than 4 weeks)

Advice for Referral

- Factors favoring referral to an allergist/immunologist include:
  - Personal history of respiratory allergies
  - Family history of early-onset asthma
  - Adult onset of asthma
  - Presumed provocation by specific environmental exposure
- Factors favoring referral to a pulmonologist include:
  - Incompletely reversible airway obstruction
  - History of smoking
  - History of respiratory failure
  - Abnormal chest radiograph

Tests to Prepare for Consult

- Radiograph, chest, PA and lateral
- CBC with differential
- Spirometry, before and after bronchodilator

Tests Not Useful Before Consult

- Immediate hypersensitivity skin testing
- RAST

Tests Consultant May Need to Do

- Spirometry, serial
- Peak flow meter for serial monitoring
- Arterial blood gas
- Skin testing
- Theophylline level
- Pulmonary function tests
- RAST
- Methacholine challenge

Follow-up Visits Generally Required

- One

Suggested Readings

Chan-Yeung M, Malo JL. Current concepts: occupational asthma. N Engl J Med 1995;333:107–112.

Venables KM, Chan-Yeung M. Occupational asthma. [Review] [36 refs]. Lancet 1997;349:1465–1469.

Bernstein DI. Occupational asthma. [Review]. Med Clin North Am 1992;76:917–934.

Bright P, Burge PS. Occupational lung disease. 8. The diagnosis of occupational asthma from serial measurements of lung function at and away from work. [Review] [49 refs]. Thorax 1996;51:857–863.

Alberts WM, Brooks SM. Advances in occupational asthma. [Review]. Clin Chest Med 1992;13:281–302.

Selected Guidelines

Chan-Yeung M. Assessment of asthma in the workplace. ACCP consensus statement. American College of Chest Physicians. [Review] [159 refs]. Chest 1995;108:1084–1117.

See Also

- Asthma, cold- and exercise-induced
- Reactive airway dysfunction syndrome
- Disability evaluation, lung disease
- Inhalation, toxic
- Lung disease, occupational
- Asthma, in the elderly
- Asthma
- Asthma, during pregnancy

Atelectasis

Indications and Timing for Referral

- Clinical suspicion of cancer

Timing: Expedited (less than 1 week)

- Atelectasis not accompanied by acute respiratory infection syndrome
- Degree of atelectasis greater than or equal to segmental section of lung for more than 6 weeks

Timing: Routine (less than 4 weeks)

Advice for Referral

- The larger the area involved, the lower the threshold for referral.

Tests to Prepare for Consult

- Radiograph, chest, PA and lateral
- Radiograph, chest, obtain old films

Tests Not Useful Before Consult

- None

Tests Consultant May Need to Do

- CT scan, thorax
- Bronchoscopy
- Sputum cytology

Follow-up Visits Generally Required

- One

Suggested Readings

Matthay RA, Arroliga AC. Localized abnormalities of lung aeration. In: Bennett JC, Plum F, eds. Cecil Textbook of Medicine. 20th ed. Philadelphia: WB Saunders, 1996:389–390.

Wilson AG. Large airway obstruction. In: Grainger RG, Allison DY, eds. Diagnostic Radiology: An Anglo-American Textbook of Imaging. 3rd ed. New York: Churchill Livingstone, 1997:343–357.

See Also

- Pulmonary consolidation

PULMONARY

Cavitary Lung Lesion

Indications and Timing for Referral

- Etiology unclear

Timing: Routine (less than 4 weeks)

Advice for Referral

- In patients producing sputum, appropriate cultures and stains, including those for TB and fungi, should be obtained.

Tests to Prepare for Consult

- Radiograph, chest
- Radiograph, chest, obtain old films
- CBC
- Electrolytes (Na, K, Cl, CO_2)
- Calcium, phosphorus
- Creatinine
- PPD

Tests Not Useful Before Consult

- None

Tests Consultant May Need to Do

- Sputum
  - Cytology
  - AFB stain
  - AFB culture
  - Routine culture
  - Fungal culture
  - Fungal stain
  - PCP stain
- CT scan, thorax
- Bronchoscopy

Follow-up Visits Generally Required

- One

Suggested Readings

Morgenthaler TI, Ryu JH, Utz JP. Cavitary pulmonary infarct in immunocompromised hosts. [Review]. Mayo Clin Proc 1995;70:66–68.

THE CONSULTATION GUIDE

Chronic Obstructive Pulmonary Disease (COPD)

Indications and Timing for Referral

- Decline in arterial pO_2 greater than 12 mm Hg
- Increase in pCO_2 greater than 12 mm Hg
- Marked increase in breathlessness
- Cyanosis
- New chest pain

Timing: Immediate

- Multiple flares of the disease requiring unscheduled primary care visits
- One or more episodes of respiratory failure requiring mechanical ventilation or with documented hypercapnia
- Symptoms uncontrolled or progression of the disease
- Need for either multiple or prolonged courses of systemic glucocorticoids

Timing: Routine (less than 4 weeks)

Advice for Referral

- Referral threshold should be lower if FEV_1 is less than 50% of predicted, or if patient requires continuous oxygen therapy (see *Cor Pulmonale*).

Tests to Prepare for Consult

- Radiograph, chest
- Spirometry, before and after bronchodilator
- CBC
- Electrolytes (Na, K, Cl, CO_2)
- Creatinine
- Arterial blood gas
- ECG

Tests Not Useful Before Consult

- CT scan, thorax

Tests Consultant May Need to Do

- Spirometry, before and after bronchodilator
- Lung volumes
- Flow volume loops
- Lung CO diffusing capacity
- Arterial blood gas
- CBC
- Electrolytes (Na, K, Cl, CO_2)
- Creatinine
- Calcium, phosphorus
- Radiograph, chest
- Exercise test for oxygen titration

PULMONARY

Chronic Obstructive Pulmonary Disease (COPD) (*continued*)

Follow-up Visits Generally Required
- Two

Suggested Readings
Celli BR. Current thoughts regarding treatment of chronic obstructive pulmonary disease. [Review] [120 refs]. Med Clin North Am 1996;80:589–609.

Ferguson GT, Cherniack RM. Management of chronic obstructive pulmonary disease [see comments]. [Review]. N Engl J Med 1993;328:1017–1022.

Kanner RE. Early intervention in chronic obstructive pulmonary disease. A review of the Lung Health Study results. Med Clin North Am 1996;80:523–547.

Murphy TF, Sethi S. Bacterial infection in chronic obstructive pulmonary disease. [Review]. Am Rev Respir Dis 1992;146:1067–1083.

McEvoy CE, Niewoehner DE. Adverse effects of corticosteroid therapy for COPD. A critical review. [Review] [95 refs]. Chest 1997;111:732–743.

Selected Guidelines
Standards for the diagnosis and care of patients with chronic obstructive pulmonary disease. American Thoracic Society. [Review] [265 refs]. Am J Respir Crit Care Med 1995;152:S77–S121.

Siafakas NM, Vermeire P, Pride NB, et al. Optimal assessment and management of chronic obstructive pulmonary disease (COPD). The European Respiratory Society Task Force [see comments]. Eur Respir J 1995;8:1398–1420.

See Also
- Synonyms: COPD, emphysema
- Cough, chronic
- Dyspnea, chronic
- Pulmonary hypertension, primary
- Cor pulmonale
- COPD, premature
- Asthma

Chronic Obstructive Pulmonary Disease (COPD), Premature

Indications and Timing for Referral

- Uncontrolled or progressive symptoms

Timing: Expedited (less than 1 week)

- Multiple flares of the disease requiring unscheduled visits
- One or more episodes of respiratory failure requiring mechanical ventilation or with documented hypercapnia

Timing: Routine (less than 4 weeks)

Advice for Referral

- Threshold for referral is lower if the patient's FEV_1 is 50% or less.
- COPD is considered premature if the patient is a smoker and under the age of 40 years or never smoked and is younger than 65 years.

Tests to Prepare for Consult

- Radiograph, chest, PA and lateral
- Spirometry, before and after bronchodilator
- α_1-antitrypsin level

Tests Not Useful Before Consult

- Alpha-1-globulin level

Tests Consultant May Need to Do

- Spirometry
- Lung volumes
- Flow volume loops
- Lung CO diffusing capacity
- Arterial blood gas
- Sputum routine culture
- Sweat chloride test
- Immunoglobulins, quantitative
- CT scan, thorax
- ECG

Follow-up Visits Generally Required

- Two

Suggested Readings

Crystal RG. Alpha-1 antitrypsin deficiency. In: Fishman AP, ed. Update: Pulmonary Diseases and Disorders. NY: McGraw-Hill, 1992:19–36.

Hutchison DC. Natural history of alpha-1-protease inhibitor deficiency. [Review]. Am J Med 1988;84(6A):3–12.

Selected Guidelines

Guidelines for the measurement of respiratory function. Recommendations of the British Thoracic Society and the Association of Respiratory Technicians and Physiologists. Respir Med 1994;88:165–194.

See Also

- Synonyms: chronic lung disease, lung disease
- α_1-antitrypsin deficiency
- Cystic fibrosis
- Chronic obstructive pulmonary disease (COPD)

PULMONARY

Cor Pulmonale

Indications and Timing for Referral
- Oxygen therapy is required
- Etiology unclear
- Progression or exacerbation of symptoms
- Multiple flares of the disease requiring unscheduled visits
- One or more episodes of respiratory failure requiring mechanical ventilation

Timing: Urgent (less than 24 hours)

Advice for Referral
- This condition often requires co-management with a pulmonologist.

Tests to Prepare for Consult
- Radiograph, chest
- Spirometry
- Electrolytes (Na, K, Cl, CO_2)
- Creatinine
- Calcium, phosphorus
- CBC
- Arterial blood gas
- ECG

Tests Not Useful Before Consult
- None

Tests Consultant May Need to Do
- Spirometry, before and after bronchodilator
- Lung volumes
- Flow volume loops
- Lung CO diffusing capacity
- Arterial blood gas
- CBC
- Electrolytes (Na, K, Cl, CO_2)
- Creatinine
- Calcium, phosphorus
- Echocardiogram with Doppler studies
- Lung scan

Follow-up Visits Generally Required
- Co-management, see *Advice for Referral*

Suggested Readings
MacNee W. Pathophysiology of cor pulmonale in chronic obstructive pulmonary disease. Part one. [Review] [332 refs]. Am J Respir Crit Care Med 1994;150:833–852.

MacNee W. Pathophysiology of cor pulmonale in chronic obstructive pulmonary disease. Part two. [Review] [187 refs]. Am J Respir Crit Care Med 1994;150:1158–1168.

Wiedemann HP, Matthay RA. Cor pulmonale in chronic obstructive pulmonary disease. Circulatory pathophysiology and management. [Review]. Clin Chest Med 1990;11:523–545.

Klinger JR, Hill NS. Right ventricular dysfunction in chronic obstructive pulmonary disease. Evaluation and management. [Review]. Chest 1991;99:715–723.

D'Alonzo GE. Survival in patients with pulmonary hypertension: results from a national prospective study. Ann Intern Med 1991;115:343–349.

See Also
- Chronic obstructive pulmonary disease (COPD)
- Pulmonary hypertension, primary

Cough, Chronic

Indications and Timing for Referral

- Cough initially associated with respiratory infection, persisting for more than 12 weeks, with normal chest radiograph
- Cough without other evidence of respiratory infection persisting for 2 weeks

Timing: Routine (less than 4 weeks)

Advice for Referral

- If chest radiograph is negative, there is no need for a chest CT scan before consultation.
- In smokers with a new cough or a persistent increase in the severity of cough, the threshhold for consultation should be lower.
- Cough occurring as a side effect to an ACE inhibitor typically subsides within 1 week of discontinuing the drug.

Tests to Prepare for Consult

- Radiograph, chest, PA and lateral

Tests Not Useful Before Consult

- CT scan, thorax

Tests Consultant May Need to Do

- Spirometry, before and after bronchodilator
- Lung CO diffusing capacity
- Methacholine challenge
- Radiographs, sinus
- CT scan, sinuses
- Esophageal pH monitoring
- CT scan, thorax, high resolution

Follow-up Visits Generally Required

- Two

Suggested Readings

Mello CJ, Irwin RS, Curley FJ. Predictive values of the character, timing, and complications of chronic cough in diagnosing its cause. Arch Intern Med 1996;156:997–1003.

Patrick H, Patrick F. Chronic cough. [Review]. Med Clin North Am 1995;79:361–372.

Rosenow EC 3rd. Persistent cough: causes and cures [see comments]. Hosp Pract (Off Ed) 1996;31:121–127.

Chung KF, Lalloo UG. Diagnosis and management of chronic persistent dry cough. [Review] [34 refs]. Postgrad Med J 1996;72:594–598.

Irwin RS, French CL, Curley FJ, Zawacki JK, Bennett FM. Chronic cough due to gastroesophageal reflux. Clinical, diagnostic, and pathogenetic aspects [see comments]. Chest 1993;104:1511–1517.

Irwin RS, Curley FJ. The treatment of cough. A comprehensive review. [Review] [68 refs]. Chest 1991;99:1477–1484.

Irwin RS, Curley FJ, French CL. Chronic cough. The spectrum and frequency of causes, key components of the diagnostic evaluation, and outcome of specific therapy. Am Rev Respir Dis 1990;141:640–647.

See Also

- Hemoptysis
- Asthma

PULMONARY

Cystic Fibrosis

Indications and Timing for Referral

- Progressive symptoms
- Frequent exacerbations

Timing: Expedited (less than 1 week)

- Patients with confirmed diagnosis of cystic fibrosis should see a pulmonologist at least once for baseline evaluation

Timing: Routine (less than 4 weeks)

Tests to Prepare for Consult

- Sputum routine culture
- Cystic fibrosis testing by DNA analysis
- CBC
- Electrolytes (Na, K, Cl, CO_2)
- Creatinine
- Calcium, phosphorus
- Radiograph, chest

Tests Not Useful Before Consult

- None

Tests Consultant May Need to Do

- Spirometry, before and after bronchodilator
- Lung volumes
- Arterial blood gas
- ECG
- Radiograph, sinus

Follow-up Visits Generally Required

- See *Advice for Referral*

Suggested Readings

Stern RC. The diagnosis of cystic fibrosis. [Review] [39 refs]. N Engl J Med 1997;336:487–491.

Ramsey BW. Management of pulmonary disease in patients with cystic fibrosis. [Review] [96 refs]. N Engl J Med 1996;335:179–188.

Bye MR, Ewig JM, Quittell LM. Cystic fibrosis. [Review]. Lung 1994;172:251–270.

Ramsey BW, Farrell PM, Pencharz P. Nutritional assessment and management in cystic fibrosis: a consensus report. The Consensus Committee. Am J Clin Nutr 1992;55:108–116.

Selected Guidelines

Jackson A. Clinical guidelines for cystic fibrosis care. Summary of guidelines prepared by a working group of the Cystic Fibrosis Trust, the British Paediatric Association and the British Thoracic Society. J R Coll Physicians Lond 1996;30:305–308.

Cystic fibrosis in adults: recommendations for care of patients in the UK. London: Royal College of Physicians of London, c1990 vii, 24 p : ill (A Report of the Royal College of Physicians) 1995.

See Also

- COPD, premature

Disability Evaluation, Lung Disease

Indications and Timing for Referral

- To define level of impairment

Timing: Routine (less than 4 weeks)

Tests to Prepare for Consult

- Radiograph, chest, PA and lateral
- Spirometry, before and after bronchodilator
- Lung volumes
- Lung CO diffusing capacity

Tests Not Useful Before Consult

- CT scan, thorax

Tests Consultant May Need to Do

- Arterial blood gas
- Pulmonary exercise test

Follow-up Visits Generally Required

- None

Suggested Readings

Ortega F, Montemayor T, Sanchez A, et al. Role of cardiopulmonary exercise testing and the criteria used to determine disability in patients with severe chronic obstructive pulmonary disease. Am J Respir Crit Care Med 1994;150:747–751.

Harber P. Assessing disability from occupational asthma. A perspective on the AMA guides. [Review]. Chest 1990;98(Suppl):232S–235S.

Harber P, Fedoruk MJ. Work placement and worker fitness. Implications of the Americans with Disabilities Act for pulmonary medicine. Chest 1994;105:1564–1571.

Prince TS, Frank AL. Causation, impairment, disability—an analysis of coal workers pneumoconiosis evaluations. J Occup Environ Med 1996;38:77–82.

Epstein PE. Impairment and disability evaluation in lung disease. In: Fishman AP, Elias JA, Fishman JA, et al., eds. Fishman's Pulmonary Diseases and Disorders. 3rd ed. New York: McGraw Hill, 1998:631–641.

Selected Guidelines

Guidelines for the evaluation of impairment/disability in patients with asthma. American Thoracic Society. Medical Section of the American Lung Association [see comments]. Am Rev Respir Dis 1993;147:1056–1061.

Dyspnea, Chronic

Indications and Timing for Referral

- Cardiac condition has been ruled out
- No clinical evidence of congestive heart failure exists
- Radiograph, chest is negative
- No obvious cause of the dyspnea can be found

Timing: Routine (less than 4 weeks)

Tests to Prepare for Consult

- CBC
- Electrolytes (Na, K, Cl, CO_2)
- Creatinine
- Calcium, phosphorus
- Radiograph, chest, PA and lateral
- Spirometry, before and after bronchodilator
- ECG

Tests Not Useful Before Consult

- CT scan, thorax

Tests Consultant May Need to Do

- Spirometry, before and after bronchodilator
- Lung volumes
- Flow volume loops
- Lung CO diffusing capacity
- Arterial blood gas
- Pulmonary exercise test
- CT scan, thorax
- Echocardiogram with Doppler studies
- V/Q scan

Follow-up Visits Generally Required

- Two

Suggested Readings

DePaso WJ, Winterbauer RH, Lusk JA, et al. Chronic dyspnea unexplained by history, physical examination, chest roentgenogram, and spirometry. Analysis of a seven-year experience. Chest 1991;100:1293–1299.

Gillespie DJ, Staats BA. Unexplained dyspnea. Mayo Clin Proc 1994;69:657–663.

Mulrow CD, Lucey CR, Farnett LE. Discriminating causes of dyspnea through clinical examination. J Gen Intern Med 1993;8:383–392.

Tobin MJ. Dyspnea. Pathophysiologic basis, clinical presentation, and management. [Review]. Arch Intern Med 1990;150:1604–1613.

Mahler DA, Horowitz MB. Clinical evaluation of exertional dyspnea. Clin Chest Med 1994;15:259–269.

Silvestri GA, Mahler DA. Evaluation of dyspnea in the elderly patient. [Review]. Clin Chest Med 1993;14:393–404.

See Also

- Asthma
- Chronic obstructive pulmonary disease

Dyspnea, Episodic

Indications and Timing for Referral

- Cardiac condition has been ruled out
- No clinical evidence of congestive heart failure exists
- Radiograph, chest is negative
- No obvious cause of the dyspnea can be found

Timing: Routine (less than 4 weeks)

Tests to Prepare for Consult

- Radiograph, chest, PA and lateral
- Spirometry, before and after bronchodilator
- CBC
- ECG

Tests Not Useful Before Consult

- CT scan, thorax

Tests Consultant May Need to Do

- Spirometry, before and after bronchodilator
- Lung volumes
- Flow volume loops
- Lung CO diffusing capacity
- Arterial blood gas
- Methacholine challenge
- Pulmonary exercise test
- V/Q scan

Follow-up Visits Generally Required

- Two

Suggested Readings

Gillespie DJ, Staats BA. Unexplained dyspnea. Mayo Clin Proc 1994;69:657–663.

Mahler DA, Horowitz MB. Clinical evaluation of exertional dyspnea. Clin Chest Med 1994;15:259–269.

Mulrow CD, Lucey CR, Farnett LE. Discriminating causes of dyspnea through clinical examination. J Gen Intern Med 1993;8:383–392.

DePaso WJ, Winterbauer RH, Lusk JA, et al. Chronic dyspnea unexplained by history, physical examination, chest roentgenogram, and spirometry. Analysis of a seven-year experience. Chest 1991;100:1293–1299.

Silvestri GA, Mahler DA. Evaluation of dyspnea in the elderly patient. [Review]. Clin Chest Med 1993;14:393–404.

Tobin MJ. Dyspnea. Pathophysiologic basis, clinical presentation, and management. [Review]. Arch Intern Med 1990;150:1604–1613.

See Also

- Asthma
- Chronic obstructive pulmonary disease

Dyspnea, Nocturnal

Indications and Timing for Referral

- Cardiac condition has been ruled out
- No clinical evidence of congestive heart failure exists
- Radiograph, chest is negative
- No obvious cause of the dyspnea can be found

Timing: Routine (less than 4 weeks)

Tests to Prepare for Consult

- Radiograph, chest, PA and lateral
- Spirometry
- ECG

Tests Not Useful Before Consult

- CT scan, thorax

Tests Consultant May Need to Do

- Spirometry
- Methacholine challenge
- Echocardiogram with Doppler studies
- Esophageal pH monitoring

Follow-up Visits Generally Required

- Two

Suggested Readings

Gillespie DJ, Staats BA. Unexplained dyspnea. Mayo Clin Proc 1994;69:657–663.

Bradley TD. Breathing disorders in sleep. Clin Chest Med 1992;13:383.

Silvestri GA, Mahler DA. Evaluation of dyspnea in the elderly patient. [Review]. Clin Chest Med 1993;14:393–404.

See Also

- Sleep apnea/snoring

Hemoptysis

Indications and Timing for Referral
- Massive hemoptysis or associated hypotension requires immediate evaluation, as may hemoptysis associated with dyspnea or tachycardia
- Hemoptysis of greater than 1/2 cup (4 oz, 125 mL) blood

Timing: Urgent (less than 24 hours)

- Hemoptysis of greater than 1 Tbs (1/2 oz, 15 mL) pure blood

Timing: Expedited (less than 1 week)

- Hemoptysis of blood streaked sputum or small amounts of clotted blood for longer than 1 week without other evidence of respiratory infection
- Hemoptysis of blood-streaked sputum persisting for longer than 2 weeks despite appropriate antibiotic therapy for respiratory infection
- Recurrent episodes of hemoptysis

Timing: Routine (less than 4 weeks)

Advice for Referral
- Expectoration of bright red blood suggests hemoptysis is more likely than hematemesis.
- Indication for consultation may be less compelling if sputum is simply blood-tinged, particularly with other features of respiratory infection.
- Chest radiograph is useful in defining the need and timing of consultation:
  - If positive, see appropriate topic for further recommendations (e.g., pulmonary nodule).
  - If negative, indication and urgency of consultation are less.
- Smoking history is useful in defining need for consultation:
  - In nonsmokers under 40 years old, hemoptysis rarely requires extensive evaluation.
  - In smokers, the threshold for consultation should be lower.

Tests to Prepare for Consult
- Radiograph, chest, PA and lateral

Hemoptysis (continued)

Tests Not Useful Before Consult
- None

Tests Consultant May Need to Do
- Sputum cytology
- Coagulation studies as appropriate
- CT scan, thorax
- Bronchoscopy
- Sputum
  - AFB culture
  - AFB stain
  - Fungal culture
  - Fungal stain
- ANCA

Follow-up Visits Generally Required
- Two

See Also
- Cough, chronic
- Pneumonia, lobar
- Lung cancer, non-small cell

Suggested Readings

Colice GL. Hemoptysis. Three questions that can direct management. [Review] [16 refs]. Postgrad Med 1996;100:227–236.

Colice GL. Detecting lung cancer as a cause of hemoptysis in patients with a normal chest radiograph: bronchoscopy vs CT [see comments]. Chest 1997;111:877–884.

McGuinness G, Beacher JR, Harkin TJ, et al. Hemoptysis: prospective high-resolution CT/bronchoscopic correlation [see comments]. Chest 1994;105:1155–1162.

Santiago S, Tobias J, Williams AJ. A reappraisal of the causes of hemoptysis. Arch Intern Med 1991;151:2449–2451.

Nelson JE, Forman M. Hemoptysis in HIV-infected patients. Chest 1996;110:737–743.

Haponik EF, Chin R. Hemoptysis: clinicians' perspectives [see comments]. Chest 1990;97:469–475.

Inhalation, Toxic

Indications and Timing for Referral

- Diagnosis uncertain after initial testing
- Symptoms poorly controlled

Timing: Routine (less than 4 weeks)

Tests to Prepare for Consult

- Radiograph, chest, PA and lateral
- CBC with differential
- Spirometry

Tests Not Useful Before Consult

- None

Tests Consultant May Need to Do

- Spirometry, serial
- Arterial blood gas
- Methacholine challenge
- Pulmonary function tests
- Theophylline level
- Skin testing

Follow-up Visits Generally Required

- One

Suggested Readings

Rorison DG, McPherson SJ. Acute toxic inhalations. [Review]. Emerg Med Clin North Am 1992;10:409–435.

Wright JL. Inhalational lung injury causing bronchiolitis. [Review]. Clin Chest Med 1993;14:635–644.

Haponik EF, Crapo RO, Herndon DN, et al. Smoke inhalation. Am Rev Respir Dis 1988;138:1060–1063.

Lung Cancer, Non-Small Cell

Indications and Timing for Referral
- Preoperative staging needed
- Assessment of operability

Timing: Expedited (less than 1 week)

Tests to Prepare for Consult
- Spirometry
- CBC
- Electrolytes (Na, K, Cl, CO_2)
- Creatinine
- Calcium, phosphorus
- CT scan, thorax with upper abdominal cuts

Tests Not Useful Before Consult
- None

Tests Consultant May Need to Do
- Arterial blood gas
- Spirometry
- Lung volumes
- V/Q scan, quantitative, split function
- Bronchoscopy

Follow-up Visits Generally Required
- One

Suggested Readings

Feld R, Borges M, Giner V, et al. Prognostic factors in non-small cell lung cancer. Lung Cancer 1994;11(Suppl 3):S19–S23.

Ferguson MK. Diagnosing and staging of non-small cell lung cancer. [Review]. Hematol Oncol Clin North Am 1990;4:1053–1068.

Patel AM, Dunn WF, Trastek VF. Staging systems of lung cancer. [Review]. Mayo Clin Proc 1993;68:475–482.

Jett JR. Current treatment of unresectable lung cancer. [Review]. Mayo Clin Proc 1993;68:603–611.

Ihde DC, Minna JD. Non-small cell lung cancer: biology, diagnosis, and staging. Curr Probl Cancer 1991;15:61–104.

Natale RB. Overview of current and future chemotherapeutic agents in non-small cell lung cancer. [Review] [59 refs]. Semin Oncol 1997;24(Suppl 7):S7–29–S7–37.

Selected Guidelines

Screening for lung cancer. In: U. S. Preventive Services Task Force Guide to Clinical Preventive Services: an Assessment of the Effectiveness of 169 Interventions: Report of the U. S. Preventive Services Task Force Baltimore: Williams & Wilkins, c1989:67–70 1995; U.S. Preventive Serv-70.

THE CONSULTATION GUIDE

Lung Disease, Air Travel with

Indications and Timing for Referral

- Concern about safety

Timing: Routine (less than 4 weeks)

Advice for Referral

- If room air arterial blood gas is less than 70 mm Hg, consider advising patient to use supplemental oxygen on the plane.
- Private planes are typically non-pressurized.
- Seldom a problem if PaO_2 is greater than 65 mm Hg and patient is not on oxygen therapy.
- If patient is on home oxygen increase oxygen by 1 liter from baseline.
- M.D. must send a letter with approval for patient to fly with oxygen.
- Advise patient not to pack medication or oxygen in checked luggage.
- Contact airline in advance of travel to arrange in-flight oxygen.

Tests to Prepare for Consult

- None

Tests Not Useful Before Consult

- None

Tests Consultant May Need to Do

- None

Follow-up Visits Generally Required

- None

Suggested Readings

Dillard TA, Beninati WA, Berg BW. Air travel in patients with chronic obstructive pulmonary disease. Arch Intern Med 1991;151:1793–1795.

Vohra KP, Klocke RA. Detection and correction of hypoxemia associated with air travel. Am Rev Respir Dis 1993;148:1215–1219.

Berg BW. Oxygen supplementation during air travel in patients with chronic obstructive lung disease. Chest 1992;101:638–641.

Lung Disease, Handicapped License Plates with

Indications and Timing for Referral
- To determine eligibility

Timing: Routine (less than 4 weeks)

Advice for Referral
- To qualify must have FEV_1 less than 1 L, or their PaO_2 decreases to inadequate level during exercise on supplemental oxygen, with the exceptions of interstitial lung disease or pulmonary vascular disease.
- May vary by state.

Tests to Prepare for Consult
- None

Tests Not Useful Before Consult
- None

Tests Consultant May Need to Do
- Spirometry
- Oxygen saturation level

Follow-up Visits Generally Required
- None

Suggested Readings
Ortega F, Montemayor T, Sanchez A, et al. Role of cardiopulmonary exercise testing and the criteria used to determine disability in patients with severe chronic obstructive pulmonary disease. Am J Respir Crit Care Med 1994;150:747–751.

Selected Guidelines
Guidelines for the evaluation of impairment/disability in patients with asthma. American Thoracic Society. Medical Section of the American Lung Association [see comments]. Am Rev Respir Dis 1993;147:1056–1061.

Lung Disease, Occupational

Indications and Timing for Referral
- Patient symptomatic
- Abnormal chest radiograph
- Determine appropriateness of job change

Timing: Routine (less than 4 weeks)

Tests to Prepare for Consult
- Radiograph, chest, PA and lateral
- Spirometry, before and after bronchodilator

Tests Not Useful Before Consult
- None

Tests Consultant May Need to Do
- Lung volumes
- Lung CO diffusing capacity
- Arterial blood gas
- Spirometry, postprovocation
- CT scan, thorax

Follow-up Visits Generally Required
- One

Suggested Readings
Schwartz DA, Peterson MW. Occupational lung disease. [Review] [161 refs]. Adv Intern Med 1997;42:269–312.

Epler GR. Clinical overview of occupational lung disease. [Review]. Radiol Clin North Am 1992;30:1121–1133.

Alberts WM, Brooks SM. Advances in occupational asthma. [Review]. Clin Chest Med 1992;13:281–302.

Whitesell PL, Drage CW. Occupational lung cancer. [Review]. Mayo Clin Proc 1993;68:183–8.

Esposito AL. Pulmonary infections acquired in the workplace. A review of occupation-associated pneumonia. [Review]. Clin Chest Med 1992;13:355–365.

See Also
- Asthma, occupational
- Disability evaluation, lung disease

PULMONARY

Lung Disease, Scuba Diving Clearance with

Indications and Timing for Referral

- Concern about safety

Timing: Routine (less than 4 weeks)

Advice for Referral

- Contraindicated if history of any previous pneumothorax or giant bullae, or
- Previous associated history of symptomatic airflow obstruction

Tests to Prepare for Consult

- None

Tests Not Useful Before Consult

- None

Tests Consultant May Need to Do

- Spirometry, before and after bronchodilator

Follow-up Visits Generally Required

- None

Suggested Readings

Neuman TS, Bove AA, O'Connor RD, Kelsen SG. Asthma and diving. [Review]. Ann Allergy 1994;73:344–350.

Wallace JM, Stein S, Au J. Special problems of the asthmatic patient. [Review] [60 refs]. Curr Opin Pulm Med 1997;3:72–79.

Smith TF. The medical problems of underwater diving [letter; comment]. N Engl J Med 1992;326:1497–1498.

THE CONSULTATION GUIDE

Pleural Effusion

Indications and Timing for Referral

- Increasing effusion with dyspnea
- Suspected empyema

Timing: Urgent (less than 24 hours)

- Need assistance with pleural tap
- Sclerosis needed to provide symptomatic relief
- Diagnostic uncertainty

Timing: Expedited (less than 1 week)

Advice for Referral

- Thoracentesis should be performed by an M.D. appropriately skilled.
- Patients with a history of previously treated malignancy may best be referred directly to oncology.

Tests to Prepare for Consult

- CBC
- Albumin, total protein
- LDH
- Creatinine
- Glucose
- ALT, AST, alkaline phosphatase
- Radiograph, chest, PA and lateral
- Thoracentesis

Tests Not Useful Before Consult

- None

Tests Consultant May Need to Do

- Radiograph, chest, lateral decubitus
- PPD
- CT scan, thorax
- Thoracentesis
- Pleural biopsy

Follow-up Visits Generally Required

- One

Suggested Readings

Berkman N, Kramer MR. Diagnostic tests in pleural effusion-an update. Postgrad Med J 1993;69:12–18.

Bartter T, Santarelli R, Akers SM, Pratter MR. The evaluation of pleural effusion [published erratum appears in Chest 1995;107:592]. [Review]. Chest 1994;106:1209–1214.

Kennedy L, Sahn SA. Noninvasive evaluation of the patient with a pleural effusion. [Review]. Chest Surg Clin North Am 1994;4:451–465.

Miles DW, Knight RK. Diagnosis and management of malignant pleural effusion. Cancer Treat Rev 1993;19:151–168.

Lynch TJ Jr. Management of malignant pleural effusions. [Review]. Chest 1993;103(Suppl):385S–389S.

Strange C, Sahn SA. Management of parapneumonic pleural effusions and empyema. [Review]. Infect Dis Clin North Am 1991;5:539–559.

Pneumonia, Immunocompromised Host

Indications and Timing for Referral

- HIV-positive patients with PaO_2 less than 70 mm Hg
- Rapidly progressive symptoms (over 1 to 3 days)

Timing: Urgent (less than 24 hours)

- Progressive symptoms (over 3 to 7 days)
- Chronic symptoms with slow progression (over 1 to 4 weeks)

Timing: Expedited (less than 1 week)

Tests to Prepare for Consult

- Radiograph, chest, PA and lateral
- CD4 count
- Sputum, induced for Gram stain and culture
- PCP, induced sputum
- Sputum, fungal culture
- Sputum, fungal stain

Tests Not Useful Before Consult

- None

Tests Consultant May Need to Do

- Arterial blood gas
- Bronchoscopy with lavage
- Transbronchial biopsy

Follow-up Visits Generally Required

- One

Suggested Readings

Santamauro JT, Stover DE. *Pneumocystis carinii* pneumonia. [Review] [102 refs]. Med Clin North Am 1997;81:299–318.

Boiselle PM, Tocino I, Hooley RJ, et al. Chest radiograph interpretation of *Pneumocystis carinii* pneumonia, bacterial pneumonia, and pulmonary tuberculosis in HIV-positive patients: accuracy, distinguishing features, and mimics. J Thorac Imaging 1997;12:47–53.

Fraser JL, Lilly C, Israel E, et al. Diagnostic yield of bronchoalveolar lavage and bronchoscopic lung biopsy for detection of *Pneumocystis carinii* [see comments]. Mayo Clin Proc 1996;71:1025–1029.

Chaisson RE. Bacterial pneumonia in patients with human immunodeficiency virus infection. [Review]. Semin Respir Infect 1989;4:133–138.

Morris DJ. Cytomegalovirus pneumonia—a consequence of immunosuppression and pre-existing lung damage rather than immunopathology? [Review]. Respir Med 1993;87:345–349.

Whimbey E, Bodey GP. Viral pneumonia in the immunocompromised adult with neoplastic disease: the role of common community respiratory viruses. [Review]. Semin Respir Infect 1992;7:122–131.

See Also

- Pulmonary consolidation
- Pneumonia, poorly resolving
- Pneumonia, lobar

Pneumonia, Lobar

Indications and Timing for Referral

- Immunocompromised patient
- Accompanied by persistent clinical evidence of systemic or local infection

Timing: Expedited (less than 1 week)

- No radiological resolution after 6 to 8 weeks despite therapy
- Poor clinical response, e.g., cough persists at 12 weeks

Timing: Routine (less than 4 weeks)

Tests to Prepare for Consult

- Radiograph, chest, PA and lateral
- Radiograph, chest, obtain old films
- CBC
- PPD

Tests Not Useful Before Consult

- None

Tests Consultant May Need to Do

- Sputum
    - Routine culture
    - PCP stain
    - AFB culture
    - AFB stain
    - Fungal stain
    - Cytology
- HIV antibody testing
- Arterial blood gas
- *Legionella* serology
- CT scan, thorax
- Bronchoscopy

Follow-up Visits Generally Required

- One

Suggested Readings

Fang GD. New and emerging etiologies for community-acquired pneumonia with implications for therapy. Medicine 1991;69:307–316.

Coley CM, Li YH, Medsger AR, et al. Preferences for home vs hospital care among low-risk patients with community-acquired pneumonia. Arch Intern Med 1996;156:1565–1571.

Musher DM. Pneumococcal pneumonia including diagnosis and therapy of infection caused by penicillin-resistant strains. [Review]. Infect Dis Clin North Am 1991;5:509–521.

Gleason PP, Kapoor WN, Stone RA, et al. Medical outcomes and antimicrobial costs with the use of the American Thoracic Society guidelines for outpatients with community-acquired pneumonia. JAMA 1997;278:32–39.

Selected Guidelines

Niederman MS, Bass JB Jr, Campbell GD, et al. Guidelines for the initial management of adults with community-acquired pneumonia: diagnosis, assessment of severity, and initial antimicrobial therapy. American Thoracic Society. Medical Section of the American Lung Association. Am Rev Respir Dis 1993;148:1418–1426.

Guidelines for the management of community-acquired pneumonia in adults admitted to hospital. The British Thoracic Society. [Review] [14 refs]. Br J Hosp Med 1993;49:346–350.

See Also

- Pneumonia, immunocompromised host
- Pulmonary consolidation
- Pneumonia, poorly resolving

PULMONARY

Pneumonia, Poorly Resolving

Indications and Timing for Referral

- Accompanied by persistent clinical evidence of systemic or local infection
- Immunocompromised patient

Timing: Expedited (less than 1 week)

- No radiological resolution after 6 to 8 weeks despite therapy
- Poor clinical response, e.g., cough persists at 12 weeks

Timing: Routine (less than 4 weeks)

Tests to Prepare for Consult

- Radiograph, chest
- Radiograph, chest, obtain old films
- CBC
- PPD

Tests Not Useful Before Consult

- None

Tests Consultant May Need to Do

- HIV antibody testing
- Sputum
    - Routine culture
    - Gram stain
    - PCP stain
    - AFB stain
    - AFB culture
    - Cytology
    - Fungal stain
- CT scan, thorax
- Bronchoscopy
- ANCA

Follow-up Visits Generally Required

- One

Suggested Readings

Corley DE, Winterbauer RH. Infectious diseases that result in slowly resolving and chronic pneumonia. [Review]. Semin Respir Infect 1993;8:3–13.

Kirtland SH, Winterbauer RH, Dreis DF, et al. A clinical profile of chronic bacterial pneumonia. Report of 115 cases. Chest 1994;106:15–22.

Fein AM, Feinsilver SH. The approach to nonresolving pneumonia in the elderly. [Review]. Semin Respir Infect 1993;8:59–72.

Geppert EF. Chronic and recurrent pneumonia. [Review]. Semin Respir Infect 1992;7:282–288.

Gross TJ, Chavis AD, Lynch JP 3d. Noninfectious pulmonary diseases masquerading as community-acquired pneumonia. [Review]. Clin Chest Med 1991;12:363–393.

See Also

- Pulmonary consolidation
- Pneumonia, lobar
- Pneumonia, immunocompromised host

THE CONSULTATION GUIDE

Pneumothorax, Recurrent

Indications and Timing for Referral

- Etiology unclear
- Identify possible underlying lung disease

Timing: Routine (less than 4 weeks)

Tests to Prepare for Consult

- Radiograph, chest, obtain old films
- Radiograph, chest, PA and lateral

Tests Not Useful Before Consult

- None

Tests Consultant May Need to Do

- Lung CO diffusing capacity
- Lung volumes
- Pulmonary function tests
- CT scan, thorax

Follow-up Visits Generally Required

- One

Suggested Readings

Bense L. Spontaneous pneumothorax [editorial]. [Review]. Chest 1992;101:891–892.

Peters JI, Sako EY. Pneumothorax. In: Fishman AP, Elias JA, Fishman JA, et al., eds. Fishman's Pulmonary Diseases and Disorders. 3rd ed. New York: McGraw Hill, 1998:1439–1451.

Selected Guidelines

Miller AC, Harvey JE. Guidelines for the management of spontaneous pneumothorax. Standards of Care Committee, British Thoracic Society [published erratum appears in Br Med J 1993;307:308] [see comments]. Br Med J 1993;307:114–116.

PULMONARY

Preoperative Pulmonary Assessment

Indications and Timing for Referral

- Patient with moderate to severe lung disease (FEV_1 less than 65%) undergoing thoracic surgery
- Patient with severe lung disease (FEV_1 less than 50%) undergoing abdominal surgery
- Patient with very severe lung disease (FEV_1 less than 35%, PaO_2 less than 55 mm Hg, or $PaCO_2$ greater than 45 mm Hg) undergoing general anesthesia
- Patient has history of asthma with need for either multiple or prolonged courses of systemic glucocorticoids

Timing: Routine (less than 4 weeks)

Advice for Referral

- Pulmonologist or qualified internist may be appropriate consultant.

Tests to Prepare for Consult

- Radiograph, chest, PA and lateral
- Spirometry, before and after bronchodilator
- Arterial blood gas

Tests Not Useful Before Consult

- None

Tests Consultant May Need to Do

- None

Follow-up Visits Generally Required

- None

Suggested Readings

Mohr DN, Lavender RC. Preoperative pulmonary evaluation. Identifying patients at increased risk for complications. [Review] [28 refs]. Postgrad Med 1996;100:241–244.

Zibrak JD, O'Donnell CR. Indications for preoperative pulmonary function testing. [Review]. Clin Chest Med 1993;14:227–236.

Lawrence VA, Page CP, Harris GD. Preoperative spirometry before abdominal operations. A critical appraisal of its predictive value. [Review]. Arch Intern Med 1989;149:280–285.

Crapo RO. Pulmonary-function testing [see comments]. [Review]. N Engl J Med 1994;331:25–30.

Reilly JJ Jr, Mentzer SJ, Sugarbaker DJ. Preoperative assessment of patients undergoing pulmonary resection. [Review]. Chest 1993;103(Suppl):342S–345S.

Pulmonary Consolidation

Indications and Timing for Referral

- Etiology is unclear
- Consolidation is slow to resolve (no improvement after more than 4 weeks)

Timing: Routine (less than 4 weeks)

Tests to Prepare for Consult

- Radiograph, chest, PA and lateral
- Radiograph, chest, obtain old films
- CBC
- PPD

Tests Not Useful Before Consult

- None

Tests Consultant May Need to Do

- CT scan, thorax
- Bronchoscopy
- Sputum cytology

Follow-up Visits Generally Required

- One

Suggested Readings

Gross TJ, Chavis AD, Lynch JP 3d. Noninfectious pulmonary diseases masquerading as community-acquired pneumonia. [Review]. Clin Chest Med 1991;12:363–393.

Gleason PP, Kapoor WN, Stone RA, et al. Medical outcomes and antimicrobial costs with the use of the American Thoracic Society guidelines for outpatients with community-acquired pneumonia. JAMA 1997;278:32–39.

Marrie TJ. Acute bronchitis and community-acquired pneumonia. In: Fishman AP, Elias JA, Fishman JA, et al., eds. Fishman's Pulmonary Diseases and Disorders. 3rd ed. New York: McGraw Hill, 1998:1985–1995.

Selected Guidelines

Niederman MS, Bass JB Jr, Campbell GD, et al. Guidelines for the initial management of adults with community-acquired pneumonia: diagnosis, assessment of severity, and initial antimicrobial therapy. American Thoracic Society. Medical Section of the American Lung Association. Am Rev Respir Dis 1993;148:1418–1426.

Guidelines for the management of community-acquired pneumonia in adults admitted to hospital. The British Thoracic Society. Br J Hosp Med 1993;49:346–350.

See Also

- Pneumonia, lobar
- Pneumonia, poorly resolving
- Atelectasis
- Pneumonia, immunocompromised host

Pulmonary Fibrosis, Interstitial

Indications and Timing for Referral

- Rapidly progressive symptoms

Timing: Expedited (less than 1 week)

- Etiology unclear
- Slowly progressive symptoms

Timing: Routine (less than 4 weeks)

Advice for Referral

- Patients with confirmed interstitial pulmonary fibrosis should see a pulmonologist at least once for baseline evaluation.

Tests to Prepare for Consult

- Radiograph, chest, PA and lateral
- Spirometry
- Lung volumes
- Lung CO diffusing capacity
- CBC

Tests Not Useful Before Consult

- None

Tests Consultant May Need to Do

- Radiograph, chest, PA and lateral
- Spirometry, before and after bronchodilator
- Lung volumes
- Lung CO diffusing capacity
- CBC with differential
- ANA
- Rheumatoid factor
- Exercise test for oxygen titration
- CT scan, thorax, high resolution
- Bronchoscopy
- Transbronchial biopsy

Follow-up Visits Generally Required

- Two

Suggested Readings

DuBois RM. Idiopathic pulmonary fibrosis. Annu Rev Med 1993;44:441–450.

Lynch JP 3d, Hunninghake GW. Pulmonary complications of collagen vascular disease. [Review]. Annu Rev Med 1992;43:17–35.

Cherniack RM. Current concepts in idiopathic pulmonary fibrosis: a road map for the future. Am Rev Respir Dis 1991;143:680–683.

Panos RJ, Mortenson RL, Niccoli SA, King TE Jr. Clinical deterioration in patients with idiopathic pulmonary fibrosis: causes and assessment. [Review]. Am J Med 1990;88:396–404.

Hunninghake GW, Kalica AR. Approaches to the treatment of pulmonary fibrosis. Am J Respir Crit Care Med 1995;151:915–918.

See Also

- Pulmonary infiltrate with eosinophilia

Pulmonary Hypertension, Primary

Indications and Timing for Referral
- Severe dyspnea

Timing: Urgent (less than 24 hours)

- Progressive symptoms

Timing: Expedited (less than 1 week)

- Etiology is unclear

Timing: Routine (less than 4 weeks)

Advice for Referral
- This condition often requires co-management with pulmonologist.
- The accuracy of home sleep studies remains to be established.

Tests to Prepare for Consult
- Radiograph, chest, PA and lateral
- CBC
- Arterial blood gas
- ECG
- Echocardiogram with Doppler studies

Tests Not Useful Before Consult
- None

Tests Consultant May Need to Do
- Spirometry, before and after bronchodilator
- Lung volumes
- Lung CO diffusing capacity
- Pulmonary exercise test
- ANA
- Noninvasive venous studies
- V/Q scan
- CT scan, thorax
- Sleep study (see *Advice for Referral*)

Follow-up Visits Generally Required
- Co-management, see *Advice for Referral*

Suggested Readings
Rubin LJ. Primary pulmonary hypertension. [Review] [53 refs]. N Engl J Med 1997;336:111–117.

Rabinovitch M. Pulmonary hypertension: updating a mysterious disease. [Review] [31 refs]. Cardiovasc Res 1997;34:268–272.

Dinh Xuan AT, Higenbottam TW, Scott JP, Wallwork J. Primary pulmonary hypertension: diagnosis, medical and surgical treatment. [Review]. Respir Med 1990;84:189–197.

Sobieraj J. Appetite-suppressant drugs and primary pulmonary hypertension [letter; comment]. N Engl J Med 1997;336:510; discussion 512–513.

Palevsky HI, Fishman AP. The management of primary pulmonary hypertension. [Review]. JAMA 1991;265:1014–1020.

D'Alonzo GE. Survival in patients with pulmonary hypertension: results from a national prospective study. Ann Intern Med 1991;115:343–349.

See Also
- Chronic obstructive pulmonary disease
- Cor pulmonale

PULMONARY

Pulmonary Infiltrate with Eosinophilia

Indications and Timing for Referral

- Diagnosis uncertain
- Progressive symptoms

Timing: Routine (less than 4 weeks)

Tests to Prepare for Consult

- Radiograph, chest, PA and lateral
- CBC with differential

Tests Not Useful Before Consult

- None

Tests Consultant May Need to Do

- Spirometry, before and after bronchodilator
- Lung volumes
- Lung CO diffusing capacity
- Stool, ova, and parasites
- Arterial blood gas

Follow-up Visits Generally Required

- Two

Suggested Readings

Allen JN, Davis WB. Eosinophilic lung diseases. [Review]. Am J Respir Crit Care Med 1994;150:1423–1438.

Ottesen EA, Nutman TB. Tropical pulmonary eosinophilia. [Review]. Annu Rev Med 1992;43:417–424.

Umeki S. Reevaluation of eosinophilic pneumonia and its diagnostic criteria [see comments]. Arch Intern Med 1992;152:1913–1919.

See Also

- Pulmonary fibrosis, interstitial

Pulmonary Nodules, Multiple

Indications and Timing for Referral
- Etiology unclear

Timing: Expedited (less than 1 week)

Advice for Referral
- Factors favoring referral to infectious diseases include:
  - Fever present
  - Elevated WBC or left shift
- Factors favoring referral to hematology/oncology include:
  - History of primary malignancy with potential for pulmonary spread
  - Nodules persist without inflammation
- Factors favoring referral to surgeon or invasive radiology include:
  - Biopsy anticipated

Tests to Prepare for Consult
- Radiograph, chest, PA and lateral
- Radiograph, chest, obtain old films
- CBC
- Electrolytes (Na, K, Cl, CO_2)
- Calcium, phosphorus
- Creatinine
- CT scan, thorax, without contrast

Tests Not Useful Before Consult
- None

Tests Consultant May Need to Do
- PPD
- ANCA
- Bronchoscopy
- Transthoracic needle biopsy

Follow-up Visits Generally Required
- One

Suggested Readings
Lillington GA, Caskey CI. Evaluation and management of solitary and multiple pulmonary nodules. [Review]. Clin Chest Med 1993;14:111–119.

Viggiano RW, Swensen SJ, Rosenow EC 3d. Evaluation and management of solitary and multiple pulmonary nodules. [Review]. Clin Chest Med 1992;13:83–95.

PULMONARY

Pulmonary Nodules, Solitary, Central

Indications and Timing for Referral

- Etiology unclear

Timing: Routine (less than 4 weeks)

Advice for Referral

- If patient has history of primary malignancy with potential for pulmonary spread, initial oncology referral may be appropriate.

Tests to Prepare for Consult

- Radiograph, chest, PA and lateral
- Radiograph, chest, obtain old films
- Sputum cytology
- CT scan, thorax, quantify lesion density

Tests Not Useful Before Consult

- Radiograph, other

Tests Consultant May Need to Do

- Bronchoscopy
- Mediastinoscopy

Follow-up Visits Generally Required

- One

Suggested Readings

Midthun DE, Swensen SJ, Jett JR. Approach to the solitary pulmonary nodule [see comments]. [Review] [62 refs]. Mayo Clin Proc 1993;68:378–385.

Lillington GA. Management of solitary pulmonary nodules. How to decide when resection is required. [Review] [10 refs]. Postgrad Med 1997;101:145–150.

Lillington GA, Caskey CI. Evaluation and management of solitary and multiple pulmonary nodules. [Review]. Clin Chest Med 1993;14:111–119.

Caskey CI, Templeton PA, Zerhouni EA. Current evaluation of the solitary pulmonary nodule. [Review]. Radiol Clin North Am 1990;28:511–512.

Viggiano RW, Swensen SJ, Rosenow EC 3d. Evaluation and management of solitary and multiple pulmonary nodules. [Review]. Clin Chest Med 1992;13:83–95.

Howard TA, Woodring JH. Clinical and imaging evaluation of the solitary pulmonary nodule. [Review]. Am Fam Physician 1992;46:1753–1759.

Selected Guidelines

Screening for lung cancer. In: U. S. Preventive Services Task Force Guide to Clinical Preventive Services: an Assessment of the Effectiveness of 169 Interventions: Report of the U. S. Preventive Services Task Force. Baltimore: Williams & Wilkins, 1989: 67–70. 1995; U.S. Preventive Serv-70.

See Also

- Pulmonary nodules, solitary, peripheral
- Pulmonary nodules, multiple

Pulmonary Nodules, Solitary, Peripheral

Indications and Timing for Referral

- Enlarging nodule, or when change in size over time cannot be determined

Timing: Expedited (less than 1 week)

Advice for Referral

- A nodule unchanged in size for 2 years is usually benign.
- Evaluation of nodules detected in the setting of respiratory infection should usually be deferred until after 2 weeks of antibiotic therapy.

Tests to Prepare for Consult

- Radiograph, chest, PA and lateral
- Radiograph, chest, obtain old films
- CT scan, thorax, quantify lesion density

Tests Not Useful Before Consult

- Sputum cytology
- Radiograph, other

Tests Consultant May Need to Do

- Spirometry
- PPD
- Transthoracic needle biopsy

Follow-up Visits Generally Required

- One

Suggested Readings

Caskey CI, Templeton PA, Zerhouni EA. Current evaluation of the solitary pulmonary nodule. [Review]. Radiol Clin North Am 1990;28:511–520.

Midthun DE, Swensen SJ, Jett JR. Clinical strategies for solitary pulmonary nodule. [Review]. Annu Rev Med 1992;43:195–208.

Dholakia S, Rappaport DC. The solitary pulmonary nodule—is it malignant or benign. Postgrad Med 1996;99:246–250.

Lillington GA. Management of solitary pulmonary nodules. How to decide when resection is required. [Review] [10 refs]. Postgrad Med 1997;101:145–150.

Lillington GA, Caskey CI. Evaluation and management of solitary and multiple pulmonary nodules. [Review]. Clin Chest Med 1993;14:111–119.

Viggiano RW, Swensen SJ, Rosenow EC 3d. Evaluation and management of solitary and multiple pulmonary nodules. [Review]. Clin Chest Med 1992;13(1):83–95.

See Also

- Pulmonary nodules, solitary, central
- Lung cancer, non-small cell
- Pulmonary nodules, multiple

PULMONARY

Reactive Airway Dysfunction Syndrome

Indications and Timing for Referral

- Diagnosis remains uncertain after initial testing
- Symptoms are poorly controlled

Timing: Routine (less than 4 weeks)

Tests to Prepare for Consult

- Radiograph, chest, PA and lateral
- CBC with differential
- Spirometry, before and after bronchodilator

Tests Not Useful Before Consult

- None

Tests Consultant May Need to Do

- Spirometry, serial
- Arterial blood gas
- Methacholine challenge
- Pulmonary function tests
- Theophylline level
- Skin testing

Follow-up Visits Generally Required

- One

Suggested Readings

Becklake MR. The relationship between acute and chronic airway responses to occupational exposures. Curr Pulmonol 1988;9:25.

Boulet LP. Increases in airway responsiveness following acute exposure to respiratory irritants. Reactive airway dysfunction syndrome or occupational asthma? Chest 1988;94:476–481.

Selected Guidelines

Allergen skin testing. Board of Directors. American Academy of Allergy and Immunology. J Allergy Clin Immunol 1993;92:636–637.

Guidelines for the measurement of respiratory function. Recommendations of the British Thoracic Society and the Association of Respiratory Technicians and Physiologists. Respir Med 1994;88:165–194.

See Also

- Asthma, occupational
- Inhalation, toxic

Sarcoidosis

Indications and Timing for Referral
- Uncontrolled symptoms
- Hemoptysis

Timing: Expedited (less than 1 week)

- Patient symptomatic with corticosteroid treatment being considered
- Asymmetric bilateral involvement noted
- Advanced or progressive physiologic impairment
- Radiographic deterioration
- Possible fungus ball

Timing: Routine (less than 4 weeks)

Advice for Referral
- To confirm the diagnosis of sarcoidosis, additional referral may be required for biopsy of conjunctiva, lymph nodes or skin lesions.
- Active sarcoidosis often requires co-management with a pulmonologist.

Tests to Prepare for Consult
- Radiograph, chest, PA and lateral
- Electrolytes (Na, K, Cl, CO_2)
- Creatinine
- Calcium, phosphorus
- CBC
- Spirometry, before and after bronchodilator
- Lung CO diffusing capacity

Tests Not Useful Before Consult
- Mediastinoscopy

Tests Consultant May Need to Do
- Spirometry, before and after (if not done in 3 months)
- Lung volumes
- Anergy intradermal skin test panel
- PPD
- CT scan, thorax
- Bronchoscopy
- Transbronchial biopsy

Follow-up Visits Generally Required
- Co-management, see *Advice for Referral*

Suggested Readings
DeRemee RA. Sarcoidosis. [Review]. Mayo Clin Proc 1995;70:177–181.

Sharma OP. Pulmonary sarcoidosis and corticosteroids. [Review]. Am Rev Respir Dis 1993;147:1598–1600.

Johns CJ, Scott PP, Schonfeld SA. Sarcoidosis. [Review]. Annu Rev Med 1989;40:353–371.

Consensus conference: activity of sarcoidosis. Third WASOG meeting, Los Angeles, USA, September 8–11, 1993. [Review]. Eur Respir J 1994;7:624–627.

See Also
- Adenopathy, hilar, bilateral

PULMONARY

Sleep Apnea/Snoring

Indications and Timing for Referral

- Polycythemia
- Severe daytime somnolence
- Cyanosis
- Clinical evidence of right heart failure

Timing: Expedited (less than 1 week)

- Clinical features suggesting sleep apnea, i.e., snoring, intermittent apnea, morning headache, daytime somnolence, severe nocturnal restlessness reported by sleep partner

Timing: Routine (less than 4 weeks)

Advice for Referral

- Patients with snoring and/or obesity alone generally do not require consultation or sleep studies.
- Sleep studies should be requested only from centers with expertise in disordered breathing during sleep.
- The accuracy of home sleep studies remains to be established.
- Premenopausal women with low body mass, small necks, and dysmenorrhea or amenorrhea may have disordered breathing during sleep.

Tests to Prepare for Consult

- Radiograph, chest, PA and lateral
- ECG
- CBC
- TSH

Tests Not Useful Before Consult

- None

Tests Consultant May Need to Do

- Flow volume loops
- Pulmonary function tests
- Arterial blood gas

- Sleep study (see *Advice for Referral*)

Follow-up Visits Generally Required

- One

Suggested Readings

Strollo PJ, Rogers RM. Current concepts—obstructive sleep apnea [review]. N Engl J Med 1996;334:99–104.

Douglas NJ. ABC of sleep disorders. The sleep apnoea/hypopnoea syndrome and snoring [see comments]. [Review]. Br Med J 1993;306:1057–1060.

Wiegand L, Zwillich CW. Obstructive sleep apnea. Dis Mon 1994;40:197–252.

Rice DH. Snoring and obstructive sleep apnea. [Review]. Med Clin North Am 1991;75:1367–1371.

ten Brock E, Shucard DW. Sleep apnea. [Review]. Am Fam Physician 1994;49:385–394.

Kryger MH. Management of obstructive sleep apnea. [Review]. Clin Chest Med 1992;13:481–492.

Selected Guidelines

Indications and standards for cardiopulmonary sleep studies. American Thoracic Society. Medical Section of the American Lung Association [see comments]. Am Rev Respir Dis 1989;139:559–568.

Guideline fifteen: guidelines for polygraphic assessment of sleep-related disorders (polysomnography). American Electroencephalographic Society. J Clin Neurophysiol 1994;11:116–124.

See Also

- Cor pulmonale
- Pulmonary hypertension, primary

Smoking Cessation

Indications and Timing for Referral

- Assistance with motivation and/or program planning

Timing: Routine (less than 4 weeks)

Advice for Referral

- Multidisciplinary programs more effective than single-option methods.
- Patient should be committed to cessation.

Tests to Prepare for Consult

- None

Tests Not Useful Before Consult

- None

Tests Consultant May Need to Do

- None

Follow-up Visits Generally Required

- None

Suggested Readings

Danis PG, Seaton TL. Helping your patients to quit smoking. [Review] [35 refs]. Am Fam Physician 1997;55:1207–1214.

Manley MW, Epps RP, Glynn TJ. The clinician's role in promoting smoking cessation among clinic patients. [Review]. Med Clin North Am 1992;76:477–494.

Schwartz JL. Methods of smoking cessation. [Review]. Med Clin North Am 1992;76:451–476.

Joseph AM, Norman SM, Ferry LH, et al. The safety of transdermal nicotine as an aid to smoking cessation in patients with cardiac disease. N Engl J Med 1996;335:1792–1798.

Fiscella K, Franks P. Cost-effectiveness of the transdermal nicotine patch as an adjunct to physicians' smoking cessation counseling [see comments]. JAMA 1996;275:1247–1251.

Selected Guidelines

The Agency for Health Care Policy and Research Smoking Cessation clinical practice guideline [see comments]. [Review] [68 refs]. JAMA 1996;275:1270–1280.

CHAPTER 11

Rheumatology

Ankylosing Spondylitis 521
Antinuclear Antibody (ANA), Positive 523
Arthritis
    Rheumatoid, Diagnosis 524
    Rheumatoid, Management 526
    with Fever 527
    with Subcutaneous Nodules 528
Bursitis: Shoulder, Elbow, Hip 529
Carpal Tunnel Syndrome 530
Dermatomyositis 531
Discoid/Cutaneous Lupus
    Diagnosis 532
    Management 533
Fasciitis, Plantar 534
Fibrositis/Fibromyalgia 535
Giant Cell/Temporal Arteritis 536
Gout 537
Pain, Chronic Soft Tissue 538
Pain in a Few Joints
    Less Than or Equal to 4 Joints 539
    Greater Than or Equal to 5 Joints 541
Painful
    Ankle, Foot, or Toe 543
    Elbow 545
    Hip 547
    Knee 549
    Lower Back/Lumbosacral Spine 551
    Neck 553
    Shoulder 555
    Upper Back/Thoracic Spine 557
    Wrist and/or Hand 559
Polymyalgia Rheumatica 561
Polymyositis 562
Pseudogout 563
Raynaud's Phenomenon 564
Reiter's Syndrome 565

(continued)

Rheumatology (continued)

Rheumatic Fever 566
Sarcoidosis with Joint Involvement 567
Scleroderma 568
Sicca Complex, Diagnosis 569
Sjögren's Syndrome, Diagnosis 570
Systemic Lupus Erythematosus (SLE)
    Diagnosis 572
    Management 574
    with Nephritis 575
    with Neurologic Involvement 576
Tendonits 578
Tendonitis, Achilles 579

RHEUMATOLOGY

Ankylosing Spondylitis

Indications and Timing for Referral
- Acute complications present, e.g., neurologic impairment or heart failure
- Minor trauma causing persistent or localized spinal pain, potentially due to occult fracture or cauda equina syndrome

Timing: Urgent (less than 24 hours)

- Diagnostic uncertainty based on clinical features or family history
- Associated with known or suspected cardiac or ocular involvement, e.g., heart block or aortic valve dysfunction
- Associated with renal involvement, e.g., amyloidosis or IgA nephropathy
- Associated with pulmonary involvement, e.g., abnormal chest radiograph or chronic pulmonary symptoms
- Extra-articular manifestations of systemic disease present

Timing: Routine (less than 4 weeks)

Advice for Referral
- Obtain old spinal radiographs before consultation.
- Co-management with a rheumatologist is often appropriate.

Tests to Prepare for Consult
- None

Tests Not Useful Before Consult
- ANA
- Rheumatoid factor
- Spinal manipulation

Tests Consultant May Need to Do
- CBC
- ESR
- ALT, AST, alkaline phosphatase
- Calcium
- Creatinine
- Globulin
- Uric acid
- HLA B27
- Urinalysis with microscopic
- Radiographs
    - Relevant peripheral joints
    - Spine
    - Sacroiliac joints
- Joint tap
- Cell count with differential, aspirated fluid
- C&S, aspirated fluid
- Glucose, aspirated fluid
- Crystal analysis, aspirated fluid
- Barium enema
- Small bowel follow through
- Echocardiogram
- Radiograph, chest
- 24-hour urine protein
- 24-hour urine creatinine for clearance
- Abdominal fat pad aspiration for amyloid

Ankylosing Spondylitis (*continued*)

Follow-up Visits Generally Required

- Co-management, see *Advice for Referral*

Suggested Readings

van der Linden S, van der Heijde DM. Clinical and epidemiologic aspects of ankylosing spondylitis and spondyloarthropathies. [Review] [48 refs]. Curr Opin Rheumatol 1996;8:269–274.

Arnett F. Ankylosing spondylitis. In: Koopman WN, ed. Arthritis and Allied Conditions. 13th ed. Baltimore: Williams & Wilkins, 1997:1197–1208.

Ramos-Remus C, Russell AS. Clinical features and management of ankylosing spondylitis. [Review]. Curr Opin Rheumatol 1993;5:408–413.

Toivanen A, Toivanen P. Epidemiologic aspects, clinical features, and management of ankylosing spondylitis and reactive arthritis. [Review]. Curr Opin Rheumatol 1994;6:354–359.

Cuellar ML, Espinoza LR. Management of spondyloarthropathies. [Review] [52 refs]. Curr Opin Rheumatol 1996;8:288–295.

See Also

- Painful, upper back/thoracic spine
- Painful, lower back/lumbosacral spine

RHEUMATOLOGY

Antinuclear Antibody (ANA), Positive

Indications and Timing for Referral
- Assist with determining clinical significance

Timing: Routine (less than 4 weeks)

Advice for Referral
- Patients with a low ANA titer and no clinical manifestations generally do not need to be referred.
- Records of previous relevant serologies, radiographs, and biopsies are vital.

Tests to Prepare for Consult
- ANA
- CBC
- Platelet count
- Creatinine
- Urinalysis with microscopic

Tests Not Useful Before Consult
- Other autoimmune serologies

Tests Consultant May Need to Do
- Anti-Ro (SS-A)
- Anti-double stranded DNA
- Anti-Smith antibody
- Anti-RNP antibody
- Anti-La (SS-B)
- Anticardiolipin antibody
- Lupus anticoagulant (LAC)
- Complement factors (C3, C4)
- RPR or VDRL

Follow-up Visits Generally Required
- One

Suggested Readings

Moder KG. Use and interpretation of rheumatologic tests: a guide for clinicians. Mayo Clin Proc 1996;71:391–396.

Slater CA, Davis RB, Shmerling RH. Antinuclear antibody testing. A study of clinical utility. Arch Intern Med 1996;156:1421–1425.

Reeves WH, Satoh M, Wang J, et al. Systemic lupus erythematosus. Antibodies to DNA, DNA-binding proteins, and histones. [Review]. Rheum Dis Clin North Am 1994;20:1–28.

Clegg DO, Williams HJ, Singer JZ, et al. Early undifferentiated connective tissue disease. II. The frequency of circulating antinuclear antibodies in patients with early rheumatic diseases. J Rheumatol 1991;18:1340–1343.

THE CONSULTATION GUIDE

Arthritis, Rheumatoid, Diagnosis

Indications and Timing for Referral

- Progressive neurologic impairment
- Suspicion of infection

Timing: Urgent (less than 24 hours)

- Associated with severe pain

Timing: Expedited (less than 1 week)

- Associated radiologic abnormalities present
- Diagnosis uncertain with persistent symptoms for longer than 4 weeks
- Failure to follow expected course with conventional therapy
- Assistance with management

Timing: Routine (less than 4 weeks)

Advice for Referral

- Tomographic studies (CT or MR) should be obtained only after preliminary communication with the appropriate consultant.
- Patients in whom a diagnosis of rheumatoid arthritis is established often benefit from co-management with a rheumatologist.

Tests to Prepare for Consult

- CBC with differential
- Platelet count
- ESR
- ALT, AST, alkaline phosphatase
- Calcium
- Creatinine
- Globulin
- Uric acid
- ANA
- Rheumatoid factor

Tests Not Useful Before Consult

- LE prep

Tests Consultant May Need to Do

- Anti-Ro (SS-A)
- Anti-La (SS-B)
- Anti-double stranded DNA
- Anti-Smith antibody
- Antihistone antibody
- Anticentromere antibody
- Anti-scl 70 antibody
- Complement factors (C3, C4)
- Anti-RNP antibody
- Lyme (*Borrelia burgdorferi*) serology
- Urinalysis with microscopic
- Radiograph, relevant joints
- Therapeutic or diagnostic injection of relevant joints
- Radiograph, chest
- Parvovirus B19 serology
- HB_sAg
- Hepatitis C antibody

Arthritis, Rheumatoid, Diagnosis (continued)

Follow-up Visits Generally Required
- One

Suggested Readings
Akil M, Amos RS. ABC of rheumatology. Rheumatoid arthritis—I: Clinical features and diagnosis. [Review]. Br Med J 1995;310:587–590.

Wollheim FA. Established and new biochemical tools for diagnosis and monitoring of rheumatoid arthritis. [Review] [42 refs]. Curr Opin Rheumatol 1996;8:221–225.

Starz TW, Miller EB. Diagnosis and treatment of rheumatoid arthritis. [Review]. Primary Care; Clin Off Pract 1993;20:827–837.

Smith CA, Arnett FC Jr. Diagnosing rheumatoid arthritis: current criteria. [Review]. Am Fam Physician 1991;44:863–870.

Krause A, Kamradt T, Burmester GR. Potential infectious agents in the induction of arthritides. [Review] [65 refs]. Curr Opin Rheumatol 1996;8:203–209.

Wolfe F, Ross K, Hawley DJ, et al. The prognosis of rheumatoid arthritis and undifferentiated polyarthritis syndrome in the clinic: a study of 1141 patients [see comments]. J Rheumatol 1993;20:2005–2009.

See Also
- Arthritis, Rheumatoid, Management
- Pain in a few joints (≤ 4)
- Pain in a few joints (≥ 5)

Arthritis, Rheumatoid, Management

Indications and Timing for Referral
- Suspect complicating infection or acute trauma to joint

Timing: Urgent (less than 24 hours)

- Disease manifestations uncontrolled after 6 weeks of conventional therapy, e.g., nonsteroidal anti-inflammatory drugs (NSAIDs)
- Need for multiple or prolonged courses of systemic glucocorticoids
- Assistance with medical management, e.g., remitting agents or immunosuppressive therapy

Timing: Routine (less than 4 weeks)

Advice for Referral
- Patient should generally be seen early in course of disease by a rheumatologist to assist with long-term management plan.
- Acquire and transfer relevant joint radiographs, previous joint fluid analyses, and serology establishing diagnosis to consultant.
- This condition often requires co-management with a rheumatologist.

Tests to Prepare for Consult
- CBC with differential
- Platelet count
- ESR
- Creatinine
- Albumin, total protein
- ALT
- AST

Tests Not Useful Before Consult
- Autoimmune serologies
- HLA class II oligotyping

Tests Consultant May Need to Do
- CBC with differential
- Platelet count
- ESR
- ANA
- Complement factors (C3, C4)
- Urinalysis with microscopic
- Radiograph, chest
- Radiograph, relevant joints
- Therapeutic or diagnostic injection of relevant joints
- HLA class II oligotyping

Follow-up Visits Generally Required
- Co-management, see *Advice for Referral*

Suggested Readings
Stucki G, Langenegger T. Management of rheumatoid arthritis. [Review] [42 refs]. Curr Opin Rheumatol 1997;9:229–235.

Massarotti EM. Medical aspects of rheumatoid arthritis. Diagnosis and treatment. [Review] [68 refs]. Hand Clin 1996;12:463–475.

O'Dell JR, Haire CE, Erikson N, et al. Treatment of rheumatoid arthritis with methotrexate alone, sulfasalazine and hydroxychloroquine, or a combination of all three medications. N Engl J Med 1996;334:1287–1291.

Felson DT, Anderson JJ, Boers M, et al. The American College of Rheumatology preliminary core set of disease activity measures for rheumatoid arthritis clinical trials. The Committee on Outcome Measures in Rheumatoid Arthritis Clinical Trials. Arthritis Rheum 1993;36:729–740.

Kremer JM, Alarcon GS, Lightfoot RW Jr, et al. Methotrexate for rheumatoid arthritis. Suggested guidelines for monitoring liver toxicity. American College of Rheumatology [see comments]. Arthritis Rheum 1994;37:316–328.

RHEUMATOLOGY

Arthritis, with Fever

Indications and Timing for Referral

- Signs of frank joint inflammation with fever

Timing: Immediate

Advice for Referral

- Patients with true joint inflammation require emergent inpatient or immediate ambulatory evaluation.

Tests to Prepare for Consult

- None

Tests Not Useful Before Consult

- None

Tests Consultant May Need to Do

- None

Follow-up Visits Generally Required

- None

Suggested Readings

Carsons SE. Fever in rheumatic and autoimmune disease. Infect Dis Clin North Am 1996;10:67–84.

Pinals RS. Polyarthritis and fever. [Review]. N Engl J Med 1994;330:769–774.

See Also

- Rheumatic fever

527

Arthritis, with Subcutaneous Nodules

Indications and Timing for Referral
- Progressive neurologic impairment
- Suspicion of infection

Timing: Urgent (less than 24 hours)

- Associated with severe pain

Timing: Expedited (less than 1 week)

- Diagnosis uncertain with persistent symptoms for more than 4 weeks
- Failure to follow expected course with conventional therapy
- Assistance with management

Timing: Routine (less than 4 weeks)

Advice for Referral
- Nodules are usually associated with chronic systemic disease and patient may benefit from co-management with a rheumatologist.

Tests to Prepare for Consult
- CBC
- Platelet count
- ESR
- ALT, AST, alkaline phosphatase
- Calcium
- Creatinine
- Globulin
- Uric acid
- Cholesterol
- Triglycerides
- ANA
- Rheumatoid factor

Tests Not Useful Before Consult
- None

Tests Consultant May Need to Do
- Lipid profile, fasting (cholesterol, HDL, TG)
- Urinalysis with microscopic
- Radiograph, chest
- Anti-Ro (SS-A)
- Anti-La (SS-B)
- Anti-double stranded DNA
- Anti-Smith antibody
- Anticentromere antibody
- Anti-scl 70 antibody
- Complement factors (C3, C4)
- Anti-RNP antibody
- Antistreptolysin O assay (ASO)
- Radiograph, relevant joints
- Cell count with differential, aspirated fluid
- Glucose, aspirated fluid
- C&S, aspirated fluid
- Crystal analysis, aspirated fluid
- Aspiration and biopsy, nodule

Follow-up Visits Generally Required
- Co-management, see *Advice for Referral*

Suggested Readings
Ziff M. The rheumatoid nodule. [Review]. Arthritis Rheum 1990;33:761–767.

Burge DJ, DeHoratius RJ. Acute rheumatic fever. [Review]. Cardiovascul Clin 1993;23:3–23.

George DL, Winer SG. Skin and rheumatic disease. In: Klippel JH, Dieppe PA, eds. Rheumatology. 2nd ed. St. Louis: Mosby, 1998:2.5.6–2.5.7.

See Also
- Rheumatic fever
- Sarcoidosis with joint involvement

RHEUMATOLOGY

Bursitis: Shoulder, Elbow, Hip

Indications and Timing for Referral
- Progressive neurologic impairment
- Suspicion of infection
- Associated with trauma

Timing: Urgent (less than 24 hours)

- Associated with severe pain
- Assistance with bursa injection or aspiration

Timing: Expedited (less than 1 week)

- Associated radiologic abnormalities present
- Diagnosis uncertain with persistent symptoms for more than 4 weeks
- Failure to follow expected course with conventional therapy

Timing: Routine (less than 4 weeks)

Advice for Referral
- Tomographic studies (CT or MR) should be obtained only after preliminary communication with the appropriate consultant.
- Rheumatologic serologies are usually inappropriate unless other symptoms of systemic disease are present.
- Factors favoring referral to a rheumatologist include:
  - Diagnostic uncertainty
  - Other evidence of systemic disease
  - Suspicion of rheumatologic disease
  - Assistance with medical management
- Factors favoring orthopedic referral include:
  - Assistance with management
  - Associated with trauma

Tests to Prepare for Consult
- None

Tests Not Useful Before Consult
- CT or MR, affected region

Tests Consultant May Need to Do
- CBC
- ESR
- ALT, AST, alkaline phosphatase
- Calcium
- Creatinine
- Globulin
- Uric acid
- Radiograph, relevant joints
- Joint or bursa tap
- Therapeutic / diagnostic injection of bursa

Follow-up Visits Generally Required
- None

Suggested Readings
Shbeeb MI, O'Duffy JD, Michet CJ Jr, et al. Evaluation of glucocorticosteroid injection for the treatment of trochanteric bursitis. J Rheumatol 1996;23:2104–2106.

Barry M, Jenner JR. ABC of rheumatology. Pain in neck, shoulder, and arm [published erratum appears in Br Med J 1995;310:311]. [Review]. Br Med J 1995;310:183–186.

Canoso JJ. Bursitis, tenosynovitis, ganglions, and painful lesions of the wrist, elbow, and hand. [Review]. Curr Opin Rheumatol 1990;2:276–281.

Larson HM, Oconnor FG, Nirschl RP. Shoulder pain—the role of diagnostic injections. Am Fam Physician 1996;53:1637–1643.

See Also
- Tendonitis
- Painful, elbow

THE CONSULTATION GUIDE

Carpal Tunnel Syndrome

Indications and Timing for Referral

- Diagnostic uncertainty
- Suspicion of systemic illness
- Neurologic complications
- Failure of conservative therapy (e.g., splinting)
- Patient education

Timing: Routine (less than 4 weeks)

Tests to Prepare for Consult

- None

Tests Not Useful Before Consult

- CT or MR, wrist

Tests Consultant May Need to Do

- CBC
- ESR
- ALT, AST, alkaline phosphatase
- Calcium
- Creatinine
- Globulin
- Uric acid
- TSH
- ANA
- Rheumatoid factor
- Immunoelectrophoresis
  - Serum
  - Urine
- Radiograph, wrist and hand
- Bone scan
- MR, wrist and hand
- EMG
- Nerve conduction study
- Therapeutic or diagnostic injection of relevant joints

Follow-up Visits Generally Required

- One

Suggested Readings

Dawson DM. Entrapment neuropathies of the upper extremities [see comments]. [Review]. N Engl J Med 1993;329:2013–2018.

Katz RT. Carpal tunnel syndrome: a practical review [see comments]. [Review]. Am Fam Physician 1994;49:1371–1379.

von Schroeder HP, Botte MJ. Carpal tunnel syndrome. [Review] [78 refs]. Hand Clin 1996;12:643–655.

Slater RR Jr, Bynum DK. Diagnosis and treatment of carpal tunnel syndrome [see comments]. [Review]. Orthopaedic Review 1993;22:1095–1105.

Hilburn JW. General principles and use of electrodiagnostic studies in carpal and cubital tunnel syndromes. With special attention to pitfalls and interpretation. [Review] [64 refs]. Hand Clin 1996;12:205–221.

Sailer SM. The role of splinting and rehabilitation in the treatment of carpal and cubital tunnel syndromes. Hand Clin 1996;12:223–241.

See Also

- Painful, wrist and/or hand

RHEUMATOLOGY

Dermatomyositis

Indications and Timing for Referral
- Symptoms rapidly progressive
- Symptoms or signs of pulmonary or cardiac involvement

Timing: Expedited (less than 1 week)

- Suspicion of underlying malignancy or connective tissue disease
- Consideration should always be given to having rheumatologic consultation on at least one occasion to confirm diagnosis and develop a treatment plan
- Consider malignancy, especially in patients over 50 years of age; with appropriately targeted testing

Timing: Routine (less than 4 weeks)

Tests to Prepare for Consult
- CBC
- CPK
- ALT
- AST
- LDH
- Aldolase
- ANA
- TSH

Tests Not Useful Before Consult
- None

Tests Consultant May Need to Do
- CPK
- PSA
- Anti-Jo-1 antibody
- Radiograph, chest
- EMG
- Mammogram
- Muscle biopsy
- Echocardiogram
- Pulmonary function tests
- CT scan, abdomen

Follow-up Visits Generally Required
- See *Advice for Referral*

Suggested Readings
Adams-Gandhi LB, Boyd AS, King LE Jr. Diagnosis and management of dermatomyositis. [Review] [83 refs]. Compr Ther 1996;22:156–164.

Euwer RL, Sontheimer RD. Dermatologic aspects of myositis. [Review]. Curr Opin Rheumatol 1994;6:583–589.

Dalakas MC. Polymyositis, dermatomyositis and inclusion-body myositis [see comments]. [Review]. N Engl J Med 1991;325:1487–1498.

Richardson JB, Callen JP. Dermatomyositis and malignancy. [Review]. Med Clin North Am 1989;73:1211–1220.

Villalba L, Adams EM. Update on therapy for refractory dermatomyositis and polymyositis. [Review] [61 refs]. Curr Opin Rheumatol 1996;8:544–551.

See Also
- Polymyositis

Discoid/Cutaneous Lupus, Diagnosis

Indications and Timing for Referral

- Diagnostic uncertainty
- Patient has signs or symptoms of systemic lupus erythematosus (SLE) or risk factors for systemic disease

Timing: Routine (less than 4 weeks)

Advice for Referral

- Records of old biopsies, complement levels, and serologies are vital.

Tests to Prepare for Consult

- CBC
- Platelet count
- Creatinine
- Urinalysis with microscopic
- ANA
- Anti-double stranded DNA

Tests Not Useful Before Consult

- None

Tests Consultant May Need to Do

- Anticardiolipin antibody
- Lupus anticoagulant (LAC)
- Skin biopsy

Follow-up Visits Generally Required

- None

Suggested Readings

Hymes SR, Jordon RE. Chronic cutaneous lupus erythematosus. [Review]. Med Clin North Am 1989;73:1055–1071.

McCauliffe DP. Cutaneous diseases in adults associated with anti-Ro/SS-A autoantibody production. [Review] [100 refs]. Lupus 1997;6:158–166.

See Also

- Systemic lupus erythematosus, diagnosis
- Systemic lupus erythematosus, management
- Systemic lupus erythematosus, with nephritis
- Systemic lupus erythematosus, with neurological involvement
- Discoid/cutaneous lupus, management
- ANA, positive

RHEUMATOLOGY

Discoid/Cutaneous Lupus, Management

Indications and Timing for Referral
- Manifestations of systemic involvement, by SLE
- Assist with management

Timing: Routine (less than 4 weeks)

Advice for Referral
- Records of old biopsies, complement levels, and serologies are vital.

Tests to Prepare for Consult
- CBC
- Platelet count
- Creatinine
- Urinalysis with microscopic
- ANA
- Complement factors (C3, C4)
- Anti-double stranded DNA
- Anti-Ro (SS-A)
- Anti-Smith antibody
- Anti-RNP antibody

Tests Not Useful Before Consult
- None

Tests Consultant May Need to Do
- Anticardiolipin antibody
- Lupus anticoagulant (LAC)

Follow-up Visits Generally Required
- Two

Suggested Readings
Callen JP. Management of skin disease in lupus. [Review] [11 refs]. Bull Rheum Dis 1997;46:4–7.

Jones SK. Treatment of cutaneous lupus erythematosus. J Dermatological Treatment 1996;7:45–49.

Hymes SR, Jordon RE. Chronic cutaneous lupus erythematosus. [Review]. Med Clin North Am 1989;73:1055–1071.

Selected Guidelines
Drake LA, Dinehart SM, Farmer ER, et al. Guidelines of care for cutaneous lupus erythematosus. J Am Acad Dermatol 1996;34:830–836.

See Also
- Discoid/cutaneous lupus, diagnosis
- Systemic lupus erythematosus, management
- ANA, positive
- Systemic lupus erythematosus, with nephritis
- Systemic lupus erythematosus, diagnosis
- Systemic lupus erythematosus, with neurologic involvement

Fasciitis, Plantar

Indications and Timing for Referral

- Progressive neurologic impairment
- Suspicion of infection
- Associated with trauma

Timing: Urgent (less than 24 hours)

- Associated with severe pain

Timing: Expedited (less than 1 week)

- Associated radiologic abnormalities present
- Diagnosis uncertain with persistent symptoms for over 4 weeks
- Failure to follow expected course with conventional therapy

Timing: Routine (less than 4 weeks)

Advice for Referral

- Tomographic studies (CT or MR) should be obtained only after preliminary communication with the appropriate consultant.
- Rheumatologic serologies are usually inappropriate unless other symptoms of systemic disease are present.
- Factors favoring referral to a rheumatologist include:
  - Diagnostic uncertainty
  - Other evidence of systemic disease
  - Suspicion of rheumatologic disease
- Factors favoring orthopedic referral include:
  - Associated with trauma
- Factors favoring podiatric referral include:
  - Assistance with management

Tests to Prepare for Consult

- None

Tests Not Useful Before Consult

- None

Tests Consultant May Need to Do

- CBC
- ESR
- ALT, AST, alkaline phosphatase
- Calcium
- Creatinine
- Globulin
- Uric acid
- ANA
- Rheumatoid factor
- HLA B27
- Anergy intradermal skin test panel
- Radiograph, chest, PA and lateral
- Radiograph, relevant joints
- Joint tap
- *Chlamydia* culture, urethral swab
- Gonorrhea culture, urethral swab

Follow-up Visits Generally Required

- None

Suggested Readings

Kwong PK, Kay D, Voner RT, White MW. Plantar fasciitis. Mechanics and pathomechanics of treatment. [Review]. Clin Sports Med 1988;7:119–126.

Batt ME, Tanji JL, Skattum N. Plantar fasciitis: a prospective randomized clinical trial of the tension night splint. Clin J Sport Med 1996;6:158–162.

Gill LH, Kiebzak GM. Outcome of nonsurgical treatment for plantar fasciitis [published erratum appears in Foot Ankle Int 1996;17:722]. Foot Ankle Int 1996;17:527–532.

Fibrositis/Fibromyalgia

Indications and Timing for Referral

- Diagnostic uncertainty
- Symptoms continue for more than 6 weeks with conventional therapy
- Assist with management of chronic pain

Timing: Routine (less than 4 weeks)

Tests to Prepare for Consult

- CBC
- ESR
- ALT, AST, alkaline phosphatase
- Calcium
- Creatinine
- Globulin
- Uric acid
- CPK
- TSH
- ANA
- Rheumatoid factor

Tests Not Useful Before Consult

- Lyme (*B. burgdorferi*) serology
- CMV antibody
- EBV antibody
- Autoimmune serologies
- EEG
- Sleep study

Tests Consultant May Need to Do

- CBC
- ESR
- CPK
- LDH
- Calcium
- Free T_4
- PTH
- TSH
- Radiograph, relevant joints
- EMG
- ALT, AST, alkaline phosphatase

Follow-up Visits Generally Required

- One

Suggested Readings

McCain GA. A cost-effective approach to the diagnosis and treatment of fibromyalgia. [Review] [80 refs]. Rheum Dis Clin North Am 1996;22:323–349.

Doherty M, Jones A. ABC of rheumatology. Fibromyalgia syndrome. [Review]. Br Med J 1995;310:386–389.

Wolfe F. When to diagnose fibromyalgia. [Review]. Rheum Dis Clin North Am 1994;20:485–501.

Bennett RM. Fibromyalgia and the facts. Sense or nonsense. [Review]. Rheum Dis Clin North Am 1993;19:45–59.

Geel SE. The fibromyalgia syndrome: musculoskeletal pathophysiology. [Review]. Semin Arthritis Rheum 1994;23:347–353.

See Also

- Pain, chronic soft tissue
- Pain in a few joints (≥ 5)
- Pain in a few joints (≤ 4)

Giant Cell/Temporal Arteritis

Indications and Timing for Referral

- Patient with neuroophthalmologic manifestations suggesting the diagnosis

Timing: Urgent (less than 24 hours)

- Diagnostic uncertainty
- Assistance with management

Timing: Expedited (less than 1 week)

Advice for Referral

- Temporal artery biopsy not recommended in patients younger than 50 years of age, unless other clinical data are compelling.
- Co-management with a rheumatologist should be considered.

Tests to Prepare for Consult

- CBC
- Platelet count
- ESR
- ALT, AST, alkaline phosphatase

Tests Not Useful Before Consult

None

Tests Consultant May Need to Do

- CBC
- ESR
- Glucose
- Creatinine
- Cholesterol
- Triglycerides
- Urinalysis with microscopic
- Temporal artery biopsy

Follow-up Visits Generally Required

- Co-management, see *Advice for Referral*

Suggested Readings

Hunder GG. Giant cell arteritis and polymyalgia rheumatica. [Review] [93 refs]. Med Clin North Am 1997;81:195–219.

Kachroo A, Tello C, Bais R, Panush RS. Giant cell arteritis: diagnosis and management. Bull Rheum Dis 1996;45:2–5.

Hellmann DB. Immunopathogenesis, diagnosis, and treatment of giant cell arteritis, temporal arteritis, polymyalgia rheumatica, and Takayasu's arteritis. [Review]. Curr Opin Rheumatol 1993;5:25–32.

Buchbinder R, Detsky AS. Management of suspected giant cell arteritis: a decision analysis. J Rheumatol 1992;19:1220–1228.

Hunder GG, Bloch DA, Michel BA, et al. The American College of Rheumatology 1990 criteria for the classification of giant cell arteritis. Arthritis Rheum 1990;33:1122–1128.

See Also

- Polymyalgia rheumatica

RHEUMATOLOGY

Gout

Indications and Timing for Referral
- Uncontrolled acute symptoms

Timing: Urgent (less than 24 hours)

- Diagnostic uncertainty
- Assistance with long-term management

Timing: Routine (less than 4 weeks)

Advice for Referral
- Persistent, uncontrolled or tophaceous gout may require co-management with a rheumatologist.
- Records of previous joint fluid analysis and radiographs are helpful before consultation.

Tests to Prepare for Consult
- CBC
- Creatinine
- ALT, AST, alkaline phosphatase
- Uric acid
- Urinalysis with microscopic

Tests Not Useful Before Consult
- None

Tests Consultant May Need to Do
- 24-hour urine creatinine for clearance
- 24-hour urine uric acid
- Serum lead
- Radiograph, relevant joints
- Joint tap
- Cell count with differential, aspirated fluid
- Crystal analysis, aspirated fluid

Follow-up Visits Generally Required
- One

Suggested Readings

Snaith ML. ABC of rheumatology. Gout, hyperuricaemia, and crystal arthritis. [Review]. Br Med J 1995;310:521–524.

Peters TD, Ball GV. Gout and hyperuricemia. [Review]. Curr Opin Rheumatol 1992;4:566–573.

Uy JP, Nuwayhid N, Saadeh C. Unusual presentations of gout. Tips for accurate diagnosis. [Review] [21 refs]. Postgrad Med 1996;100:253–254.

Wolfe F. Gout and hyperuricemia [see comments]. [Review]. Am Fam Physician 1991;43:2141–2150.

Emmerson BT. The management of gout [see comments]. [Review] [85 refs]. N Engl J Med 1996;334:445–451.

See Also
- Pseudogout
- Pain in a few joints ($\leq$ 4 joints)
- Pain in a few joints ($\geq$ 5 joints)
- Painful ankle, foot, or toe

Pain, Chronic Soft Tissue

Indications and Timing for Referral
- Diagnostic uncertainty
- Pain continues for more than 6 weeks with conventional therapy
- Assist with management of chronic pain

Timing: Routine (less than 4 weeks)

Tests to Prepare for Consult
- CBC
- ESR
- ALT, AST, alkaline phosphatase
- Calcium
- Creatinine
- Globulin
- Uric acid
- CPK
- TSH
- ANA
- Rheumatoid factor

Tests Not Useful Before Consult
- Lyme (*B. burgdorferi*) serology
- CMV antibody
- EBV antibody
- Other autoimmune serologies

Tests Consultant May Need to Do
- CBC
- ESR
- CPK
- ALT, AST, alkaline phosphatase
- Calcium
- Free T_4
- PTH
- TSH
- Radiograph, relevant joints
- EMG
- Hepatitis C antibody

Follow-up Visits Generally Required
- One

Suggested Readings

Doherty M, Jones A. ABC of rheumatology. Fibromyalgia syndrome. [Review]. Br Med J 1995;310:386–389.

McCain GA. A cost-effective approach to the diagnosis and treatment of fibromyalgia. [Review] [80 refs]. Rheum Dis Clin North Am 1996;22:323–349.

Wallace DJ. The fibromyalgia syndrome. [Review] [83 refs]. Ann Med 1997;29:9–21.

Wolfe F. When to diagnose fibromyalgia. [Review]. Rheum Dis Clin North Am 1994;20:485–501.

RHEUMATOLOGY

Pain in a Few Joints, Less Than or Equal to 4 Joints

Indications and Timing for Referral
- Progressive neurologic impairment
- Suspicion of infection
- Associated with trauma

Timing: Urgent (less than 24 hours)

- Associated with severe pain
- Associated with known or suspected malignancy
- Need assistance with joint aspiration

Timing: Expedited (less than 1 week)

- Associated radiologic abnormalities present
- Diagnosis uncertain with persistent symptoms for longer than 4 weeks
- Failure to follow expected course with conventional therapy
- Assistance with management

Timing: Routine (less than 4 weeks)

Advice for Referral
- Tomographic studies (CT or MR) should be obtained only after preliminary communication with the appropriate consultant.
- Testing beyond ANA and RF not recommended (e.g., comprehensive autoantibody panels).
- Records of previous radiographs are helpful before consultation.
- Factors favoring referral to a rheumatologist include:
  - Diagnostic uncertainty
  - Other evidence of systemic disease
  - Suspicion of rheumatologic disease
  - Assistance with medical management
- Factors favoring orthopedic referral include:
  - Associated with trauma
  - Neurologic compromise

Tests to Prepare for Consult
- CBC
- ESR
- Rheumatoid factor

Tests Not Useful Before Consult
- Anti-Ro (SS-A)
- Anti-La (SS-B)
- Anti-double stranded DNA
- Anti-scl 70 antibody
- Anticentromere antibody
- ANCA
- C reactive protein

THE CONSULTATION GUIDE

Pain in a Few Joints, Less Than or Equal to 4 Joints (continued)

Tests Consultant May Need to Do
- CBC
- ESR
- ALT, AST, alkaline phosphatase
- Calcium
- Creatinine
- Globulin
- Uric acid
- ANA
- Rheumatoid factor
- Radiograph, chest
- HLA B27
- Lyme (*B. burgdorferi*) serology
- Urinalysis with microscopic
- Bone scan
- Radiograph, relevant joints
- Therapeutic or diagnostic injection of relevant joints
- Cell count with differential, aspirated fluid
- C&S, aspirated fluid
- Crystal analysis, aspirated fluid
- Glucose, aspirated fluid
- *Chlamydia* culture, urethral swab
- Gonorrhea culture, urethral swab
- Parvovirus B19 serology
- HB$_s$Ag
- Hepatitis C antibody

Follow-up Visits Generally Required
- Two

Suggested Readings

Phillips PE. Viral arthritis. [Review] [48 refs]. Curr Opin Rheumatol 1997;9:337–344.

Smith CA, Arnett FC, Jr. Diagnosing rheumatoid arthritis: current criteria. [Review]. Am Fam Physician 1991;44:863–870.

Wolfe F, Ross K, Hawley DJ, et al. The prognosis of rheumatoid arthritis and undifferentiated polyarthritis syndrome in the clinic: a study of 1141 patients [see comments]. J Rheumatol 1993;20:2005–2009.

Krause A, Kamradt T, Burmester GR. Potential infectious agents in the induction of arthritides. [Review] [65 refs]. Curr Opin Rheumatol 1996;8:203–209.

Sergent JS. In: Kelly WN, ed. Approach to the Patient with More than One Painful Joint. Philadelphia: WB Saunders, 1997:381–387.

See Also
- Gout
- Pain in a few joints (≥ 5)
- Arthritis, rheumatoid, diagnosis

RHEUMATOLOGY

Pain in a Few Joints, Greater Than or Equal to 5 Joints

Indications and Timing for Referral
- Progressive neurologic impairment
- Suspicion of infection

Timing: Urgent (less than 24 hours)

- Associated with severe pain
- Associated with known or suspected malignancy

Timing: Expedited (less than 1 week)

- Associated radiologic abnormalities present
- Diagnosis uncertain with persistent symptoms for more than 4 weeks
- Failure to follow expected course with conventional therapy
- Assistance with management

Timing: Routine (less than 4 weeks)

Advice for Referral
- Tomographic studies (CT or MR) should be obtained only after preliminary communication with the appropriate consultant.
- Testing beyond ANA and RF is not recommended (e.g., comprehensive autoantibody panels).
- Records of previous radiographs are helpful before consultation.
- Factors favoring referral to a rheumatologist include:
  - Diagnostic uncertainty
  - Other evidence of systemic disease
  - Suspicion of rheumatologic disease
  - Assistance with medical management
- Factors favoring neurology or orthopedic referral include:
  - Associated with trauma
  - Neurologic compromise

Tests to Prepare for Consult
- CBC
- ESR
- Rheumatoid factor

Tests Not Useful Before Consult
- Anti-Ro (SS-A)
- Anti-La (SS-B)
- Anti-double stranded DNA
- Anti-scl 70 antibody
- Anticentromere antibody
- ANCA
- C reactive protein
- Anti-Smith antibody
- Anti-RNP antibody

THE CONSULTATION GUIDE

Pain in a Few Joints, Greater Than or Equal to 5 Joints (*continued*)

Tests Consultant May Need to Do
- CBC
- ESR
- ALT, AST, alkaline phosphatase
- Calcium
- Creatinine
- Globulin
- Uric acid
- ANA
- Rheumatoid factor
- Radiograph, chest
- HLA B27
- Lyme (*B. burgdorferi*) serology
- Urinalysis with microscopic
- Bone scan
- Radiograph, relevant joints
- Therapeutic or diagnostic injection of relevant joints
- Cell count with differential, aspirated fluid
- C&S, aspirated fluid
- Crystal analysis, aspirated fluid
- Glucose, aspirated fluid
- *Chlamydia* culture, urethral swab
- Gonorrhea culture, urethral swab
- Parvovirus B19 serology

Follow-up Visits Generally Required
- Two

Suggested Readings

Akil M, Amos RS. ABC of rheumatology. Rheumatoid arthritis—I: Clinical features and diagnosis. [Review]. Br Med J 1995;310:587–590.

Smith CA, Arnett FC Jr. Diagnosing rheumatoid arthritis: current criteria. [Review]. Am Fam Physician 1991;44:863–870.

Phillips PE. Viral arthritis. [Review] [48 refs]. Curr Opin Rheumatol 1997;9:337–344.

Wolfe F, Ross K, Hawley DJ, et al. The prognosis of rheumatoid arthritis and undifferentiated polyarthritis syndrome in the clinic: a study of 1141 patients [see comments]. J Rheumatol 1993;20:2005–2009.

McCain GA. A cost-effective approach to the diagnosis and treatment of fibromyalgia. [Review] [80 refs]. Rheum Dis Clin North Am 1996;22:323–349.

Sergent JS. In: Kelly WN, ed. Approach to the Patient with More than One Painful Joint. Philadelphia: WB Saunders, 1997:381–387.

See Also
- Arthritis, rheumatoid
- Pain in a few joints (≤ 4 joints)
- Arthritis, rheumatoid, diagnosis
- Gout

RHEUMATOLOGY

Painful Ankle, Foot, or Toe

Indications and Timing for Referral
- Progressive neurologic impairment
- Suspicion of infection
- Associated with trauma

Timing: Urgent (less than 24 hours)

- Associated with severe pain
- Associated with known or suspected malignancy
- Assistance with joint aspiration or injection

Timing: Expedited (less than 1 week)

- Diagnosis uncertain with persistent symptoms for more than 4 weeks
- Failure to follow expected course with conventional therapy
- Associated radiologic abnormalities present

Timing: Routine (less than 4 weeks)

Advice for Referral
- Tomographic studies (CT or MR) should be obtained only after preliminary communication with the appropriate consultant.
- Rheumatologic serologies are usually inappropriate unless other symptoms of systemic disease are present.
- Factors favoring referral to a rheumatologist include:
  - Other evidence of systemic disease
  - Suspicion of rheumatologic disease
- Factors favoring orthopedic referral include:
  - Associated with trauma
  - Neurologic compromise
- Factors favoring podiatric referral include:
  - Diagnostic uncertainty
  - Assistance with management

Tests to Prepare for Consult
- Radiograph, affected region

Tests Not Useful Before Consult
- MR, relevant region

THE CONSULTATION GUIDE

Painful Ankle, Foot, or Toe (continued)

Tests Consultant May Need to Do

- CBC
- ESR
- ALT, AST, alkaline phosphatase
- Calcium
- Creatinine
- Glucose
- Globulin
- Uric acid
- TSH
- ANA
- Rheumatoid factor
- HLA B27
- Immunoelectrophoresis
  - Serum
  - Urine
- Vitamin B_{12}, serum
- Lyme (*B. burgdorferi*) serology
- *Chlamydia* culture, urethral swab
- Gonorrhea culture, urethral swab
- Radiograph, affected region
- Bone scan
- Doppler ultrasound flow study
- CT or MR, affected region
- EMG
- Nerve conduction study
- Joint tap
- Cell count with differential, aspirated fluid
- C&S, aspirated fluid
- Crystal analysis, aspirated fluid
- Glucose, aspirated fluid

Follow-up Visits Generally Required

- One

Suggested Readings

West SG, Woodburn J. ABC of rheumatology. Pain in the foot. [Review]. Br Med J 1995;310:860–864.

Jahss MH. Foot and ankle pain resulting from rheumatic conditions. [Review]. Curr Opin Rheumatol 1992;4:233–240.

Plattner PF. Tendon problems of the foot and ankle. The spectrum from peritendinitis to rupture. [Review]. Postgrad Med 1989;86:155–162.

Stern SH. Ankle and foot pain. [Review]. Primary Care 1988;15:809–826.

See Also

- Gout
- Reiter's syndrome

RHEUMATOLOGY

Painful Elbow

Indications and Timing for Referral

- Progressive neurologic impairment
- Suspicion of infection
- Associated with trauma

Timing: Urgent (less than 24 hours)

- Associated with severe pain
- Associated with known or suspected malignancy
- Assistance with elbow injection or aspiration

Timing: Expedited (less than 1 week)

- Associated radiologic abnormalities present
- Diagnosis uncertain with persistent symptoms for more than 4 weeks
- Failure to follow expected course with conventional therapy

Timing: Routine (less than 4 weeks)

Advice for Referral

- Tomographic studies (CT or MR) should be obtained only after preliminary communication with the appropriate consultant.
- Rheumatologic serologies are usually inappropriate unless other symptoms of systemic disease are present.
- Factors favoring referral to a rheumatologist include:
  - Diagnostic uncertainty
  - Other evidence of systemic disease
  - Suspicion of rheumatologic disease
  - Assistance with medical management
- Factors favoring neurology or orthopedic referral include:
  - Neurologic compromise
  - Associated with trauma, acute or repetitive

Tests to Prepare for Consult

- None

Tests Not Useful Before Consult

- MR, elbow
- Thermography

Painful Elbow (*continued*)

Tests Consultant May Need to Do
- CBC
- ESR
- ALT, AST, alkaline phosphatase
- Calcium
- Creatinine
- Uric acid
- Radiograph, elbow
- EMG
- Nerve conduction study
- Joint tap
- Soft tissue aspiration
- Therapeutic or diagnostic injection of elbow
- Lyme (*B. burgdorferi*) serology

Follow-up Visits Generally Required
- None

Suggested Readings

Gellman H. Tennis elbow (lateral epicondylitis). [Review]. Orthop Clin North Am 1992;23:75–82.

Barry M, Jenner JR. ABC of rheumatology. Pain in neck, shoulder, and arm [published erratum appears in Br Med J 1995;310:311]. [Review]. Br Med J 1995;310:183–186.

Barton NJ, Hooper G, Noble J, Steel WM. Occupational causes of disorders in the upper limb [see comments]. [Review]. Br Med J 1992;304:309–311.

Nirschl RP. Elbow tendinosis/tennis elbow. [Review]. Clin Sports Med 1992;11:851–870.

See Also
- Bursitis: shoulder, elbow, hip
- Tendonitis

RHEUMATOLOGY

Painful, Hip

Indications and Timing for Referral

- Progressive neurologic impairment
- Suspicion of infection
- Associated with trauma
- History of medical condition known to compromise structural integrity of central nervous system (CNS) and cord

Timing: Urgent (less than 24 hours)

- Associated with severe pain
- Associated with known or suspected malignancy
- Assistance with aspiration or injection of hip joint

Timing: Expedited (less than 1 week)

- Diagnosis uncertain with persistent symptoms for longer than 4 weeks
- Failure to follow expected course with conventional therapy
- Associated radiologic abnormalities present

Timing: Routine (less than 4 weeks)

Advice for Referral

- Tomographic studies (CT or MR) should be obtained only after preliminary communication with the appropriate consultant.
- Rheumatologic serologies are usually inappropriate unless other symptoms of systemic disease are present.
- Factors favoring referral to a rheumatologist include:
  - Diagnostic uncertainty
  - Other evidence of systemic disease
  - Patient age under 60 years
  - Assistance with medical management
- Factors favoring neurology or orthopedic referral include:
  - Neurologic compromise
  - Known disease with failed medical therapy warranting consideration of joint replacement
  - Associated with trauma

Tests to Prepare for Consult

- Radiograph, hip
  - PA (weight-bearing) and lateral
  - PA and frog lateral

Tests Not Useful Before Consult

- MR, hip

Tests Consultant May Need to Do

- CBC
- ESR
- ALT, AST, alkaline phosphatase
- Calcium
- Creatinine
- Globulin
- Uric acid
- HLA B27
- Lyme (*B. burgdorferi*) serology
- Radiograph, L-spine
- Radiograph, sacroiliac joints
- Bone scan
- MR, hip

Painful Hip (*continued*)

Follow-up Visits Generally Required
- One

See Also
- Reiter's syndrome

Suggested Readings

Paice E. ABC of rheumatology. Pain in the hip and knee. [Review]. Br Med J 1995;310:319–322.

Roberts WN, Williams RB. Hip pain. [Review]. Primary Care; Clin Off Pract 1988;15:783–793.

Shbeeb MI, Matteson EL. Trochanteric bursitis (greater trochanter pain syndrome). [Review] [26 refs]. Mayo Clin Proc 1996;71:565–569.

Traycoff RB. "Pseudotrochanteric bursitis": the differential diagnosis of lateral hip pain [see comments]. J Rheumatol 1991;18:1810–1812.

Harris WH, Sledge CB. Total hip and total knee replacement. N Engl J Med 1990;323:725–731.

RHEUMATOLOGY

Painful Knee

Indications and Timing for Referral
- Progressive neurologic impairment
- Suspicion of infection
- Associated with trauma

Timing: Urgent (less than 24 hours)

- Associated with severe pain
- Associated with known or suspected malignancy
- Need for diagnostic or therapeutic joint tap

Timing: Expedited (less than 1 week)

- Associated radiologic abnormalities present
- Diagnosis uncertain with persistent symptoms for more than 4 weeks
- Failure to follow expected course with conventional therapy

Timing: Routine (less than 4 weeks)

Advice for Referral
- Tomographic studies (CT or MR) should be obtained only after preliminary communication with the appropriate consultant.
- Rheumatologic serologies are usually inappropriate unless other symptoms of systemic disease are present.
- Factors favoring referral to a rheumatologist include:
    - Diagnostic uncertainty
    - Known systemic disease including osteoarthritis
    - Patient age under 60 years
    - Assistance with medical management
- Factors favoring orthopedic referral include:
    - Neurologic compromise
    - History of significant trauma
    - Arthroscopic or surgical intervention contemplated

Tests to Prepare for Consult
- Radiograph, knee, standing, AP, and lateral

Tests Not Useful Before Consult
- MR, knee

Painful Knee (continued)

Tests Consultant May Need to Do
- CBC
- ESR
- ALT, AST, alkaline phosphatase
- Calcium
- Creatinine
- Globulin
- Uric acid
- ANA
- Rheumatoid factor
- HLA B27
- Lyme (*B. burgdorferi*) serology
- *Chlamydia* culture, urethral swab
- Gonorrhea culture, urethral swab
- Radiographs
  - Knee, special views
  - Hip
  - Spinal
- Bone scan
- CT or MR, knee
- EMG
- Nerve conduction study
- Joint tap
- Aspirated fluid
  - Cell count with differential
  - C&S
  - Glucose
  - Crystal analysis

Follow-up Visits Generally Required
- One

Suggested Readings

McCune WJ, Matteson EL, MacGuire A. Evaluation of knee pain. [Review]. Prim Care 1988;15:795–808.

Ike RW. The role of arthroscopy in the differential diagnosis of osteoarthritis of the knee. [Review]. Rheum Dis Clin North Am 1993;19:673–696.

Mody EA, Greene JM. In: Noble J, ed. Primary Care Medicine. 2nd ed. St. Louis: Mosby, 1996:1055–1063.

See Also
- Reiter's syndrome

RHEUMATOLOGY

Painful Lower Back/Lumbosacral Spine

Indications and Timing for Referral
- Progressive neurologic impairment
- Suspicion of infection
- Associated with trauma
- History of medical condition known to compromise structural integrity of CNS and cord
- Minor trauma causing persistent pain or localized spinal pain in setting of cauda equina syndrome

Timing: Urgent (less than 24 hours)

- Associated with severe pain
- Associated with known or suspected malignancy

Timing: Expedited (less than 1 week)

- Diagnosis uncertain with persistent symptoms for more than 4 weeks
- Failure to follow expected course with conventional therapy
- Associated radiologic abnormalities present

Timing: Routine (less than 4 weeks)

Advice for Referral
- Gynecologic examination within 6 months is important in women over 30 years with unexplained low back pain.
- Tomographic studies (CT or MR) should be obtained only after preliminary communication with the appropriate consultant.
- Rheumatologic serologies are usually inappropriate unless other symptoms of systemic disease are present.
- Factors favoring referral to a rheumatologist include:
  - Diagnostic uncertainty
  - Other evidence of systemic disease
  - Suspicion of rheumatologic disease
  - Assistance with medical management
- Factors favoring orthopedic or neurosurgery referral include:
  - Neurologic compromise
  - Unstable spine, e.g., caused by spondylolisthesis, fracture, or tumor
  - Associated with trauma
  - Consideration of spinal stenosis

Tests to Prepare for Consult
- Radiograph, LS-spine; PA and lateral

Tests Not Useful Before Consult
- None

THE CONSULTATION GUIDE

Painful Lower Back/Lumbosacral Spine (*continued*)

Tests Consultant May Need to Do

- Radiograph, LS-spine; PA, lateral and oblique
- CBC
- ESR
- ALT, AST, alkaline phosphatase
- Calcium
- Creatinine
- Globulin
- Uric acid
- Urinalysis with microscopic
- HLA B27
- Immunoelectrophoresis
  - Serum
  - Urine
- PSA, in men
- Radiograph, sacroiliac joints
- Radiograph, pelvis, AP
- Bone scan
- CT or MR, lumbosacral spine
- EMG
- Nerve conduction study

Follow-up Visits Generally Required

- One

Suggested Readings

Deyo RA, Rainville J, Kent DL. What can the history and physical examination tell us about low back pain? [see comments]. [Review]. JAMA 1992;268:760–765.

Borenstein D. Epidemiology, etiology, diagnostic evaluation, and treatment of low back pain. [Review]. Curr Opin Rheumatol 1992;4:226–232.

Haldeman S. Diagnostic tests for the evaluation of back and neck pain. [Review] [52 refs]. Neurol Clin 1996;14:103–117.

Jensen MC, Brant-Zawadzki MN, Obuchowski N, et al. Magnetic resonance imaging of the lumbar spine in people without back pain [see comments]. N Engl J Med 1994;331:69–73.

Selected Guidelines

Bowyer BS, Braen G. Acute low back problems in adults. Clinical Practice Guideline No. 14 [Anonymous]. Rockville, MD: Agency for Health Care Policy and Research, 1994: Report nr 95-0642.

See Also

- Painful, upper back/thoracic spine
- Ankylosing spondylitis
- Reiter's syndrome

RHEUMATOLOGY

Painful Neck

Indications and Timing for Referral

- Progressive neurologic impairment
- Suspicion of infection
- Associated with trauma
- History of medical condition known to compromise structural integrity of CNS and cord, e.g., cancer with potential metastatic spread

Timing: Urgent (less than 24 hours)

- Associated with severe pain
- Associated with known or suspected malignancy

Timing: Expedited (less than 1 week)

- Associated neurological complaints present
- Diagnosis uncertain with persistent symptoms for more than 4 weeks
- Failure to follow expected course with conventional therapy
- Associated relevant radiologic abnormalities present

Timing: Routine (less than 4 weeks)

Advice for Referral

- Tomographic studies (CT or MR) should be obtained only after preliminary communication with the appropriate consultant.
- Rheumatologic serologies are usually inappropriate unless other symptoms of systemic disease are present.
- Factors favoring referral to a rheumatologist include:
    - Diagnostic uncertainty
    - Other evidence of systemic disease
    - Suspicion of rheumatologic disease
    - Assistance with medical management
- Factors favoring neurology or orthopedic referral include:
    - Neurologic compromise
    - Unstable spine
    - Associated with trauma
    - Consideration of spinal stenosis

Tests to Prepare for Consult

- CBC
- ESR
- Radiograph, C-spine; PA, lateral and oblique views

Tests Not Useful Before Consult

- None

Tests Consultant May Need to Do

- CBC
- ESR
- Creatinine
- ALT, AST, alkaline phosphatase
- Calcium
- Uric acid
- Radiograph, C-spine, special views
- Bone scan
- Electromyogram
- Nerve conduction study
- CT or MR, C-spine
- CT or MR, cranial

Painful Neck (*continued*)

Follow-up Visits Generally Required
- One

Suggested Readings

Swezey RL. Chronic neck pain. [Review] [72 refs]. Rheum Dis Clin North Am 1996;22:411–437.

Haldeman S. Diagnostic tests for the evaluation of back and neck pain. [Review] [52 refs]. Neurol Clin 1996;14:103–117.

Barry M, Jenner JR. ABC of rheumatology. Pain in neck, shoulder, and arm [published erratum appears in Br Med J 1995;310:311]. [Review]. Br Med J 1995;310:183–186.

Newman PK. Whiplash injury [editorial] [see comments]. [Review]. Br Med J 1990;301:395–396.

Goodman BW Jr. Neck pain. [Review]. Primary care; Clin Off Pract 1988;15:689–708.

RHEUMATOLOGY

Painful Shoulder

Indications and Timing for Referral
- Progressive neurologic infection
- Suspicion of infection
- Associated with trauma

Timing: Urgent (less than 24 hours)

- Associated with severe pain
- Associated with known or suspected malignancy

Timing: Expedited (less than 1 week)

- Diagnosis uncertain with persistent symptoms for more than 4 weeks
- Failure to follow expected course with conventional therapy
- Associated radiologic abnormalities present
- Assistance with shoulder injection

Timing: Routine (less than 4 weeks)

Advice for Referral
- Tomographic studies (CT or MR) should be obtained only after preliminary communication with the appropriate consultant.
- Rheumatologic serologies are usually inappropriate unless other symptoms of systemic disease are present.
- Factors favoring referral to a rheumatologist include:
  - Diagnostic uncertainty
  - Other evidence of systemic disease
  - Suspicion of rheumatologic disease
  - Assistance with medical management
- Factors favoring neurology or orthopedic referral include:
  - Neurologic compromise
  - Associated with trauma (e.g., suspicion of acute tendon or ligament tear, dislocation or fracture)
  - Weakness of shoulder rotation

Tests to Prepare for Consult
- None

Tests Not Useful Before Consult
- CT or MR, shoulder

Tests Consultant May Need to Do
- CBC
- ESR
- ALT, AST, alkaline phosphatase
- Calcium
- Creatinine
- Uric acid
- ANA
- Rheumatoid factor
- Radiograph, cervical spine
- Radiograph, shoulder, Y view
- Electromyogram
- Nerve conduction study
- Therapeutic / diagnostic injection of shoulder
- Joint or bursa tap
- Cell count with differential, aspirated fluid
- C&S, aspirated fluid
- Crystal analysis, aspirated fluid
- Glucose, aspirated fluid
- Lyme (*B. burgdorferi*) serology

Painful Shoulder (continued)

Follow-up Visits Generally Required

- None

Suggested Readings

Barry M, Jenner JR. ABC of rheumatology. Pain in neck, shoulder, and arm [published erratum appears in Br Med J 1995 Feb 4;310:311]. [Review]. Br Med J 1995;310:183–186.

Turner-Stokes L. Clinical differential diagnosis of shoulder pain. [Review] [3 refs]. Br J Hosp Med 1996;56:73–77.

Uhthoff HK, Sarkar K. Periarticular soft tissue conditions causing pain in the shoulder. [Review]. Curr Opin Rheumatol 1992;4:241–246.

Zuckerman JD, Mirabello SC, Newman D, et al. The painful shoulder: Part II. Intrinsic disorders and impingement syndrome. [Review]. Am Fam Physician 1991;43:497–512.

Zuckerman JD, Mirabello SC, Newman D, et al. The painful shoulder: Part I. Extrinsic disorders [see comments]. [Review]. Am Fam Physician 1991;43:119–128.

Vanderwindt DAWM, Koes BW, Dejong BA, Bouter LM. Shoulder disorders in general practice-incidence, patient characteristics, and management. Ann Rheum Dis 1995;54:959–964.

Binder A. Management of common shoulder problems. [Review] [22 refs]. Br J Hosp Med 1996;56:66–72.

RHEUMATOLOGY

Painful Upper Back/Thoracic Spine

Indications and Timing for Referral
- Progressive neurologic infection
- Suspicion of infection
- Associated with trauma
- History of medical condition known to compromise structural integrity of CNS and cord

Timing: Urgent (less than 24 hours)

- Associated with severe pain
- Associated with known or suspected malignancy

Timing: Expedited (less than 1 week)

- Diagnosis uncertain with persistent symptoms for more than 4 weeks
- Failure to follow expected course with conventional therapy
- Associated radiologic abnormalities present

Timing: Routine (less than 4 weeks)

Advice for Referral
- Lateral chest radiograph may be acceptable, if not preferable if extra-spine issues are suspected.
- Tomographic studies (CT or MR) should be obtained only after preliminary communication with the appropriate consultant.
- Rheumatologic serologies are usually inappropriate unless other symptoms of systemic disease are present.
- Factors favoring referral to a rheumatologist include:
    - Diagnostic uncertainty
    - Other evidence of systemic disease
    - Suspicion of rheumatologic disease
    - Assistance with medical management
- Factors favoring neurosurgery or orthopedic referral include:
    - Neurologic compromise
    - Unstable spine, e.g., caused by spondylolisthesis, fracture, or tumor
    - Associated with trauma
    - Consideration of rare thoracic spinal stenosis

Tests to Prepare for Consult
- Radiograph, T-spine, lateral

Tests Not Useful Before Consult
- None

Tests Consultant May Need to Do
- CBC
- ESR
- ALT, AST, alkaline phosphatase
- Calcium
- Creatinine
- Globulin
- Uric acid
- Glucose
- HLA B27
- Radiograph, T-spine, lateral and AP
- Bone scan
- CT or MR, T-spine

Painful Upper Back/Thoracic Spine (*continued*)

Follow-up Visits Generally Required
- One

Suggested Readings
Bland JH. Cervical and thoracic pain. [Review]. Curr Opin Rheumatol 1991;3:218–225.
Rosenbloom SA. Thoracic disc disease and stenosis. Radiol Clin North Am 1991;29:765–775.
Haldeman S. Diagnostic tests for the evaluation of back and neck pain. [Review] [52 refs]. Neurol Clin 1996;14:103–117.
Martin DS, Awwad EE, Pittman T, et al. Current imaging concepts of thoracic intervertebral disks. [Review]. Crit Rev Diagnostic Imaging 1992;33:109–181.

See Also
- Painful, lower back/lumbosacral spine
- Ankylosing spondylitis

RHEUMATOLOGY

Painful Wrist and/or Hand

Indications and Timing for Referral
- Progressive neurologic infection
- Suspicion of infection
- Associated with trauma

Timing: Urgent (less than 24 hours)

- Associated with severe pain

Timing: Expedited (less than 1 week)

- Diagnosis uncertain with persistent symptoms for longer than 4 weeks
- Failure to follow expected course with conventional therapy
- Assistance with management
- Associated radiologic abnormalities present

Timing: Routine (less than 4 weeks)

Advice for Referral
- Tomographic studies (CT or MR) should be obtained only after preliminary communication with the appropriate consultant.
- Rheumatologic serologies are usually inappropriate unless other symptoms of systemic disease are present.
- Factors favoring referral to a rheumatologist include:
  - Diagnostic uncertainty
  - Other evidence of systemic disease
- Suspicion of rheumatologic disease
- Assistance with medical management or therapeutic injection
- Factors favoring neurology or orthopedic referral include:
  - Neurologic compromise
  - Associated with trauma, acute or repetitive

Tests to Prepare for Consult
- None

Tests Not Useful Before Consult
- CT or MR, hand

Tests Consultant May Need to Do
- CBC
- ESR
- ALT, AST, alkaline phosphatase
- Calcium
- Creatinine
- Globulin
- Uric acid
- ANA
- Rheumatoid factor
- TSH
- Radiograph, chest, PA and lateral
- Radiograph, affected region
- Electromyogram
- Nerve conduction study
- Doppler ultrasound flow study
- Bone scan
- MR, relevant region
- Therapeutic or diagnostic injection to relevant joints

Painful Wrist and/or Hand (*continued*)

Follow-up Visits Generally Required
- One

Suggested Readings
Shipley M. ABC of rheumatology. Pain in the hand and wrist. [Review]. Br Med J 1995;310:239–243.

Koman LA, Smith TL, Smith BP, Li Z. The painful hand. [Review] [34 refs]. Hand Clin 1996;12:757–764.

Kuschner SH, Lane CS. Evaluation of the painful wrist. [Review] [66 refs]. Am J Orthop 1997;26:95–102.

Chidgey LK. Chronic wrist pain. [Review]. Orthop Clin North Am 1992;23:49–64.

Shmerling RH. Finger pain. [Review]. Primary Care; Clin Off Pract 1988;15:751–766.

Czop C, Smith TL, Rauck R, Koman LA. The pharmacologic approach to the painful hand. [Review] [42 refs]. Hand Clin 1996;12:633–642.

See Also
- Carpal tunnel syndrome

RHEUMATOLOGY

Polymyalgia Rheumatica

Indications and Timing for Referral
- Diagnostic uncertainty
- Assistance with management
- Age 50 years or older

Timing: Expedited (less than 1 week)

Advice for Referral
- If headache or neurologic symptoms are present, consider giant cell/temporal arteritis.

Tests to Prepare for Consult
- CBC
- ESR
- Electrolytes (Na, K, Cl, CO_2)
- Calcium, phosphorus
- ALT, AST, alkaline phosphatase
- Creatinine
- Cholesterol
- Triglycerides
- TSH

Tests Not Useful Before Consult
- Temporal artery biopsy

Tests Consultant May Need to Do
- CPK
- ESR
- CBC
- Cholesterol
- Triglycerides
- Rheumatoid factor
- ANA
- Radiograph, chest
- Temporal artery biopsy

Follow-up Visits Generally Required
- Two

Suggested Readings
Salvarani C, Macchioni P, Boiardi L. Polymyalgia rheumatica. [Review] [60 refs]. Lancet 1997;350:43–47.

Hunder GG. Giant cell arteritis and polymyalgia rheumatica. [Review] [93 refs]. Med Clin North Am 1997;81:195–219.

Brooks RC, McGee SR. Diagnostic dilemmas in polymyalgia rheumatica. [Review] [78 refs]. Arch Intern Med 1997;157:162–168.

Dwolatzky T, Sonnenblick M, Nesher G. Giant cell arteritis and polymyalgia rheumatica: clues to early diagnosis. Geriatrics 1997;52:38–40.

Cohen MD, Ginsburg WW. Polymyalgia rheumatica. [Review]. Rheum Dis Clin North Am 1990;16:325–339.

Michet CJ. Polymyalgia rheumatica/giant cell arteritis and other vasculitides. [Review]. Rheum Dis Clin North Am 1990;16:667–680.

See Also
- Giant cell/temporal arteritis

THE CONSULTATION GUIDE

Polymyositis

Indications and Timing for Referral
- Symptoms rapidly progressive
- Symptoms or signs of pulmonary or cardiac involvement

Timing: Expedited (less than 1 week)

- Suspicion of underlying malignancy or connective tissue disease
- Diagnostic uncertainty
- Assistance with management

Timing: Routine (less than 4 weeks)

Advice for Referral
- Consideration should always be given to having rheumatologic consultation on at least one occasion to confirm diagnosis and develop a treatment plan.
- Consider malignancy, especially in patients over 50 years of age with appropriately targeted testing.
- A complete medication history is vital before consultation.

Tests to Prepare for Consult
- CBC
- CPK
- ALT
- AST
- Sodium
- Potassium
- Phosphorus
- LDH
- ANA
- TSH
- Creatinine
- Urinalysis with microscopic

Tests Not Useful Before Consult
- None

Tests Consultant May Need to Do
- CPK
- Anti-Jo-1 antibody
- ESR
- Aldolase
- Anti-tRNA synthetases
- Anti-SRP c signal recognition particle
- Radiograph, chest
- Electromyogram
- Muscle biopsy
- ECG
- Echocardiogram
- Pulmonary function tests

Follow-up Visits Generally Required
- See *Advice for Referral*

Suggested Readings
Dalakas MC. Polymyositis, dermatomyositis and inclusion-body myositis [see comments]. [Review]. N Engl J Med 1991;325:1487–1498.

Snaith ML. How assiduously should one investigate for occult malignancy in an elderly or middle-aged patient with dermatomyositis or polymyositis? Br J Rheumatol 1990;29:334.

Plotz PH, Rider LG, Targoff IN, et al. NIH conference. Myositis: immunologic contributions to understanding cause, pathogenesis, and therapy. Ann Intern Med 1995;122:715–724.

Villalba L, Adams EM. Update on therapy for refractory dermatomyositis and polymyositis. [Review] [61 refs]. Curr Opin Rheumatol 1996;8:544–551.

See Also
- Dermatomyositis

RHEUMATOLOGY

Pseudogout

Indications and Timing for Referral
- Diagnostic uncertainty
- Diagnostic joint aspiration
- Assistance with management

Timing: Routine (less than 4 weeks)

Advice for Referral
- Records of previous joint fluid analysis and relevant joint radiographs are helpful before consultation.
- In patients younger than 60 years old, primary care physician should order calcium, and iron/TIBC and ferritin levels.

Tests to Prepare for Consult
- None

Tests Not Useful Before Consult
- None

Tests Consultant May Need to Do
- Calcium
- Magnesium
- Iron/TIBC
- Ferritin
- Genotyping for hemochromatosis
- PTH
- Ceruloplasmin
- Therapeutic / diagnostic inj., relevant joints
- Aspirated fluid
  - Cell count with differential
  - C&S
  - Crystal analysis
  - Glucose
  - Gram stain
- Radiograph, relevant joints

Follow-up Visits Generally Required
- One

Suggested Readings
Pritzker KP. Calcium pyrophosphate dihydrate crystal deposition and other crystal deposition diseases. [Review]. Curr Opin Rheumatol 1994;6:442–447.

Snaith ML. ABC of rheumatology. Gout, hyperuricaemia, and crystal arthritis. [Review]. Br Med J 1995;310:521–524.

Wolfe F, Cathey MA. The misdiagnosis of gout and hyperuricemia. J Rheumatol 1991;18:1232–1234.

Raynaud's Phenomenon

Indications and Timing for Referral
- Signs of digital ischemia present (e.g., ulcers, puffy fingers, demarcation)

Timing: Urgent (less than 24 hours)

- Symptoms of systemic disease present (e.g., Buerger's)
- New onset at over 30 years of age
- Intense Raynaud's attacks

Timing: Routine (less than 4 weeks)

Tests to Prepare for Consult
- None

Tests Not Useful Before Consult
- Cold challenge test

Tests Consultant May Need to Do
- ANA
- ANCA
- Anti-scl 70 antibody
- Anti-Ro (SS-A)
- Anti-La (SS-B)
- Anti-Smith antibody
- Anti-RNP antibody
- Anti-double stranded DNA
- Anticardiolipin antibody
- Lupus anticoagulant (LAC)
- PTT
- Lung CO diffusing capacity
- Lung volumes
- Spirometry
- Cryoglobulins
- SPEP with immunofixation

Follow-up Visits Generally Required
- One

Suggested Readings
Wigley FM, Flavahan NA. Raynaud's phenomenon. [Review] [121 refs]. Rheum Dis Clin North Am 1996;22:765–781.

Belch J. Raynaud's phenomenon. [Review] [41 refs]. Cardiovasc Res 1997;33:25–30.

Isenberg DA, Black C. ABC of rheumatology. Raynaud's phenomenon, scleroderma, and overlap syndromes. [Review]. Br Med J 1995;310:795–798.

Adee AC. Managing Raynaud's phenomenon: a practical approach. [Review]. Am Fam Physician 1993;47:823–829.

Luggen M, Belhorn L, Evans T, et al. The evolution of Raynaud's phenomenon—a longterm prospective study. J Rheumatol 1995;22:2226–2232.

See Also
- Sicca complex, diagnosis
- Sjögren's syndrome, diagnosis

RHEUMATOLOGY

Reiter's Syndrome

Indications and Timing for Referral
- Acute joint inflammation present
- Other serious systemic infection present

Timing: Urgent (less than 24 hours)

- Need to confirm diagnosis
- Assistance with management
- Extra-articular manifestations present

Timing: Routine (less than 4 weeks)

Advice for Referral
- Co-management with a rheumatologist is often required.
- Gynecologic examination in females and genital examination in males are important.

Tests to Prepare for Consult
- None

Tests Not Useful Before Consult
- Spinal manipulation

Tests Consultant May Need to Do
- CBC
- ESR
- ALT, AST, alkaline phosphatase
- Calcium
- Creatinine
- Globulin
- Uric acid
- HLA B27
- Urinalysis with microscopic
- Radiographs, relevant peripheral joints
- Radiographs, spinal
- *Chlamydia* culture
  - Cervical
  - Urethral swab
- Gonococcal culture, cervical
- Gonorrhea culture, urethral swab
- VDRL
- HIV antibody testing
- Joint tap
- Aspirated fluid
  - Cell count with differential
  - C&S
  - Glucose
  - Crystal analysis
- PCR for bacterial DNA, joint aspirate
- Synovial biopsy
- Serology for:
  - *Chlamydia*
  - *Campylobacter*
  - *Salmonella*
  - *Shigella*
  - *Yersinia*

Follow-up Visits Generally Required
- Co-management, see *Advice for Referral*

Suggested Readings
Keat A, Rowe I. Reiter's syndrome and associated arthritides. [Review]. Rheum Dis Clin North Am 1991;17:25–42.

Mielants H, Veys EM. Clinical and radiographic features of Reiter's syndrome and inflammatory bowel disease related to arthritis. [Review]. Curr Opin Rheumatol 1990;2:570–576.

See Also
- Painful, lower back/lumbosacral spine
- Painful, hip
- Painful, knee
- Painful, ankle, foot, or toe

Rheumatic Fever

Indications and Timing for Referral
- Diagnostic uncertainty
- Assistance with management

Timing: Urgent (less than 24 hours)

- Prophylaxis of contacts

Timing: Expedited (less than 1 week)

- Prevention of recurrences

Timing: Routine (less than 4 weeks)

Tests to Prepare for Consult
- CBC with differential
- ESR
- Creatinine
- Globulin
- Uric acid
- ASLO titer
- ANA
- Rheumatoid factor
- Throat culture
- Blood cultures × 3
- Urinalysis with microscopic

Tests Not Useful Before Consult
- None

Tests Consultant May Need to Do
- Anti-DNase antibody
- Anti-DNase B antibody
- Anti-streptozyme antibody
- Radiograph, chest
- ECG
- Echocardiogram

Follow-up Visits Generally Required
- Two

Suggested Readings
Bisno AL. Group A streptococcal infections and acute rheumatic fever. [Review]. N Engl J Med 1991;325:783–793.

Burge DJ, DeHoratius RJ. Acute rheumatic fever. [Review]. Cardiovasc Clin 1993;23:3–23.

Pinals RS. Polyarthritis and fever. [Review]. N Engl J Med 1994;330:769–774.

Selected Guidelines
Guidelines for the diagnosis of rheumatic fever. Jones Criteria, 1992 update. Special Writing Group of the Committee on Rheumatic Fever, Endocarditis, and Kawasaki Disease of the Council on Cardiovascular Disease in the Young of the American Heart Association [published erratum appears in JAMA 1993;269:476] [see comments]. JAMA 1992;268:2069–2073.

See Also
- Arthritis, with subcutaneous nodules
- Arthritis, with fever

RHEUMATOLOGY

Sarcoidosis with Joint Involvement

Indications and Timing for Referral
- Rapidly progressive symptoms
- Associated with Lofgren's syndrome

Timing: Expedited (less than 1 week)

- Diagnostic uncertainty
- Assistance with management

Timing: Routine (less than 4 weeks)

Advice for Referral
- Obtain records of previous biopsies and radiographs of relevant joints before consultation.
- Patients with this condition benefit from co-management with a rheumatologist.

Tests to Prepare for Consult
- CBC
- Radiograph, chest
- ESR
- ALT, AST, alkaline phosphatase

Tests Not Useful Before Consult
- None

Tests Consultant May Need to Do
- ACE
- Calcium
- ANA
- Rheumatoid factor
- Anti-double stranded DNA
- Anti-Smith antibody
- Anti-Ro (SS-A)
- Anti-La (SS-B)
- Anti-RNP antibody
- ANCA
- Lyme (*B. burgdorferi*) serology
- Radiograph, chest
- Radiograph, relevant joints
- Bone radiographs
- Lung CO diffusing capacity
- Lung volumes
- Spirometry
- Therapeutic or diagnostic injection of relevant joints
- Lumbar puncture
- CSF
    - Cell count
    - C&S
    - Glucose
    - Gram stain
    - Protein

Follow-up Visits Generally Required
- Co-management, see *Advice for Referral*

Suggested Readings
Pettersson T. Rheumatic features of sarcoidosis. [Review] [42 refs]. Curr Opin Rheumatol 1997;9:62–67.

Glennas A, Kvien TK, Melby K, et al. Acute sarcoid arthritis: occurrence, seasonal onset, clinical features and outcome. Br J Rheumatol 1995;34:45–50.

Tozman EC. Sarcoidosis. [Review]. Curr Opin Rheumatol 1989;1:540–544.

See Also
- Hilar adenopathy, bilateral
- Sarcoidosis

Scleroderma

Indications and Timing for Referral

- Digital ischemia present

Timing: Immediate

- Hypertension present
- Progressive renal dysfunction present

Timing: Urgent (less than 24 hours)

- Diagnostic uncertainty
- Patients with a definite diagnosis generally benefit from a rheumatology consultation to assess their status and develop a treatment plan
- Co-management is often appropriate

Timing: Routine (less than 4 weeks)

Tests to Prepare for Consult

- CBC
- Platelet count
- ALT, AST, alkaline phosphatase
- Calcium
- Creatinine
- Albumin, total protein
- Globulin
- CPK
- TSH
- Urinalysis with microscopic

Tests Not Useful Before Consult

- Cold challenge test

Tests Consultant May Need to Do

- ANA
- Anticentromere antibody
- Anti-RNP antibody
- Anti-scl 70 antibody
- 24-hour urine creatinine for clearance
- 24-hour urine protein
- Radiograph, chest
- Spirometry
- Lung CO diffusing capacity
- Lung volumes
- Echocardiogram with Doppler studies
- Barium swallow
- CT scan, thorax, high resolution

Follow-up Visits Generally Required

- Co-management, see *Advice for Referral*

Suggested Readings

Mitchell H, Bolster MB, LeRoy EC. Scleroderma and related conditions. [Review] [112 refs]. Med Clin North Am 1997;81:129–149.

Isenberg DA, Black C. ABC of rheumatology. Raynaud's phenomenon, scleroderma, and overlap syndromes. [Review]. Br Med J 1995;310:795–798.

Wigley FM. Clinical aspects of systemic and localized scleroderma. [Review]. Curr Opin Rheumatol 1994;6:628–636.

Moder KG. Use and interpretation of rheumatologic tests: a guide for clinicians. Mayo Clin Proc 1996;71:391–396.

Rothfield NF. Autoantibodies in scleroderma. [Review]. Rheum Dis Clin North Am 1992;18:483–498.

Sjögren RW. Gastrointestinal features of scleroderma. [Review] [57 refs]. Curr Opin Rheumatol 1996;8:569–575.

Wigley FM. Raynaud's phenomenon and other features of scleroderma, including pulmonary hypertension. [Review] [92 refs]. Curr Opin Rheumatol 1996;8:561–568.

See Also

- Raynaud's phenomenon

RHEUMATOLOGY

Sicca Complex, Diagnosis

Indications and Timing for Referral

- Diagnostic uncertainty
- Assistance with management

Timing: Routine (less than 4 weeks)

Advice for Referral

- Opthamalogic evaluation for dry eye is essential.
- Dental evaluation is important to detect and prevent complications of xerostomia.

Tests Not Useful Before Consult

- EBV antibody
- CMV antibody
- Lip biopsy

Tests Consultant May Need to Do

- CBC
- Platelet count
- Electrolytes (Na, K, Cl, CO_2)
- Creatinine
- Globulin
- Urinalysis with microscopic
- Immunoelectrophoresis, serum
- ANA
- Rheumatoid factor
- Anti-Ro (SS-A)
- Anti-La (SS-B)
- Triglycerides
- HIV antibody testing
- Radiograph, chest
- Lip biopsy

Follow-up Visits Generally Required

- One

Suggested Readings

Van Bijsterveld OP. Diagnosis and differential diagnosis of keratoconjunctivitis sicca associated with tear gland degeneration. [Review]. Clin Exper Rheumatol 1990;(Suppl 5):3–6.

Friedlaender MH. Ocular manifestations of Sjögren's syndrome: keratoconjunctivitis sicca. [Review]. Rheum Dis Clin North Am 1992;18:591–608.

Fox RI, Saito I. Criteria for diagnosis of Sjögren's syndrome. [Review]. Rheum Dis Clin North Am 1994;20:391–407.

Fox RI. Sjögren's syndrome. In: Kelly WN, ed. Approach to the Patient with More than One Painful Joint. Textbook of Rheumatology. 5th ed. Philadelphia: WB Saunders, 1997:955–968.

See Also

- Sjögren's syndrome, diagnosis

Sjögren's Syndrome, Diagnosis

Indications and Timing for Referral
- Assist with differential diagnosis of underlying etiology
- Assist with management

Timing: Routine (less than 4 weeks)

Advice for Referral
- Opthamalogic evaluation of significantly dry eyes is essential before or concurrent with rheumatology evaluation.
- Dental evaluation is important to detect and prevent complications of xerostomia.

Tests to Prepare for Consult
- CBC
- Platelet count
- Electrolytes (Na, K, Cl, CO_2)
- Creatinine
- Globulin
- Urinalysis with microscopic
- ANA
- Rheumatoid factor

Tests Not Useful Before Consult
- EBV antibody
- CMV antibody

Tests Consultant May Need to Do
- CPK
- TSH
- HIV antibody testing
- T lymphocyte subsets
- FTA-ABS
- Anticardiolipin antibody
- Lupus anticoagulant (LAC)
- Anti-ribosomal p antibody
- Anti-Ro (SS-A)
- Anti-La (SS-B)
- Immunoelectrophoresis, serum
- Radiograph, chest
- Anergy intradermal skin test panel
- Lip biopsy
- Lung CO diffusing capacity
- Lung volumes
- Spirometry
- EEG
- CT or MR, cranial
- Lumbar puncture
- CSF
  - Cell count
  - C&S
  - Cryptococcal antigen
  - Glucose
  - Gram stain
  - Protein
  - Cryptococcal stain

Follow-up Visits Generally Required
- One

Sjögren's Syndrome, Diagnosis (continued)

Suggested Readings

Fox RI, Saito I. Criteria for diagnosis of Sjögren's syndrome. [Review]. Rheum Dis Clin North Am 1994;20:391–407.

Talal N. Sjögren's syndrome: historical overview and clinical spectrum of disease. [Review]. Rheum Dis Clin North Am 1992;18:507–515.

Moder KG. Use and interpretation of rheumatologic tests: a guide for clinicians. Mayo Clin Proc 1996;71:391–396.

Xu KP, Katagiri S, Takeuchi T, Tsubota K. Biopsy of labial salivary glands and lacrimal glands in the diagnosis of Sjögren's syndrome [see comments]. J Rheumatol 1996;23:76–82.

Yoshiura K, Yuasa K, Tabata O, et al. Reliability of ultrasonography and sialography in the diagnosis of Sjögren's syndrome. Oral Surg Oral Med Oral Pathol Oral Radiol Endod 1997;83:400–407.

See Also

- Raynaud's phenomenon
- Sicca complex, diagnosis

Systemic Lupus Erythematosus (SLE), Diagnosis

Indications and Timing for Referral

- Progressive neurologic infection
- Suspicion of infection
- Progressive renal involvement or severe rash

Timing: Urgent (less than 24 hours)

- Associated with severe pain
- Active polyarthritis

Timing: Expedited (less than 1 week)

- Diagnosis uncertain with persistent symptoms for over 4 weeks
- Failure to follow expected course with conventional therapy
- Associated radiologic abnormalities present
- Assistance with management

Timing: Routine (less than 4 weeks)

Advice for Referral

- Tomographic studies (CT or MR) should be obtained after preliminary communication with the appropriate consultant.
- Patients in whom diagnosis of SLE is established often benefit from co-management with a rheumatologist.

Tests to Prepare for Consult

- CBC
- Platelet count
- ESR
- ALT, AST, alkaline phosphatase
- Calcium
- Creatinine
- Globulin
- Uric acid
- ANA
- Rheumatoid factor
- Urinalysis with microscopic

Tests Not Useful Before Consult

- LE prep

Tests Consultant May Need to Do

- PTT
- RPR or VDRL
- 24-hour urine creatinine for clearance
- 24-hour urine protein
- Anti-Ro (SS-A)
- Anti-La (SS-B)
- Anti-Smith antibody
- Anti-RNP antibody
- Anti-double stranded DNA
- Anti-ribosomal p antibody
- Anticardiolipin antibody
- Lupus anticoagulant (LAC)
- Complement factors (C3, C4)
- Skin biopsy
- Radiograph, relevant joints

Follow-up Visits Generally Required

- See *Advice for Referral*

Systemic Lupus Erythematosus (SLE), Diagnosis (continued)

Suggested Readings

Pisetsky DS, Gilkeson G, St.Clair EW. Systemic lupus erythematosus. Diagnosis and treatment. [Review] [47 refs]. Med Clin North Am 1997;81:113–128.

Moder KG. Use and interpretation of rheumatologic tests: a guide for clinicians. Mayo Clin Proc 1996;71:391–396.

Mills JA. Systemic lupus erythematosus [see comments]. [Review]. N Engl J Med 1994;330:1871–1879.

Venables PJ. Diagnosis and treatment of systemic lupus erythematosus [see comments]. [Review]. Br Med J 1993;307:663–666.

See Also

- ANA, positive
- Systemic lupus erythematosus, management
- Systemic lupus erythematosus, with nephritis
- Systemic lupus erythematosus, with neurological involvement
- Discoid/cutaneous lupus, management
- Discoid/cutaneous lupus, diagnosis

THE CONSULTATION GUIDE

Systemic Lupus Erythematosus (SLE), Management

Indications and Timing for Referral

- Assistance with management of neurological involvement or associated infection

Timing: Immediate

- Assistance with management of serositis

Timing: Urgent (less than 24 hours)

- Assistance with management of other manifestations

Timing: Expedited (less than 1 week)

Advice for Referral

- Patients with this confirmed diagnosis generally benefit from co-management by a rheumatologist

Tests to Prepare for Consult

- CBC
- Platelet count
- Albumin, total protein
- ALT, AST, alkaline phosphatase
- Creatinine
- ESR
- Anti-double stranded DNA
- Complement factors (C3, C4)
- Urinalysis with microscopic

Tests Not Useful Before Consult

- ANA, sequential

Tests Consultant May Need to Do

- CBC
- Platelet count
- Urinalysis with microscopic
- 24-hour urine creatinine for clearance
- 24-hour urine protein
- PTT
- Anticardiolipin antibody
- Lupus anticoagulant (LAC)
- Anti-ribosomal p antibody
- ECG
- Radiograph, relevant joints

Follow-up Visits Generally Required

- Co-management, see *Advice for Referral*

Suggested Readings

Gladman DD. Indicators of disease activity, prognosis, and treatment of systemic lupus erythematosus. [Review]. Curr Opin Rheumatol 1994;6:487–492.

Gladman DD. Prognosis and treatment of systemic lupus erythematosus. [Review] [60 refs]. Curr Opin Rheumatol 1996;8:430–437.

Mills JA. Systemic lupus erythematosus [see comments]. [Review]. N Engl J Med 1994;330:1871–1879.

Stoll T, Stucki G, Malik J, et al. Association of the Systemic Lupus International Collaborating Clinics/American College of Rheumatology Damage Index with measures of disease activity and health status in patients with systemic lupus erythematosus. J Rheumatol 1997;24:309–313.

Miller ML. Treatment of systemic lupus erythematosus. [Review]. Curr Opin Rheumatol 1992;4:693–699.

See Also

- Systemic lupus erythematosus, with nephritis
- Systemic lupus erythematosus, with neurological involvement
- Discoid/cutaneous lupus, diagnosis
- Discoid/cutaneous lupus, management
- ANA, positive
- Systemic lupus erythematosus, diagnosis

RHEUMATOLOGY

Systemic Lupus Erythematosus (SLE), with Nephritis

Indications and Timing for Referral
- Confirm etiology of renal dysfunction
- Plan management strategy

Timing: Urgent (less than 24 hours)

Advice for Referral
- Old records are vital (e.g., renal function tests; complement levels; old biopsies, especially of kidney).
- Renal biopsy may be required.
- Condition generally requires co-management with a rheumatologist and/or nephrologist.
- Factors favoring referral to a nephrologist include:
  - Uncertain etiology of renal disease
  - Manifestations of acute or chronic renal failure
  - Need for dialysis or renal biopsy
- Factors favoring referral to a rheumatologist include:
  - Extrarenal manifestations of disease

Tests to Prepare for Consult
- CBC with differential
- Creatinine
- Complement factors (C3, C4)
- Anti-double stranded DNA
- Urinalysis with microscopic
- 24-hour urine creatinine for clearance
- 24-hour urine protein

Tests Not Useful Before Consult
- Renal biopsy

Tests Consultant May Need to Do
- ESR
- Complement factors (C3, C4)

Follow-up Visits Generally Required
- Co-management, see *Advice for Referral*

Suggested Readings
Golbus J, McCune WJ. Lupus nephritis. Classification, prognosis, immunopathogenesis, and treatment. [Review]. Rheum Dis Clin North Am 1994;20:213–242.

Appel GB, Valeri A. The course and treatment of lupus nephritis. [Review]. Annu Rev Med 1994;45:525–537.

Sloan RP, Schwartz MM, Korbet SM, Borok RZ. Long-term outcome in systemic lupus erythematosus membranous glomerulonephritis. J Am Soc Nephrol 1996;7:299–305.

Salach RH, Cash JM. Managing lupus nephritis—algorithms for conservative use of renal biopsy [review]. Cleve Clin J Med 1996;63:106–115.

Ward MM, Studenski S. Clinical prognostic factors in lupus nephritis. The importance of hypertension and smoking. Arch Intern Med 1992;152:2082–2088.

See Also
- ANA, positive
- Systemic lupus erythematosus, with neurological involvement
- Systemic lupus erythematosus, management
- Systemic lupus erythematosus, diagnosis
- Discoid/cutaneous lupus, diagnosis
- Discoid/cutaneous lupus, management

Systemic Lupus Erythematosus (SLE), with Neurologic Involvement

Indications and Timing for Referral

- Confirm cause of neurologic dysfunction
- Assist with management plan

Timing: Urgent (less than 24 hours)

Advice for Referral

- This condition generally requires co-management with a rheumatologist.
- Reports of previous biopsies, complements and serologies are vital.

Tests to Prepare for Consult

- CBC
- Platelet count
- ESR
- Calcium
- Albumin, total protein
- ALT, AST, alkaline phosphatase
- Magnesium
- TSH (assay sensitivity <0.1 mU/L)
- RPR or VDRL

Tests Not Useful Before Consult

- None

Tests Consultant May Need to Do

- FTA-ABS
- RPR or VDRL
- Anticardiolipin antibody
- Lupus anticoagulant (LAC)
- Anti-ribosomal p antibody
- Anti-Ro (SS-A)
- CT or MR, cranial
- EEG
- Lumbar puncture
- CSF
  - Glucose
  - Cell count
  - C&S
  - Protein
  - Gram stain
  - Cryptococcal stain
- Cryptococcal antigen, serum
- HIV antibody testing
- MR, spine

Follow-up Visits Generally Required

- Co-management, see *Advice for Referral*

Suggested Readings

Sibley JT, Olszynski WP, Decoteau WE, Sundaram MB. The incidence and prognosis of central nervous system disease in systemic lupus erythematosus. J Rheumatol 1992;19:47–52.

West SG. Neuropsychiatric lupus. [Review]. Rheum Dis Clin North Am 1994;20:129–158.

Utset TO, Golden M, Siberry G, et al. Depressive symptoms in patients with systemic lupus erythematosus: association with central nervous system lupus and Sjögren's syndrome. J Rheumatol 1994;21:2039–2045.

Sailer M, Burchert W, Ehrenheim C, et al. Positron emission tomography and magnetic resonance imaging for cerebral involvement in patients with systemic lupus erythematosus. J Neurol 1997;244:186–193.

Systemic Lupus Erythematosus (SLE), with Neurologic Involvement (*continued*)

Selected Guidelines

Magnetic resonance imaging of the brain and spine: a revised statement. American College of Physicians [comment] [see comments]. Ann Intern Med 1994;120:872–875.

See Also

- ANA, positive
- Systemic lupus erythematosus, with nephritis
- Systemic lupus erythematosus, management
- Systemic lupus erythematosus, diagnosis
- Discoid/cutaneous lupus, diagnosis
- Discoid/cutaneous lupus, management

Tendonitis

Indications and Timing for Referral
- Progressive neurologic infection
- Suspicion of infection
- Associated with trauma

Timing: Urgent (less than 24 hours)

- Associated with severe pain
- Assistance with injection

Timing: Expedited (less than 1 week)

- Diagnosis uncertain with persistent symptoms for more than 4 weeks
- Failure to follow expected course with conventional therapy
- Associated radiologic abnormalities present

Timing: Routine (less than 4 weeks)

Advice for Referral
- Tomographic studies (CT or MR) should be obtained only after preliminary communication with the appropriate consultant.
- Rheumatologic serologies are usually inappropriate unless other symptoms of systemic disease are present.
- Factors favoring referral to a rheumatologist include:
  - Diagnostic uncertainty
  - Other evidence of systemic disease
  - Suspicion of rheumatologic disease
  - Assistance with medical management
- Factors favoring neurology or orthopedic referral include:
  - Associated with trauma

Tests to Prepare for Consult
- None

Tests Not Useful Before Consult
- None

Tests Consultant May Need to Do
- CBC
- ESR
- ALT, AST, alkaline phosphatase
- Calcium
- Creatinine
- Globulin
- Uric acid
- ANA
- Rheumatoid factor
- HLA B27
- Anergy intradermal skin test panel
- Radiograph, chest, PA and lateral
- Radiograph, relevant joints
- Joint tap

Follow-up Visits Generally Required
- None

Suggested Readings
Nirschl RP. Elbow tendinosis/tennis elbow. [Review]. Clin Sports Med 1992;11:851–870.

Kiefhaber TR, Stern PJ. Upper extremity tendinitis and overuse syndromes in the athlete. [Review]. Clin Sports Med 1992;11:39–55.

Soma CA, Mandelbaum BR. Achilles tendon disorders. [Review]. Clin Sports Med 1994;13:811–823.

Biundo JJ Jr, Mipro RC Jr, Fahey P. Sports-related and other soft-tissue injuries, tendinitis, bursitis, and occupation-related syndromes [see comments]. [Review] [20 refs]. Curr Opin Rheumatol 1997;9:151–154.

See Also
- Bursitis: shoulder, elbow, hip
- Painful, elbow

Tendonitis, Achilles

Indications and Timing for Referral
- Progressive neurologic infection
- Suspicion of infection
- Associated with trauma

Timing: Urgent (less than 24 hours)

- Associated with severe pain

Timing: Expedited (less than 1 week)

- Associated radiologic abnormalities present
- Diagnosis uncertain with persistent symptoms for longer than 4 weeks
- Failure to follow expected course with conventional therapy

Timing: Routine (less than 4 weeks)

Advice for Referral
- Tomographic studies (CT or MR) should be obtained only after preliminary communication with the appropriate consultant.
- Rheumatologic serologies are usually inappropriate unless other symptoms of systemic disease are present.
- Factors favoring referral to a rheumatologist include:
  - Diagnostic uncertainty
  - Other evidence of systemic disease
  - Suspicion of rheumatologic disease
  - Assistance with medical management
- Factors favoring orthopedic referral include:
  - Associated with trauma
  - Weakness of plantar flexion of the foot

Tests to Prepare for Consult
- None

Tests Not Useful Before Consult
- None

Tests Consultant May Need to Do
- CBC
- ESR
- ALT, AST, alkaline phosphatase
- Calcium
- Creatinine
- Globulin
- Uric acid
- ANA
- Rheumatoid factor
- HLA B27
- Anergy intradermal skin test panel
- Radiograph, chest, PA and lateral
- Radiograph, relevant joints
- Joint tap
- *Chlamydia* culture, urethral swab
- Gonorrhea culture, urethral swab

Follow-up Visits Generally Required
- None

Suggested Readings
Scioli MW. Achilles tendinitis. [Review]. Orthop Clin North Am 1994;25:177–182.

Soma CA, Mandelbaum BR. Achilles tendon disorders. [Review]. Clin Sports Med 1994;13:811–823.

Shrier I, Matheson GO, Kohl HW 3rd. Achilles tendonitis: are corticosteroid injections useful or harmful? [see comments]. Clin J Sport Med 1996;6:245–250.

Index

Abdominal mass
  epigastric, 177
  left lower quadrant, 178
  left upper quadrant, 237
  midabdominal, 179
  right lower quadrant, 180
  right upper quadrant, 219
Abdominal pain, chronic, 181
Achilles tendonitis, 579
Acidosis with renal insufficiency, 347
Acromegaly, 105
Adenopathy
  cervical, 295
  generalized, 296
  hilar, bilateral, 473
  supraclavicular, 451
Adrenal glands
  Cushing's syndrome, 112–113
  insufficiency, 106–107
    glucocorticoid taper, 126
  neoplasia, 108
  pheochromocytoma, 161–162
Air travel with lung disease, 498
Alanine aminotransferase (ALT) elevation, 240
Alcohol and liver disease, 223
Aldosterone
  elevated, 131
  low, 140
Alkaline phosphatase, elevated, 182
Allergen disease, environmental controls for, 2
Allergy, 2–29. (*see also* Sinusitis)
  anaphylaxis, 3
  beesting, 3
  chemical sensitivity syndrome, multiple, 17
  common variable hypogammaglobulinemia, 5
  dermatitis, 6–8
    atopic, 6–8
    contact, 7
    occupational contact, 8, 16
  drug reactions, 9
    desensitization, 10
    idiosyncratic, 11
  environmental controls, 2
  eosinophilia and, 261

  food and additive, 12
  insect sting, 4, 15
  latex sensitivity, 16
  nasal polyposis, 18
  pneumonitis, hypersensitivity, 20
  postnasal drainage, 21
  pruritus, 22
  pulmonary infections, recurrent, 22, 23
  rhinitis
    perennial, 25
    seasonal, 24
  urticaria and angioedema
    acute, 27
    chronic, 28
  vasculitis, 29
Alpha-1-antitrypsin (a_1-antitrypsin) deficiency, 474
ALT elevation, 240
Alzheimer's disease. (*see also* Mental status change)
  diagnosis, 391–392
  management, 393
Amenorrhea, secondary, 109
Amylase, elevated serum, 220
ANA, positive, 523
Anaphylaxis, 3
Anemia, 247
  aplastic, 248
  hemolytic, 249, 250
  macrocytic, 253–254
  microcytic, 255–256
  normocytic, 257–258
  pregnancy, 252
  renal failure, chronic, 251
  sickle cell, 259
Aneurysm, ventricular, 33–34
Angina, 43–44
Angioedema, 27–28
Ankle pain, 543–544
  tendonitis, Achilles, 579
Ankylosing spondylitis, 521–522
Anosmia, 19, 25
Anovulatory syndrome, chronic, 110
Antinuclear antibody (ANA), positive, 523

581

INDEX

Antitrypsin deficiency, 474
Aortic valve, calcified, 35
Aplastic anemia, 248
Arrhythmias. (*see also* Cardiology)
   atrial fibrillation, 36–37
   atrial flutter, 38
   bradycardia, 39
   premature ventricular complexes (PVCs), 92
   tachycardia
      supraventricular, 97–98, 102
      ventricular, 99–100
   Wolff-Parkinson-White (WPW) syndrome, 102
Arteritis, giant cell/temporal, 536
Arthritis. (*see also* Pain, joint)
   with fever, 527
   Reiter's syndrome, 565
   rheumatoid, diagnosis, 524–525
   rheumatoid, management, 526
   with subcutaneous nodules, 528
Asbestos lung disease, 475
Ascites, 183
Aspergillus, 20
Aspirin
   intolerance, 19
   peptic distress, 231
Asthma. (*see also* Allergy)
   cold and exercise-induced, 478
   dyspnea, 54–56
   in the elderly, 480
   general, 476–477
   nasal polyposis, 19
   occupational, 481
   postnasal drainage, 21
   during pregnancy, 479
   pulmonary infections, recurrent, 23
   rhinitis, 24–25
Atelectasis, 482. (*see also* Consolidation, pulmonary)
Atopic dermatitis, 6
Atrial fibrillation, 36–37
Atrial flutter, 38
Autoimmune disease
   adrenal insufficiency, 106–107
   Graves' disease, 168
   Graves' ophthalmopathy, 168
   hepatitis, 214
   hypothyroidism, 148
   myasthenia gravis, diagnosis, 424
   polymyositis, 562
   systemic lupus erythematosus (SLE), 572

Back pain
   with history of cancer, 452
   lower, 551–552
   upper, 557–558
Bacterial diseases. (*see* Infectious diseases; *specific diseases*)
Barlow's syndrome, 81
Barrett's esophagus, 184
Beesting allergy, 4
Bleeding disorder, 260
Blood. (*see* Hematology)
Blood pressure
   hypertension, 138, 357–360, 510
   hypotension, 77
Bloody cough, 494–495
Boils, recurrent, 297
Bone lesion, lytic, 453
Bone marrow aspirate. (*see* Hematology)
Bradycardia, 39
Brain mass, 395–396
Breast cancer
   family history of, 455
   history of, 456
Breast mass, 454
Bursitis, 529. (*see also* Tendonitis)

Calcification of renal parenchyma, 381
Calcium
   elevated, 132, 133, 135–136
   hyperparathyroidism, 135–136
   hypocalcemia, 141, 142
   low parathyroid hormone, 133
Calcium oxalate stones, 382
Cancer. (*see* Neoplasia; Oncology)
Candidiasis, urinary, 341
Carbuncles, recurrent, 297
Carcinoid syndrome, 111
Cardiac catheterization. (*see specific diseases/disorders*)
Cardiac evaluation, preoperative, 93
Cardiology, 33–102
   aneurysm, ventricular, 33–34

INDEX

aortic valve, calcified, 35
atrial fibrillation, 36–37
atrial flutter, 38
bradycardia, 39
cardiomyopathy, 40–41
cerebrovascular accident (CVA), 42
chest discomfort
   anginal, 43–44
   nonanginal, 45–46
   possible anginal, 47–48
conduction defect
   left anterior fascicular block, 51
   left bundle branch block, 49
   right bundle branch block, 50
cor pulmonale, 487
coronary artery disease, 52–53
dyspnea
   chronic, 54
   episodic, 55
   nocturnal, 56
edema, dependent, 57
electrocardiogram (ECG)
   abnormal, 58–59
   abnormal stress, 60–61
fenfluramine/dexfenfluramine use, 62
heart block
   first-degree atrioventricular, 63
   second-degree atrioventricular
      Mobitz 1, 64
      Mobitz 2, 65
   third-degree atrioventricular, 66–67
heart failure
   cardiomyopathy, 40–41
   etiology uncertain, new onset, 68–69
   management, 70–71
heart murmur
   aortic, 35, 72
   diastolic, 73–74
   mitral, 75–76, 81–82
hypotension, orthostatic, 77
lightheadedness/near syncope, 78–79
mitral annulus calcification, 80
mitral valve prolapse
   ECG confirmed, 82
   suspected, 81
myocardial infarction
   recent, uncomplicated, 83–84
   silent, ECG evidence of, 85–86
palpitations, 87
percutaneous transluminal coronary angioplasty (PTCA), 52–53, 90–91
pericardial effusion, 88
pericarditis, 89
precoronary bypass grafting, 90
premature ventricular complexes (PVCs), 92
preoperative cardiac evaluation, 93
Q-T interval abnormality, 94
rheumatic fever, 566
syncope, 95–96
tachycardia
   supraventricular, 97–98, 102
   ventricular, nonsustained, 99–100
transient ischemic attack (TIA), 42
valve replacement, 101
Wolff-Parkinson-White (WPW) syndrome, 102
Cardiomyopathy, 40–41
Carotid stenosis, asymptomatic, 397
Carpal tunnel syndrome, 530
Catheters, infection with indwelling urinary, 343
Cavitary lung lesion, 483
Cerebrovascular accident (CVA), 42
Cervical adenopathy, 295
Cervical bruit, asymptomatic, 398
Cervical pain, 553–554
Cervical spondylosis with myelopathy, 399
Chemical sensitivity syndrome, multiple, 18
Chest pain
   anginal, 43–44
   gastrointestinal origin, 185
   nonanginal, 45–46
   possible anginal, 47–48
Chicken pox, 313
Chlamydia
   pyuria, 326
   sore throat, recurrent, 334–335
   urethral discharge, 340
Cholangitis, sclerosing, 236
Cholesterol
   HDL, low, 129
   hypercholesterolemia, 134
   hypertriglyceridemia, 139

INDEX

Chronic obstructive pulmonary disease (COPD), 54–56, 484–486
Cirrhosis
   with complications, 189
   etiology unknown, 186–187
   primary biliary, 188
Click-murmur syndrome, 83
Clostridium difficile, 190, 198
Coagulation disorders
   bleeding disorder, 260
   lupus anticoagulant, 274
Coin lesion, 513–514
Cold-induced asthma, 476
Colitis
   Crohn's disease, 196
   infectious, 190
   ulcerative, 191
   ulcerative, history of, 192
Colon cancer, family history of, 193
Colonic polyposis, 105
Colorectal cancer, history of, 194
Colorectal polyps, 234
Common variable hypogammaglobulinemia, 5
Conduction defect
   left anterior fascicular block, 51
   left bundle branch block, 49
   right bundle branch block, 50
Congestive heart failure. (*see* Heart failure)
Consciousness loss, 403–404
Consolidation, pulmonary, 508. (*see also* Atelectasis)
Constipation, 195
Contact dermatitis, 7
   latex sensitivity, 16
   occupational, 8
Coombs' test. (*see* Anemia)
COPD (chronic obstructive pulmonary disease), 54–56, 484–486
Cor pulmonale, 487
Coronary angiography, 43, 47, 52, 60, 83–85
Coronary artery disease (CAD), 52–53
   chest discomfort, 43–48
Coronary bypass grafting, 52–53, 90
Cough
   chronic, 488
   hemoptysis, 494–495
   in HIV-positive patient, 298

Cranial neuropathy, immunocompromised patient, 400
Creatinine elevation, 348
Crohn's disease, 196–197
Cushing's syndrome, 112–113
Cutaneous lupus, 532–533
Cystic fibrosis, 489

Daytime somnolence, 517
Dementia, in HIV-positive patient, 299
Dermatitis
   atopic, 6–8
   contact, 7
   occupational contact, 8, 16
Dermatological conditions
   cutaneous lupus, 532–533
   dermatitis, 6–8, 16
   dermatomyositis, 531
   fever with rash, 310
Dermatomyositis, 531
Desensitization, 11
Dexfenfluramine, 62
Diabetes insipidus, 116
Diabetes mellitus
   gastrointestinal complications, 119
   glycemic control, 117–118
   hypertension, 357
   nephropathy, 120–121
   neuropathy, 122
Diarrhea
   chronic, 198–199
   history of recent foreign travel, 302
   in HIV-positive patient, 300–301
Diplopia, 401
Disability evaluation, lung disease, 490
Discoid lupus, 532–533
Diverticulitis, 200
Dizziness, nonvertiginous, 402
Drug reactions
   allergic, 9
   desensitization, 11
   idiosyncratic, 10
   nephritis, chronic tubulointerstitial, 368
   vasculitis, 29
Duodenal ulcer, recurrent, 204

INDEX

Dyspepsia
  indigestion, 201
  nonulcer and *H. pylori*-positive, 202
Dysphagia, 203, 441
  in HIV-positive patient, 303
Dyspnea. (*see also* Asthma)
  chronic, 56, 491
  COPD, 484–486
  episodic, 57, 492
  nocturnal, 58, 493

Edema
  angioedema, 27–28
  dependent, 59
Effusion, pericardial, 88
Elbow
  bursitis, 529
  pain, 545–546
  tendonitis, 578
Electrocardiogram (ECG). (*see also specific diseases/disorders*)
  abnormal, 60–61
  abnormal stress, 62–63
Electrophysiologic study, 78, 95, 97, 102
Emphysema. (*see* COPD [chronic obstructive pulmonary disease])
Empty sella syndrome, 123
Endocarditis
  aortic valve, calcified, 35
  heart murmur, 72–75
Endocrinology and metabolism, 105–173
  acromegaly, 105
  adrenal insufficiency, 106–107
  adrenal mass, 108
  amenorrhea, secondary, 109
  anovulatory syndrome, chronic, 110
  carcinoid syndrome, 111
  Cushing's syndrome, 112–113
  delayed puberty
    female, 114
    male, 115
  diabetes insipidus, 116
  diabetes mellitus
    gastrointestinal complications, 119
    glycemic control, 117–118
    nephropathy, 120–121
    neuropathy, 122

empty sella syndrome, 123
flushing, 124
galactorrhea, 125
glucocorticoid taper, 126
goiter, 127
gynecomastia, 128
HDL (high-density lipoprotein) cholesterol, low, 129
hirsutism, 130
hyperaldosteronism, primary, 131
hypercalcemia, 132
  low parathyroid hormone, 133
hypercholesterol, 134
hyperparathyroidism, 135–136
hyperprolactinemia, 137
hypertension, 138
hypertriglyceridemia, 139
hypoaldosteronism, 140
hypocalcemia, 141
  elevated parathyroid hormone, 142
hypoglycemia
  fasting, 144
  reactive, 145
hypogonadism, male, 143
hypoparathyroidism, 146
hypopituitarism, 147
hypothyroidism, 148
impotence, 149
menopause
  hormone replacement, 150
  premature, 151
multiple endocrine neoplasia
  type 1, 152
  type 2, 153
obesity, 154
osteodystrophy, renal, 155
osteomalacia, 156
osteopenia, 157
osteoporosis, 158–159
Paget's disease, 160
pheochromocytoma, 161–162
pituitary tumor, 163–164
polycystic ovaries, 165
sella turcica, enlarged, 166
thyroid gland
  function tests, abnormal, 170
  nodule, 167

INDEX

Endocrinology and metabolism—*Continued*
  ophthalmopathy, 168
  painful, 169
  thyroiditis, subacute, 171
  thyrotoxicosis, 172–173
Eosinophilia, 261–262
  pulmonary infiltrate, 511
Episodic loss of consciousness, seizure versus syncope, 403
Esophagus
  Barrett's, 184
  esophagitis, 205
  gastric reflux, 184, 208
Exercise-induced asthma, 476

Facial weakness, 405
Fasciitis, plantar, 534
Fatigue
  afebrile, chronic, 305
  febrile, chronic, 306–307
Fenfluramine, 64
Fever
  with arthritis, 527
  with rash, 310
  of unknown origin (FUO), 308–309
Fibrosis, pulmonary interstitial, 509
Fibrositis/fibromyalgia, 535
First-degree heart block, 63
Flatulence, persistent or recurrent, 206
Flushing, 124
  carcinoid syndrome, 111
  medullary thyroid cancer, history of, 469
  menopause, hormone replacement, 150
Folate deficiency, 263. (*see also* Anemia)
Food and additive reactions
  allergic, 12
  nonallergic, 13
Foot pain, 543–544
  plantar fasciitis, 534
Fungal diseases. (*see also* Infectious diseases; *specific diseases*)
  cough in HIV-positive patient, 298
  eosinophilia, 261–262
  urinary candidiasis, 341

Gait disorders, 406
Galactorrhea, 125

Gastric ulcer, by upper gastrointestinal series (UGIS), 207
Gastroenterology
  abdominal mass
    epigastric, 177
    left lower quadrant, 178
    left upper quadrant, 237
    midabdominal, 179
    right lower quadrant, 180
    right upper quadrant, 219
  abdominal pain, chronic, 181
  alkaline phosphatase, elevated, 182
  ascites, 183
  Barrett's esophagus, 184
  chest pain, 185
  cirrhosis
    with complications, 189
    etiology unknown, 186–187
    primary biliary, 188
  colitis
    Crohn's disease, 196
    infectious, 190
    ulcerative, 191
    ulcerative, history of, 192
  colon cancer, family history of, 193
  colorectal cancer, family history of, 194
  constipation, 195
  Crohn's disease
    colitis, 196
    ileitis, regional, 197
  diabetic complications, 119
  diarrhea, chronic, 198–199
  diverticulitis, 200
  duodenal ulcer, recurrent, 204
  dyspepsia
    indigestion, 201
    dyspepsia, nonulcer and *H. pylori* positive, 202
  dysphagia, 203
  esophagitis, 205
  flatulence, persistent or recurrent, 206
  gastric ulcer, by UGIS, 207
  gastroesophageal reflux, 184, 208
  heartburn, 184, 208
  hematochezia, 209
  hemochromatosis, 210
  hepatic cyst

INDEX

multiple, 211
solitary, 212
hepatic mass, solid, on imaging, 213
hepatitis
   autoimmune, 214
   exposure to, 215
   hepatitis B, 216
   hepatitis C, 217
   hepatitis D, 218
hepatomegaly, 219
hyperamylasemia, 220
irritable bowel syndrome, 221
jaundice/hyperbilirubinemia, 222
liver disease in the alcohol drinker, 223
malabsorption, 224
melena, 225
nausea, persistent or recurrent, 226
odynophagia, 227
pancreatic mass
   cystic, on radiograph, 228
   solid, on radiograph, 229
pancreatitis, chronic or recurrent, 230
peptic distress, on NSAIDs, 231
peptic ulcer disease
   H. pylori-negative, persistent symptoms, 232
   refractory, 232–233
polyps, family history of, 234
right upper quadrant pain, intermittent, 235
sclerosing cholangitis, 236
splenomegaly, 237
steatorrhea, 238
tenesmus, 239
transaminase elevation, 240
vomiting, persistent or recurrent, 241
weight loss, despite good appetite, 242
Wilson's disease, 243
Gastroesophageal reflux, 184
Geriatric patients and asthma, 478
Giant cell arteritis, 536
Globulin levels, elevated, 267
Glomerulonephritis
   history of, 349
   in scleroderma, 350
   in systemic lupus erythematosus, 351
Glucocorticoid taper, 126

Glucose, blood. (*see* Diabetes mellitus; Hypoglycemia)
Glucose-6-phosphate dehydrogenase (G6PD) deficiency, 264
Goiter, 127
Gonorrhea
   asymptomatic partner with, 321
   pyuria, 326
   sore throat, recurrent, 334–335
   urethral discharge, 340
Gout, 537
G6PD deficiency, 249, 250
Graves' disease, 168
Gynecomastia, 128

Hand, painful, 559–560
Handicapped license plates with lung disease, 499
Head and neck irradiation, childhood, 457
Headache
   acute, 407
   chronic recurrent, 4–8
   in HIV-positive patient, 311
   migraine, 409
   post-traumatic, 410
Heart block
   first-degree atrioventricular, 65
   left anterior fascicular block, 51
   left bundle branch block, 49
   right bundle branch block, 50
   second-degree atrioventricular
      Mobitz 1, 66
      Mobitz 2, 67
   third-degree atrioventricular, 68
Heart failure
   cardiomyopathy, 40–41
   etiology uncertain, new onset, 70–71
   management, 72–73
   right. (*see* Corpulmonale)
Heart murmur
   aortic, 35, 74
   diastolic, 75–76
   mitral, 77–78, 83–84
Heartburn, 208
Heinz body test. (*see* Hematology)
Helicobacter pylori
   duodenal ulcer, 204

INDEX

Helicobacter pylori—Continued
   dyspepsia, 202
   peptic ulcer, 207, 232–233
Hematochezia, 209
Hematocrit, elevated, 265
Hematology
   anemia, 247
      aplastic, 248
      hemolytic, 249, 250
      macrocytic, 253–254
      microcytic, 255–256
      normocytic, 257–258
      pregnancy, 252
      renal failure, chronic, 251
      sickle cell, 259
   bleeding disorder, 260
   eosinophilia, 261–262
   folate deficiency, 263
   glucose-6-phosphate dehydrogenase (G6PD) deficiency, 264
   hematocrit, elevated, 265
   hypercoagulable state, 266
   hyperglobulinemia, 267
   hypersplenism, 268
   iron deficiency, 269
   leukemia, 270–271
   leukocytosis, 272–273
   lupus anticoagulant, 274
   lymphocytosis, 275
   lymphoma, 276
   monocytosis, 277
   myelodysplastic syndromes, 278
   myeloma, multiple, 279
   neutropenia, 280
   pancytopenia, 281–282
   paroxysmal nocturnal hemoglobinuria, 283
   polycythemia vera, 284
   porphyria, acute, intermittent, 285
   splenomegaly, 286
   thalassemia, 287
   thrombocytopenia, 288–289
   thrombocytosis, 290
   vitamin B_{12} deficiency, 291
Hematuria
   gross, 352–353
   microscopic, 354–355

red blood cell casts, 380
red urine, 388
Hemochromatosis, 210
Hemoglobinuria, paroxysmal nocturnal, 283.
   (*see also* Anemia, hemolytic)
Hemolytic anemia, 249, 250
Hemoptysis, 494–495
Hepatic cysts
   multiple, 211
   solitary, 212
Hepatic mass, solid, on imaging, 213
Hepatitis
   autoimmune, 214
   exposure to, 215
   hepatitis B, 216
   hepatitis C, 217
   hepatitis D, 218
   serology, positive, rejected by blood bank, 312
Hepatomegaly, 219
Herpes simplex, partner with, 322
Herpes zoster, 313
High density lipoprotein (HDL) cholesterol, low, 129
Hilar adenopathy, bilateral, 473
Hip
   bursitis, 529
   pain, 547–548
Hirsutism, 130
Hormonal disorders. (*see* Endocrinology and metabolism)
Human immunodeficiency virus (HIV)
   HIV-positive patient
      cough, 298
      cranial neuropathy, 400
      dementia, 299
      diarrhea, 300–301
      dysphagia or odynophagia, 303
      headache, 311
      mental status change, 421
      pneumonia, 503
   needlesticks, 319
   partner positive, 320
   western blot, indeterminant, 314
   western blot, positive, 315
Hydrocephalus, 411
Hygroma, 412
Hyperadrenocorticism, 112–113

INDEX

Hyperaldosteronism, primary, 131
Hyperamylasemia, 220
Hyperandrogenemia. (*see* Hirsutism)
Hyperbilirubinemia, 222
Hypercalcemia, 132
   hyperparathyroidism, 135–136
   low parathyroid hormone, 133
Hypercholesterolemia, 134
Hypercoagulable state, 266
Hyperglobulinemia, 267. (*see also* Myeloma, multiple)
Hyperkalemia, 356
Hyperparathyroidism, 135–136
Hyperprolactinemia, 125, 137
   galactorrhea, 125
Hypersensitivity. (*see* Allergy)
Hypersplenism, 268
Hypertension, 138
   diabetes mellitus, 357
   in diabetes mellitus, 357
   labile/paroxysmal, 358
   pulmonary, primary, 510
   renovascular, 359
   secondary, 360
Hyperthyroidism
   Graves' ophthalmology, 168
   thyrotoxicosis, 172–173
Hypertriglyceridemia, 139
Hyperuricemia, 537
Hypoaldosteronism, 140
Hypocalcemia, 141
   elevated parathyroid hormone, 142
Hypogammaglobulinemia, common variable, 5
Hypoglycemia
   fasting, 144
   reactive, 145
Hypogonadism, male, 143
Hyponatremia, 362
Hypoparathyroidism, 146
Hypopituitarism, 147
Hypotension, orthostatic, 77
Hypothyroidism, 148
   bradycardia, 39

Ileitis, regional, 197
Imaging abnormality, cranial
   hydrocephalus, 411

hygroma, 412
   subdural, asymptomatic, 413
   unidentified bright objects, 414
Immunoglobulin A deficiency, 14
Immunology. (*see also* Allergy; Human immunodeficiency virus [HIV])
   hepatitis, autoimmune, 214
   hypogammaglobulinemia, common variable, 5
   immunoglobulin A deficiency, 14
   mast cell disorders, 17
Impotence, 149
Indigestion, 202
Infectious diseases, 293–343. (*see also specific diseases*)
   adenopathy
      cervical, 295
      generalized, 296
   carbuncles or boils, recurrent, 297
   cough in HIV-positive patient, 298
   dementia in HIV-positive patient, 299
   diarrhea
      foreign travel, history of recent, 302
      in HIV-positive patient, 300–301
   dysphagia or odynophagia in HIV-positive patient, 303
   dysuria, nonpyuric, 304
   fatigue
      afebrile, chronic, 305
      febrile, chronic, 306–307
   fever
      with rash, 310
      of unknown origin (FUO), 308–309
   headache in HIV-positive patient, 311
   hepatitis serology, positive, 311
   herpes zoster, 313
   human immunodeficiency virus (HIV)
      western blot indeterminant, 314
      western blot positive, 315
   lower leg ulcers, poorly resolving, 316
   Lyme titer, positive, 317–318
   needlestick, 319
   partners
      with gonorrhea, asymptomatic, 321
      with herpes simplex, 322
      HIV-positive, 320
   pneumonia, recurrent, 324
   pyuria, 326

INDEX

Infectious diseases—*Continued*
  rapid plasma reagin (RPR) test positive, 325
  rubella exposure, 327
  sinusitis
    persistent, 328–329
    recurrent, 330–331
  soft tissue infection
    poorly resolving, 332
    recurrent, 333
  sore throat
    recurrent, 334–335
    severe, Streptococcus-negative, 336
  tick bite, asymptomatic, 339
  tuberculosis skin test
    positive, uncertain duration, 337
    recent conversion, 338
  urethral discharge, 340
  urinary candidiasis, 341
  urinary tract infections
    with indwelling catheter, 343
    recurrent, 342
  venereal disease research laboratories test (VDRL) positive, 325
Inflammatory bowel disease. (*see* Colitis)
Inhalation, toxic, 496, 515
Inherited disorders
  hemolytic anemia, 250
  polycystic kidneys, 371–373
Insect sting, 4, 15
Intestinal disorders. (*see* Gastroenterology)
Iron deficiency, 269. (*see also* Anemia)
Irradiation of head and neck, childhood, 457
Irritable bowel syndrome, 221
Ischemia. (*see* Transient ischemic attack [TIA] or Chest pain, anginal)

Jaundice, 222
Joint pain
  4 or fewer, 539–540
  5 or more, 541–542
  bursitis, 529
  carpal tunnel syndrome, 530
  gout, 537
Joints
  pseudogout, 563
  Reiter's syndrome, 565
  sarcoidosis, 567

Kidneys. (*see also* Nephrology)
  cancer, history of renal cell, 465
  diabetic nephropathy, 120–121
  glomerulonephritis, 349–351
  medullary cystic disease, 366
  nephritis, 367–369, 575
  parenchymal calcification, 381
  polycystic, 371–373
  size
    enlarged, bilateral, 363
    enlarged by imaging, 364
    small, unilateral, 365
  stones, 382–386
Knee pain, 549–550

Lactose intolerance, 206
Latex sensitivity, 16
Left anterior fascicular block, 51
Left bundle branch block, 49
Leg ulcers, 316
Leukemia
  lymphocytic, 270
  myelogenous, 271
Leukocytosis, 272–273
Lightheadedness/near syncope, 80–81
Lipoproteins, low HDL cholesterol, 129
Liver
  alcohol drinkers and disease, 223
  cirrhosis
    with complications, 189
    etiology unknown, 186–187
    primary biliary, 188
  cysts
    multiple, 211
    solitary, 212
  hepatitis
    autoimmune, 214
    exposure to, 215
    hepatitis B, 216
    hepatitis C, 217
    hepatitis D, 218
  hepatomegaly, 219
  jaundice/hyperbilirubinemia, 222
  mass, solid, on imaging, 213
  transferase elevation, 240
  Wilson's disease, 243

INDEX

Lower back pain, 551–552
Lower leg ulcers, poorly resolving, 316
Lumbosacral pain, 551–552
Lung disease. (*see also* Pulmonary)
    air-travel with, 498
    cancer
        non-small cell, 497
        small cell, history of, 458
        squamous cell, history of, 459
    handicapped license plates, 499
    occupational, 500
    premature
        alpha-1-antitrypsin deficiency, 474
        cystic fibrosis, 489
        preoperative assessment, 507
    scuba diving clearance with, 501
Lupus. (*see* Systemic lupus erythematosus [SLE])
Lupus anticoagulant, 274
Lyme titer
    neurological disorders, 415
    positive, 317–318
    tick bite, asymptomatic, 339
Lymphocytosis, 275
Lymphoma, 276
    history of, 460

Macrocytic anemia, 253–254
Magnetic resonance imaging (MRI) (*see* Imaging abnormality, cranial) and kidney enlargement, 364
Malabsorption, 224
Mammary gland
    cancer, family history of, 455
    cancer, history of, 456
    mammogram, suspicious, 461
    mass, 454
Mammogram, suspicious, 461
Mass
    abdominal, 177–180, 219, 237
    adrenal, 108
    brain, 219, 237
    breast, 454
    extremity, 462
    hepatic, 213
    kidney, 363–364
    pancreatic, 228–229

Mast cell disorders, 17
Medullary cystic disease, 366
Melanoma, history of, 463
Melena, 225
Memory loss, 416
Menopause
    flushing, 124
    hormone replacement, 150
    premature, 151
Menstruation
    amenorrhea, secondary, 109
    hematuria, 352, 354
Mental status change
    acute or subacute, 417–418
    Alzheimer's disease, 391–393
    chronic dementia, 419–420
    dementia in HIV-positive patient, 299
    immunocompromised patient, 421
    memory loss, 416
Metabolism. (*see* Endocrinology and metabolism)
Methacholine, 481, 488, 492, 496
Microcytic anemia, 255–256
Migraine headache, 409
Mitral annulus calcification, 82
Mitral valve prolapse
    echocardiographically confirmed, 84
    suspected, 83
Monocytosis, 277
Multiple chemical sensitivity syndrome, 18
Multiple endocrine neoplasia
    type 1, 152
    type 2, 153
Multiple sclerosis
    diagnosis, 422
    management, 423
Murmur, heart. (*see* Heart murmur)
Myasthenia gravis, diagnosis, 424
Myelodysplastic syndromes, 278. (*see also* Leukemia)
Myeloma, multiple, 279. (*see also* Hyperglobulinemia)
Myelopathy, 399
Myocardial infarction
    recent, uncomplicated, 85–86
    silent, ECG evidence of, 87–88
Myopathic weakness, 425

INDEX

Myositis
 dermatomyositis, 531
 polymyositis, 562
Myxedema, 148

Nasal conditions
 polyposis, 18
 postnasal drainage, 21
 rhinitis
  perennial, 25
  seasonal, 24
 rhinorrhea, 26
Nasal polyposis, 19
Nausea, persistent or recurrent, 226
Neck pain, 553–554
Needlestick, 319
Neoplasia. (*see also* Oncology)
 abdominal
  epigastric, 177
  left lower quadrant, 178
  left upper quadrant, 237
  midabdominal, 179
  right lower quadrant, 180
  right upper quadrant, 219
 adrenal, 108
 carcinoid syndrome, 111
 colon, 193
 colorectal, 193
 dermatomyositis and, 531
 flushing, 124
 liver, 213
 lung cancer
  non-small cell, 497
  small cell, history of, 458
  squamous cell, history, 459
 multiple endocrine
  type 1, 152
  type 2, 153
 pheochromocytoma, 161–162
 pituitary, 163–164
 pulmonary nodules, 512–514
Nephritis
 chronic tubulointerstitial, 367
 chronic tubulointerstitial, drug-induced, 368
 chronic tubulointerstitial with industrial exposure, 369
 systemic lupus erythematosus (SLE), 515, 575
Nephrolithiasis. (*see* Renal stones)

Nephrology, 345–388
 acidosis with renal insufficiency, 347
 creatinine elevation, 348
 diabetic nephropathy, 120–121
 glomerulonephritis
  history of, 349
  in scleroderma, 350
  in systemic lupus erythematosus, 351
 hematuria
  gross, 352–353
  microscopic, 354–355
 hyperkalemia, 356
 hypertension
  diabetes mellitus, 357
  labile/paroxysmal, 358
  renovascular, 359
  secondary, 360
 kidney size
  enlarged, bilateral, 363
  enlarged by imaging, 364
  small, unilateral, 365
 medullary cystic disease, 366
 nephritis
  chronic tubulointerstitial, 367
  chronic tubulointerstitial, drug-induced, 368
  chronic tubulointerstitial with industrial exposure, 369
 oliguria, 370
 polycystic kidneys
  history of, with abnormal renal function, 371
  history of, with normal renal function, 372
  incidentally detected, 373
 polyuria, 374
 proteinuria
  nephrotic range, 377–378
  trace to 1+ positive, 375–376
 pyelonephritis. chronic, 379
 red blood cell casts, 380
 renal cell cancer, history of, 465
 renal parenchymal calcification, 381
 renal stones
  calcium oxalate, 382
  initial, 383
  recurrent, 384

INDEX

struvite, 385
uric acid, 386
uremia, 387
urine, red, 388
Neurology, 389–448
   Alzheimer's disease
      diagnosis, 391–392
      management, 393
   amyotrophic lateral sclerosis (ALS), 394
   brain mass, 395–396
   carotid stenosis, asymptomatic, 397
   cervical bruit, asymptomatic, 398
   cervical spondylosis with myelopathy, 399
   cranial neuropathy in immunocompromised patient, 400
   diabetic neuropathy, 122
   diplopia, 401
   dizziness, nonvertiginous, 402
   episodic loss of consciousness, seizure versus syncope, 403–404
   facial weakness, 405
   gait disorders, 406
   headache
      acute, 407
      chronic recurrent, 4–8
      migraine, 409
      post-traumatic, 410
   imaging abnormality
      hydrocephalus, 411
      hygroma, 412
      subdural, asymptomatic, 413
      unidentified bright objects, 414
   Lyme disease, 415
   memory loss, 416
   mental status change
      acute or subacute, 417–418
      chronic dementia, 419–420
      immunocompromised patient, 421
   multiple sclerosis
      diagnosis, 422
      management, 423
   myasthenia gravis, 424
   myopathic weakness, 425
   neuropathy
      diabetic, 122
      peripheral, 426
      systemic lupus erythematosus (SLE), 576–577
   paresthesias
      feet, 427
      hands, 428
   Parkinsonian syndrome, atypical, 429
   Parkinson's disease, 430
   postconcussion syndrome, 431
   ptosis, 432
   radiculopathy
      cervical, 433
      thoracic, 434
   seizures
      generalized, 435
      new onset in adults, 436–437
      partial, 438
   speech disorder, 439
   spells, 440
   swallowing disorder, 441
   tics, 442
   transient ischemic attacks (TIAs), 443–444
   tremor, 445
   vertigo, 446
   visual loss, monocular, 447
   weakness, generalized, 448
Neuropathy
   diabetic, 122
   peripheral, 426
   systemic lupus erythematosus (SLE), 576–577
Neutropenia, 280
Nocturnal dyspnea, 56
Nodules, subcutaneous, 528
Nonsteroidal anti-inflammatory drugs and peptic distress, 231
Normocytic anemia, 257–258

Obesity, 154
Occupational disorders
   asthma, 481
   contact dermatitis, 8
   lung disease, 500
      asbestos, 475
      disability evaluation, 490
   nephritis, chronic tubulointerstitial, 369
   pneumonitis, hypersensitivity, 20
   reactive airway dysfunction syndrome, 515
Odynophagia, 227
   in HIV-positive patient, 303

INDEX

Oliguria, 370
Oncology, 450–469. (*see also* Neoplasia)
  adenopathy, supraclavicular, 451
  back pain, history of cancer, 452
  bone lesion, lytic, 453
  brain mass, 395–396
  breast cancer
    family history of, 455
    history of, 456
  breast mass, 454
  head and neck irradiation, childhood, 457
  lung cancer
    non-small cell, 497
    small cell, history of, 458
    squamous cell, history of, 459
  lymphoma, 276, 460
  mammogram, suspicious, 461
  mass, extremity, 462
  melanoma, history of, 463
  prostate cancer, history of, 464
  renal cell cancer, history of, 465
  sarcoma, history of, 466
  thyroid cancer
    history of, 468
    medullary, family history of, 469
Ophthalmology
  diplopia, 401
  Graves' ophthalmopathy, 168
  ptosis, 432
  sicca complex, 569
  Sjögren's syndrome, 570–571
  visual loss, monocular, 447
Orthostatic, hypotension, 77
Osteodystrophy, renal, 155
Osteomalacia, 156
Osteopenia, 157
Osteoporosis, 158–159
Ovaries, polycystic, 165

Pacemaker, temporary transvenous, 66
Paget's disease, 160
Pain
  abdominal, chronic, 181
  arthritis, 524–528
  chest, 43–48, 185
  elbow, 545–546
  fibrositis/fibromyalgia, 535
  hand, 559–560
  hip, 547–548
  joint
    4 or fewer, 539–540
    5 or more, 541–542
    bursitis, 529
    carpal tunnel syndrome, 530
    gout, 537
    knee, 549–550
    lower back/lumbosacral, 551–552
    neck, 553–554
    shoulder, 555–556
    soft tissue, chronic, 538
    tendonitis, 578–579
    upper back/thoracic, 557–558
    wrist, 559–560
Palpitations, 89
Pancreas
  mass, cystic, 228
  mass, solid, 229
Pancreatitis, chronic or recurrent, 230
Pancytopenia, 281–282. (*see also* Anemia)
Parasites, internal and eosinophilia, 261–262
Parathyroid gland
  hyperparathyroidism, 135–136
  hypocalcemia, 142
  hypoparathyroidism, 146
Paresthesias
  feet, 427
  hands, 428
Parkinsonian syndrome, atypical, 429
Parkinson's disease, 430
Paroxysmal nocturnal hemoglobinuria, 283
Partners
  with gonorrhea, asymptomatic, 321
  with herpes simplex, 322
  positive HIV, 320
  with syphilis, 323
PCV (packed cell volume), elevated, 265
Peptic distress, on NSAIDs, 231
Percutaneous transluminal coronary angioplasty (PTCA), 52–53, 90–91
Pericardial effusion, 90
Pericarditis, 91
Pharyngitis. (*see* Sore throat)

INDEX

Pheochromocytoma, 161–162
Pickwickian syndrome, 517
Pituitary gland
    Cushing's syndrome, 112–113
    empty sella syndrome, 123
    hyperprolactinemia, 137
    hypopituitarism, 147
    neoplasia, 137
    sella turcica, enlarged, 166
    tumor, 163–164
Plantar fasciitis, 534
Platelets. (*see* Hematology)
Pleural effusion, 502
Pneumocystosis. (*see* Cough, in HIV-positive patient)
Pneumonia
    consolidation, 508
    immunocompromised host, 503
    lobar, 504
    poorly resolving, 505
    recurrent, 324
Pneumonitis, hypersensitivity, 20
Pneumothorax, recurrent, 506
Polycystic kidneys
    history of, with abnormal renal function, 371
    history of, with normal renal function, 372
    incidentally detected, 373
Polycystic ovaries, 165
Polycythemia vera, 284
Polymyalgia rheumatica, 561
Polymyositis, 562
Polyps, family history of, 234
Polyuria, 374
Porphyria, acute, intermittent, 285
Postconcussion syndrome, 431
Postnasal drainage, perennial, 21
Potassium
    hyperkalemia, 356
    hypokalemia, 361
Precoronary bypass grafting, 90
Pregnancy
    anemia in, 252
    asthma during, 477
    herpes varicella-zoster exposure, 313
    leukocytosis in, 273
    rubella exposure, 327

Premature ventricular complexes (PVCs), 92
Preoperative cardiac evaluation, 93
Preoperative lung disease assessment, 507
Prolactin, elevated, 137
Prostate cancer, history of, 464
Proteinuria
    nephrotic range, 377–378
    trace to 1+ positive, 375–376
Pruritus, 22
Pseudogout, 563
PTCA (percutaneous transluminal coronary angioplasty), 52–53, 90–91
Ptosis, 432
Puberty, delayed
    female, 114
    male, 115
Pulmonary, 471–518
    adenopathy, hilar, bilateral, 473
    alpha-1 antitrypsin deficiency, 474
    asbestos lung disease, 475
    asthma
        cold and exercise-induced, 476
        in the elderly, 478
        general, 479–480
        occupational, 481
        during pregnancy, 477
    atelectasis, 482
    cavitary lung lesion, 483
    chronic obstructive pulmonary disease (COPD), 484–486
    consolidation, 508. (*see also* atelectasis)
    cor pulmonale, 487
    cough, chronic, 488
    cystic fibrosis, 489
    disability evaluation, lung disease, 490
    dyspnea
        chronic, 491
        episodic, 492
        nocturnal, 493
    hemoptysis, 494–495
    infections, recurrent, 23
    inhalation, toxic, 496
    lung cancer
        non-small cell, 491
        small cell, history of, 458
        squamous cell, history of, 459

INDEX

Pulmonary—*Continued*
  lung disease
    air-travel with, 498
    handicapped license plates, 499
    occupational, 500
    scuba diving clearance with, 501
  pleural effusion, 502
  pneumonia
    immunocompromised host, 503
    lobar, 504
    poorly resolving, 505
  pneumothorax, recurrent, 506
  preoperative pulmonary assessment, 507
  pulmonary consolidation, 508
  pulmonary fibrosis, interstitial, 509
  pulmonary hypertension, primary, 510
  pulmonary infiltrate with eosinophilia, 511
  pulmonary nodules
    multiple, 512
    solitary, central, 513
    solitary, peripheral, 514
  reactive airway dysfunction syndrome, 515
  sarcoidosis, 516
  sleep apnea/snoring, 517
  smoking cessation, 518
PVCs (premature ventricular complexes), 92
Pyuria, 325

Q-T interval abnormality, 94

Radiculopathy
  cervical, 433
  thoracic, 434
Rapid plasma reagin (RPR) test, 326
Raynaud's phenomenon, 564
Reactive airway dysfunction syndrome, 515
Red blood cell casts, 380
Reiter's syndrome, 565
Renal disorders. (*see also* Kidneys; Nephrology)
  anemia in chronic, 251
  cancer, history of renal cell, 465
  parenchymal calcification, 381
Renal osteodystrophy, 155
Renal stones
  calcium oxalate, 384

  initial, 382
  recurrent, 383
  struvite, 385
  uric acid, 386
Reproductive system disorders
  amenorrhea, secondary, 109
  anovulatory syndrome, 110
  gynecomastia, 128
  hirsutism, 130
  hypogonadism, male, 143
  impotence, 149
  menopause
    hormone replacement, 150
    premature, 151
  polycystic ovaries, 165
  puberty delay
    female, 114
    male, 115
Respiratory disorders, 482
Reticulocyte count. (*see* Hematology)
Rheumatic fever, 566
Rheumatoid arthritis
  diagnosis, 524–525
  management, 526
Rheumatology, 519–579
  ankylosing spondylitis, 521–522
  antinuclear antibody (ANA), positive, 523
  arthritis
    with fever, 527
    rheumatoid, diagnosis, 524–525
    rheumatoid, management, 526
    with subcutaneous nodules, 528
  bursitis, 529
  carpal tunnel syndrome, 530
  dermatomyositis, 531
  discoid/cutaneous lupus
    diagnosis, 532
    management, 533
  fasciitis, plantar, 534
  fibrositis/fibromyalgia, 535
  giant cell/temporal arteritis, 536
  gout, 537
  pain
    ankle, foot or toe, 543–544
    elbow, 545–546
    hip, 547–548
    joints, multiple, 539–542

INDEX

knee, 549–550
lower back/lumbosacral, 551–552
neck, 553–554
shoulder, 555–556
soft tissue, chronic, 538
upper back/thoracic spine, 557–558
wrist and/or hand, 559–560
polymyalgia rheumatica, 561
polymyositis, 562
pseudogout, 563
Raynaud's phenomenon, 564
Reiter's syndrome, 565
rheumatic fever, 566
sarcoidosis with joint involvement, 567
scleroderma, 568
sicca complex, diagnosis, 569
Sjögren's syndrome, diagnosis, 570–571
systemic lupus erythematosus (SLE)
    diagnosis, 572–573
    management, 574
    with nephritis, 575
    with neurological involvement, 576–577
tendonitis, 578
    Achilles, 579
Rhinitis
    perennial, 25
    seasonal, 24
Rhinorrhea, 26
Right bundle branch block, 50
Right upper quadrant pain, intermittent, 235
RPR (rapid plasma reagin) test, 326
Rubella exposure, 327

Sarcoidosis, 516
    with joint involvement, 567
Sarcoma, history of, 466
Schilling test, 253, 263
Scleroderma, 568
    and glomerulonephritis, 350
Sclerosing cholangitis, 236
Scuba diving clearance with lung disease, 501
Second-degree heart block, 64–65
Seizures
    episodic loss of consciousness, 403–404
        seizure comparison, 403–404
    generalized, 435
    new onset in adults, 436–437

    partial, 438
    syncope comparison, 403–404
    transient ischemic attack (TIA) compared, 440
Sella turcica
    empty sella syndrome, 123
    enlarged, 166
Serum sickness, 4, 15
Sexually transmitted diseases. (*see specific diseases*)
Shingles exposure, 313
Shortness of breath. (*see* Dyspnea)
Shoulder
    bursitis, 529
    pain, 555–556
Sicca complex, diagnosis, 569
Sickle cell anemia, 259
Sinusitis
    nasal polyposis, 19
    persistent, 328–329
    postnasal drainage, 21
    recurrent, 330–331
    rhinitis, 24–25
Sjögren's syndrome, 570–571
Skin disease. (*see* Dermatological conditions)
Sleep apnea, 56, 517
Smoke inhalation, 496
Smokers
    asthma, 481
    cessation, 518
    cough, chronic, 488
    hemoptysis, 494–495
Snoring, 517
Sodium, low, 362
Soft tissue
    infection
        poorly resolving, 332
        recurrent, 333
    pain, chronic, 538
Sore throat
    recurrent, 334–335
    severe, Streptococcus-negative, 336
Spells, 440
Spine
    ankylosing spondylitis, 521–522
    painful
        cervical, 553–554

INDEX

Spine—*Continued*
    lumbosacral, 551–552
    thoracic, 557–558
Spleen disorders
    hypersplenism, 268
    splenomegaly, 286
Splenomegaly, 237, 286
Spondylitis, ankylosing, 521–522
Spondylosis, cervical, 399
Steatorrhea, 238
Stings, allergy to, 4, 15
Struvite renal stones, 385
Subcutaneous nodules with arthritis, 528
Supraventricular tachycardia, 97–98, 102
Swallowing disorder, 441
Syncope, 95–96
    lightheadedness, 78–79
    orthostatic hypotension, 77
    seizure comparison, 403–404
Syphilis
    partner with, 323
    rapid plasma reagin (RPR) test positive, 325
    Venereal Disease Research Laboratories Test (VDRL) positive, 325
Syspepsia, 202
Systemic lupus erythematosus (SLE)
    diagnosis, 572–573
    discoid/cutaneous lupus, 532–533
    glomerulonephritis, 351
    management, 574
    with nephritis, 575
    with neurological involvement, 576–577

Tachycardia
    supraventricular, 97–98, 102
    ventricular, nonsustained, 99–100
Tarry stools, 225
Temporal arteritis, 536
Tendonitis, 578
    Achilles, 579
Tenesmus, 239
Testicular cancer, history of, 467
Testosterone
    gynecomastia, 128
    hirsutism, 130

hypogonadism, 143
impotence, 149
Thalassemia, 287
Third-degree heart block, 66–67
Thoracic spinal pain, 557–558
Throat
    sore, 334–336
    swallowing disorder, 441
Thrombocytopenia, 288–289
Thrombocytosis, 290
Thromboses, 266
Thyroid gland
    cancer
        history of, 468
        history of medullary, 469
    function tests, abnormal, 170
    goiter, 127
    hypothyroidism, 148
    nodule, 167
    ophthalmopathy, Graves', 168
    painful, 169
    thyroiditis, subacute, 171
    thyrotoxicosis, 172–173
Thyroiditis, subacute, 171
Thyrotoxicosis, 172–173
Tick bite, 337. (*see also* Lyme titer)
Tics, 442
Toe pain, 543–544
Transaminase elevation, 240
Transient ischemic attack (TIA), 42, 443–444
    carotid stenosis, asymptomatic, 397
    cervical bruit, asymptomatic, 398
    seizures compared, 440
Tremors, 445
    Parkinsonian syndrome, atypical, 429
    Parkinson's disease, 430
Triglycerides, elevated, 139
Tuberculosis
    cough in HIV-positive patient, 298
    skin test
        positive, uncertain duration, 338
        recent conversion, 339
Tumors. (*see* Mass; Neoplasia; Oncology)

Ulcers
    duodenal, 204

gastric, 207
lower leg, 316
Ultrasound and kidney enlargement, 364
Upper back pain, 557–558
Urethral discharge, 340
Uric acid renal stones, 386
Urinalysis
  hematuria, 352–355, 388
  proteinuria, 375–379
  red blood cell casts, 380
  stones, 382–386
Urinary candidiasis, 341
Urinary disorders. (*see also* Nephrology)
  diabetes insipidus, 116
  dysuria, nonpyuric, 304
  hematuria, 352–355
  pyuria, 326
  urethral discharge, 340
  UTI (urinary tract infections)
    with indwelling catheter, 343
    recurrent, 342
Urolithiasis. (*see* Renal stones)
Urticaria, 27–28

Valvular heart disease
  fenfluramine/dexfenfluramine, 62
mitral annulus calcification, 80
murmurs, 72–76
valve replacement, 101
Varicella-zoster, 313
Vasculitis and cutaneous lesions, 29
Venereal Disease Research Laboratories Test (VDRL) positive, 326
Ventricular tachycardia, 99–100
Vertigo, 446
Viral diseases. (*see* Infectious diseases; *specific diseases*)
Visual loss, monocular, 447
Vitamin B_{12} deficiency, 291. (*see also* Anemia)
Vomiting, persistent or recurrent, 241

Weakness
  amylotrophic lateral sclerosis (ALS), 394
  generalized, 448
  myasthenia gravis, 424
  myopathic, 425
  neuropathy, peripheral, 426
  paresthesias, 427–428
Weight loss, 242
Wilson's disease, 243
Wolff-Parkinson-White (WPW) syndrome, 102
Wrist pain, 559–560